R Dalen, MD
1983

Protein Abnormalities, Volume 1

PHYSIOLOGY OF IMMUNOGLOBULINS
DIAGNOSTIC AND CLINICAL ASPECTS

Protein Abnormalities

Volume 1
Physiology of Immunoglobulins: Diagnostic and Clinical Aspects
Stephan E. Ritzmann, *Editor*

Volume 2
Pathology of Immunoglobulins: Diagnostic and Clinical Aspects
Stephan E. Ritzmann, *Editor*

Protein Abnormalities, Volume 1

PHYSIOLOGY OF IMMUNOGLOBULINS

DIAGNOSTIC AND CLINICAL ASPECTS

Editor

Stephan E. Ritzmann, MD

Department of Pathology
Baylor University Medical Center
Dallas, Texas

ALAN R. LISS, INC., NEW YORK

About the Editor

Director, Clinical Chemistry and Proteinology
Department of Pathology
Baylor University Medical Center
Dallas, Texas

Clinical Professor of Pathology
The University of Texas Southwestern Medical School
Dallas, Texas

Adjunct Professor of Biology
Baylor University
Waco, Texas

Formerly, Professor of Internal Medicine and Pathology
The University of Texas Medical Branch
Galveston, Texas

Address all Inquiries to the Publisher
Alan R. Liss, Inc., 150 Fifth Avenue, New York, NY 10011

Library of Congress Cataloging in Publication Data

Main entry under title:

Physiology of immunoglobulins: diagnostic and
clinical aspects.

(Protein abnormalities; v. 1)
Includes bibliographical references and index.
1. Immunodiagnosis. 2. Immunoglobulins —
Diagnostic use. 3. Immunoglobulins — Analysis.
I. Ritzmann, Stephan E. II. Series. [DNLM:
1. Immunoglobulins. W1 PR787 v.1/QW 601 P578]
RB46.5.P49 1982   616.07'9   82-13101
ISBN 0-8451-2800-0

Contents

v

Contributors

James J. Aguanno, PhD, Clinical Chemistry and Proteinology, Department of Pathology, Baylor University Medical Center, 3500 Gaston Avenue, Dallas, TX 75246 **[139]**

John F. Chapman, Dr PH, Department of Pathology, University of North Carolina School of Medicine, Chapel Hill, NC 27514 **[65]**

Gerald B. Dermer, PhD, Department of Pathology, University of North Carolina School of Medicine, Chapel Hill, NC 27154 **[65]**

William R. Dito, MD, Adjunct Associate Professor of Pathology, University of California at San Diego. Laboratory Medicine, Green Hospital of Scripps Clinic, La Jolla, CA 92037 **[119]**

Melodie A. Finney, MEd, MT (ASCP), Clinical Chemistry and Proteinology, Department of Pathology, Baylor University Medical Center, 3500 Gaston Avenue, Dallas, TX 75246 **[139]**

Gary S. Hahn, MD, Immunology and Allergy Division, Department of Pediatrics and Biology, University of California at San Diego, La Jolla, CA 92093 **[193]**

R. Condon Hughes III, MD, Department of Pathology, Baylor University Medical Center, 3500 Gaston Avenue, Dallas, TX 75246 **[139]**

Carol E. Killingsworth, BS, Clinical Chemistry and Immunology Laboratories, Sacred Heart Medical Center, West 101 Eighth Avenue, TAF-C9, Spokane, WA 99220 **[89]**

L. M. Killingsworth, PhD, Clinical Chemistry and Immunology Laboratories, Sacred Heart Medical Center, West 101 Eighth Avenue, TAF-C9, Spokane, WA 99220 **[89]**

Joachim Kohn, MD, Guildhay Protein Unit, Royal Marsden Hospital and University of Surrey. Protein Reference Unit, Department of Chemical Pathology, Westminster Hospital, 17 Page Street, London, SW 1, England **[15]**

Glenn Palomaki, Foundation for Blood Research, P.O. Box 426, Scarborough, ME 04074 **[159]**

Pamela G. Riches, PhD, Protein Reference Unit, Department of Chemical Pathology, Westminster Hospital, 17 Page Street, London, SW 1, England **[15]**

The number in brackets following each contributor's affiliation is the first page number of that contributor's chapter.

Robert F. Ritchie, MD, Foundation for Blood Research, P.O. Box 426, Scarborough, ME 04074 **[159]**

Stephan E. Ritzmann, MD, Clinical Professor of Pathology, The University of Texas Southwestern Medical School at Dallas. Adjunct Professor of Biology, Baylor University, Waco, TX. Clinical Chemistry and Proteinology, Department of Pathology, Baylor University Medical Center, 3500 Gaston Avenue, Dallas, TX 75246 **[ix,1,139]**

Lawrence M. Silverman, PhD, Departments of Pathology and Biochemistry, University of North Carolina School of Medicine, Chapel Hill, NC 27514 **[65]**

Dwight E. Smith, Foundation for Blood Research, P.O. Box 426, Scarborough, ME 04074 **[159]**

Tsieh Sun, MD, Department of Laboratories, North Shore University Hospital, 300 Community Drive, Manhasset, NY 11030. Professor of Clinical Pathology, Cornell University Medical College, New York, NY **[29,97]**

Mary M. Tyllia, BS, Clinical Chemistry and Immunology Laboratories, Sacred Heart Medical Center, West 101 Eighth Avenue TAF-C9, Spokane, WA 99220 **[89]**

Wilfred P. Turgeon, Foundation for Blood Research, P.O. Box 426, Scarborough, ME 04074 **[159]**

Konrad J. Wicher, DM Sc, PhD, Professor of Microbiology, School of Medicine, SUNY at Buffalo. Clinical Microbiology & Immunology Laboratory, Division of Laboratories and Research, New York Department of Health, Albany, NY 12201 **[305]**

Preface

The history of many classic biological disciplines has shown periods of extraordinary ferment accompanied by logarithmic increases in verifiable knowledge. A decade ago it became evident that biochemistry, cell physiology, genetics, endocrinology, and immunology were in such a garguantuan growth phase. Clinical and laboratory proteinology is emerging now as a functional discipline in its own right. It has provided insight into the biological roles of numerous proteins, such as the immunoglobulins, complement, oncofetal proteins, carrier proteins, and protease inhibitors. Together with immunological approaches, it has produced the modern diagnostic tools that aid in the detection and characterization of numerous proteins and their clinical effects. Many of the major advances of the past 10 years are presently in clinical use for the benefit of the patient, and many more are potentially applicable. This progress reflects the state of flux of a growing field.

In a series of books on protein abnormalities the multifaceted spectrum of proteinology will be presented by experts in basic, laboratory, and clinical fields. Volumes 1 and 2 deal with the various physiologic, pathologic, diagnostic, and clinical aspects of the immunoglobulins. Subsequent volumes will be concerned with proteins in the numerous body compartments other than blood, as well as with carrier proteins, complement, protease inhibitors, oncofetal placental proteins, coagulation proteins, hemoglobinopathies, and certain enzyme abnormalities.

The increasing awareness of nutritional deficiencies and the affliction by parasitic infections of hundreds of millions of individuals worldwide have necessitated the inclusion of these subjects. Likewise, the growing need for solid, basic information supportive of the diagnosis and treatment of pediatric and geriatric diseases warrants their special consideration. Further, the ever-increasing need for clinically relevant information concerning the amino acids and peptides and, in particular, their abnormalities in newborns has necessitated the addition of these relatively new topics.

This series reflects a concerted effort to present updated material in emerging areas of importance, without necessarily superseding the information presented in the earlier book *Serum Protein Abnormalities: Diagnostic and Clinical Aspects* [1]. These volumes are intended to provide the personnel involved in health care delivery with a distillation of current information on serum proteins and their counterparts in other biological fluids, as well as their relation to clinical and immunological aspects, in a practical and selective, rather than encyclopedic, fashion. The textual material is supplemented generously with illustrations and tables, and provisions are made for convenient source-finding by inclusion of cumulative indices.

Foremost among the potential audience of this series are the clinician, clinical pathologist, clinical chemist, medical technologist, and other laboratory personnel, but a broader audience—medical students, house officers, practicing physicians, and educators—may find in it a spectrum of useful information. Emphasis has been placed on the complex relationship between human disease and protein pathophysiology, as it relates to diagnosis, therapy, and prevention. It is hoped that this attempt at bridging the widening gap between "bench" and "bed" will provide for the busy professional charged with the responsibility for patient care a valuable addition to his armamentarium and a reliable companion in times of need.

1. Ritzmann SE, Daniels JC: "Serum Protein Abnormalities: Diagnostic and Clinical Aspects," 2nd printing. New York: Alan R. Liss, Inc., 1982.

Stephan E. Ritzmann, MD

Acknowledgments

Acknowledgments are due the contributing authors for their cooperation and for sharing their expertise with their colleagues in the medical community. The publisher's extraordinary commitment to this project and the expeditious processing of its complex material are commendable. Special gratitude is expressed to Sandra K. Ritzmann, the editorial secretary, for her dedicated, resourceful, and diligent supervision of the laborious task of manuscript preparation, collation, communications with contributors and publisher, proofreading, and revisions. Without her dedication, this publishing endeavor would not have come to fruition.

Physiology of Immunoglobulins: Diagnostic and
Clinical Aspects, pages 1–11
© 1982 Alan R. Liss, Inc., 150 Fifth Avenue, New York, NY 10011

Introduction

Stephan E. Ritzmann, MD

The term *protein* was coined by Berzelius in 1838: "Protein (from Greek—proteios—of the first rank) is that important component of living matter without which life would not be possible." Berzelius assumed that there was only one protein in all living matter—i.e. in all plants and animals. With modern advances in analytical methodology, however, an increasing number of different proteins has been recognized, and the application of modern separation techniques [2,48,51] has vaulted the potential number of proteins in body fluids and cellular elements exponentially to at least 1,000 and possibly more than 10,000. Sophisticated identification and recognition procedures, including computerized "libraries," are now required to exploit fully the burgeoning and promising field of protein analysis. It is difficult to overemphasize its clinically and genetically relevant applications to recognition of lanthanic disease, monitoring of therapeutic effects, and taxonomy of proteins.

Protein methodology[1]—like the life sciences in general—requires a recognition of its historical evolution and the appropriate context for its optimal application. Clinically useful techniques for the determination of the total serum protein concentrations were introduced by modified Kjeldahl's assays for nitrogen [3,4,14]. Howe's precipitation technique and its modifications [5,6] allowed the salting-out of several protein fractions and facilitated the systematic original study of serum proteins. By employing various concentrations of sodium sulfate, three fractions were identified: albumin, euglobulin (i.e., globulin precipitable with distilled water [6]), and pseudoglobulins [7].

---

[1]Ed. note: These techniques will be discussed in this and the following volumes in the series by authorities in their respective fields.

The two globulin fractions identified by this technique are now of historical interest only, but occasionally these terms still arise in clinical discussions, in the literature, and as part of problem-solving requirements in the clinical laboratory (e.g., euglobulin lysis test, euglobulin or Sia test [1,8]). The albumin-globulin (A/G) ratio is also based on this precipitation technique. The introduction and further development of the moving boundary or "free" electrophoresis device by Tiselius [9] allowed the delineation of four major serum protein groups: albumin, α_1-globulin, β-globulin, and γ-globulin. The pseudoglobulin fraction identified by Howe's technique was found to be predominantly composed of β- and γ-globulins. The subsequent application of electrophoretic analysis in the clinical laboratory and its clinical importance cannot be overemphasized; the use of zone electrophoresis on paper [10,11,44–47] and cellulose acetate [12–14,42,43] has led to further distinctions among the serum protein fractions. These methods allowed the subdivision into α_1- and α_2-globulins, thereby increasing the number of recognized major fractions to five (i.e., albumin, α_1-globulin, α_2-globulin, β-globulin, and γ-globulin). Acrylamide gel electrophoresis [18,66] further separated serum protein mixtures. Recent refinements of electrophoretic techniques, including high-resolution agarose electrophoresis [15,16,49], isoelectrofocusing electrophoresis [17,87], and immunofixation electrophoresis [19,20,50,53], have provided an analytical armamentarium for the clinical chemist and pathologist that represents the most advanced yet practical and economic spectrum of diagnostic procedures for routine use on a day-to-day basis.

By means of the techniques of analytical ultracentrifugation [21,54], serum proteins have been categorized on the basis of their molecular weight into 4S ($\sim$ 65,000 daltons), 7S ($\sim$ 150,000 daltons), and 19S ($\sim$ 900,000 daltons). The γ-globulin fraction, which has been defined as such by its electrophoretic characteristics, can be separated ultracentrifugally into 7S and 19S components, the former containing the IgG, IgA, and IgD, and the latter the IgM.

The application of single and double immunodiffusion [52,55–57,62] and of combined separation techniques, such as electrophoresis and immunodiffusion, is the basis for numerous qualitative and quantitative, highly sensitive, and powerful approaches that provide specificity for the characterization of individual proteins. These qualitative [22–24,62] and quantitative [25,26,58,62] immunoelectrophoresis techniques utilize antigen-antibody precipitation reactions to further separate and categorize serum proteins. With this approach, more than 40 normal serum proteins can be demonstrated routinely. Quantitative immunodiffusion techniques, such as radial immunodiffusion [27–29] and electroimmunodiffusion [30,31,62], and as an extension, nephelometric and turbidimetric techniques [1,34–41,52,59–62] have revolutionized the field of protein quantitation in biological fluids by virtue of their specificity, sensitivity, and practicality. Techniques with exquisite sensitivity and specificity include the radio (immuno) assay techniques [33,52,59,62,63] and the various nonisotopic quantitative (immuno) fluorescence assays [34–40,52,62–65]. Further refinements of these principles have led to techniques that may extend the sensitivity limits into the attomole range, i.e. to a few hundred molecules of analyte [32,81][2].

A perplexing and potentially misleading system of nomenclature for serum proteins has evolved as a consequence of the different analytical separation methods employed. Most new methods of separation have led to the recognition of additional fractions and the renaming of previously described protein groups. For example, the 19S γ-globulin that is determined by ultracentrifugation is identical with IgM and α_2-macroglobulin as characterized by immunoelectrophoresis; the β1C/A globulins that are identified by immunoelectrophoresis are analogous to moieties of the third component of complement, or C_3, which are also defined by their specific biologic activity. Clearly, the application of newer analytic approaches and their expected yield of new proteins and their moieties [48,51] requires careful consideration of a challenging new taxonometric common denominator. Table I summarizes the evolution of clinically applicable techniques for the analysis of proteins in blood and other biological fluids. The major proteins, which will be the subject of discussion in this and subsequent volumes in the series, are summarized in Table II.

The chapters that follow will consider some of the presently available techniques and their applications in the clinical laboratory and in clinical medicine. Other techniques will be presented in subsequent volumes in the series, supplementing and updating the diagnostic methodology for protein separation, characterization, and quantitation presented in Ritzmann and Daniels (eds.), "Serum Protein Abnormalities, Diagnostic and Clinical Aspects" [1].

---

[2]Ed. note: To convey fully the exquisite degree of sensitivity provided by some of these immunoassays, the following analogy has been offered: "If a sugar cube were to be dissolved in the combined waters of the five Great Lakes, a few drops of the solution would be sufficient to determine the amount of analyte."

TABLE I. Selected Methodology of Serum Protein Analysis in the Clinical Laboratory

Techniques	Authors (references)	Year	Fractions, terminology, comments	Approx[a] sensitivity (per dL)	Approx time required (h)
Total serum protein (TSP)					
Modified Kjeldahl Method	Cullen and Van Slyke [3]	1920		0.1 g	
	Kabat and Mayer [4]	1961			
Biuret Method	Kingsley [67]	1939	1 fraction: TSP	0.1 g	< 1
	Kingsley and Getchell [68]	1957		0.01 g	
Refractometry	Reiss [69]	1902		0.1 g	<0.01
	Naumann [70]	1964		0.1 g	
Precipitation techniques					
Sodium Sulfate Precipitation	Howe [5]	1921	2 fractions: albumin and globulin (TSP minus albumin)	0.1 g	
Ethanol Precipitation	Cohn [72]	1946	> 5 fractions	< 0.1 g	
Analytical ultracentrifugation	Svedberg and Pederson [21]	1940	3 fractions: 4.5S, 7S, 19S	0.1 g	2–3
Protein electrophoresis (PE)					
Free boundary electrophoresis	Tiselius [9]	1937	4 fractions: albumin, α-, β-, and γ-globulins	0.1 g	
Paper electrophoresis	König [10]	1937		0.1 g	
	Durrum [11]	1958		0.1 g	
Cellulose acetate electrophoresis	Kohn [12]	1957	5 fractions: albumin, α_1-, α_2-, β-, and γ-globulins	0.1 g	< 2
High resolution agarose	Laurell [15]	1972	12 fractions	< 0.1 g	< 2
High resolution two-dimensional electrophoresis (ISO-DALT)	O'Farrell [79]	1975	> 1000 proteins	< 100 ng	24
	Anderson and Anderson [84]	1977			
Ouchterlony double immunodiffusion (OT)	Ouchterlony [56]	1949	Numerous proteins	< 0.1 mg	6–24

Method	Reference	Year	Proteins	Sensitivity	Units	Time
Counter immunoelectrophoresis	Gocke and Howe [71]	1970	Numerous anodic proteins	<100	μg	0.5–1
Cross immunoelectrophoresis	Pesendörfer [73]	1970	proteins			
Qualitative immunoelectrophoresis (IEP)	Poulik [22,74]	1952	>40 serum proteins	5–10	mg	24
	Grabar and Williams [23]	1953	proteins			
Oudin single immunodiffusion	Oudin [55,75]	1942	Numerous proteins	1	mg	24
Radial immunodiffusion (RID)	Fahey-McKelvey [27]	1965	Numerous proteins	1	mg	8–72
	Mancini-Heremans [28]	1965				
Electroimmunodiffusion (EID)	Laurell [30]	1966	Numerous proteins	<1	mg	2–3
	Hartley et al [31]	1966				
Two-dimensional immunoelectrophoresis (2D-IEP)	Ressler [25]	1960	Numerous proteins	<5	mg	24–48
	Clark-Freeman [26]	1968				
Immunonephelometry and turbidimetry assays						
Turbidity assays	Schultze and Schwick [76]	1959	} Numerous proteins	<1	mg	0.1–2.0
	Ritchie [39]	1973		<1	mg	0.1–0.2
Automated immunoprecipitation (AIP)	Killingsworth and Savory [85]	1972		<1	mg	0.1–2.0
	Buffone et al. [86]	1974				
Endpoint and rate nephelometry						
Radioimmunoassays (RIA)	Berson-Yalow [33,77,78]	1959	>50 proteins	<100	pg	1–24
Enzyme immunoassays (EIA)	Engvall and Perlman [82]	1971	>50 serum proteins	<1,	μg	2–24
	Van Weemen and Schuurs [83]	1971				
Immunofixation (IFX)	Alper and Johnson [50]	1969	>40 proteins	5–10	mg	1
Isoelectric focusing (IEF)	Kolin [80]	1955	>50 proteins	<100	mg	8

[a]The quoted figures are minimal values, which can be improved by optimizing the assay conditions. The sensitivity levels depend upon several factors, including reaction volumes, reaction times, antiserum avidity, and instrumental sensitivity.

TABLE II. Functional Classes of Proteins

Functional groups	Proteins	Functions
Immunoglobulins (Ig)	Immunoglobulin G (IgG) Immunoglobulin A (IgA) Immunoglobulin M (IgM) Immunoglobulin D (IgD) Immunoglobulin E (IgE)	Provide diverse antibody functions
Complement factors (C)		Provide amplifying functions in inflammatory responses
Classical pathway	$C1q,r,s$ C_2 C_4 C_3	
Alternative pathway	C_3 Factor B Factor D Properdin	
Common pathway	C_5 C_6 C_7 C_8 C_9	
Regulators	$C\overline{1}s$ inhibitor C_4 binding protein C_{3b} inactivator $\beta_1 H$ Anaphylatoxin inactivator S protein	Regulate C-functions and inhibit certain enzymes, kinins, etc.
Transport proteins	Albumin	General transport and oncotic functions
	Prealbumin	Transports T3 and some T4
	Transferrin	Iron carrier
	Haptoglobin	Hemoglobin carrier
	Hemopexin	Heme carrier
	Ceruloplasmin	Copper carrier
	Retinol-binding globulin	Vitamin A carrier
	Gc-group specific protein	Vitamin D carrier
	Steroid-binding β-globulin	Binds steroids

(*Continued on next page*)

TABLE II (Continued)

Functional groups	Proteins	Functions
	Thyroxin-binding globulin	Binds thyroxin
	Ferritin	Binds iron
	Transcortin	Cortisol transport
	Transcobalamine II	Binds and transports vitamin B_{12}
	Hemoglobins	Oxygen transport
	Lipoproteins	Transport fatty acids, cholesterol, phospholipids, glycerides
Protease inhibitors	α_1-Antitrypsin	Inhibitor of trypsin, kallikrein, acute phase protein, etc.
	α_2-Macroglobulin	Inhibitor of trypsin, plasmin, etc.
	Antithrombin III	Inhibitor of thrombin
	α_2-Plasmin Inhibitor	Inhibitor of plasmin
	α_1-Antichymotrypsin	Inhibitor of chymotrypsin, acute phase protein
	Inter-α-trypsin inhibitor	Inhibitor of trypsin, plasmin, acute phase protein
Onco-fetal-placental proteins	α_1-Fetoprotein	Fetal protein, also associated with hepatomas, teratomas, etc.
	Carcinoembryonic antigen	Fetal protein, also associated with gastrointestinal carcinomas, etc.
	Placental and pregnancy-specific proteins	Functions unknown
Miscellaneous proteins	β_2-microglobulin	Related to HLA moieties
	α_1-Acid glycoprotein	Binds certain drugs, acute phase protein
	Fibronectin	Promotes cellular interaction
	α_1-, α_2-, and β-glycoproteins	Varied but largely unknown functions
	AA-protein, PAPP-A_1B	Acute phase response proteins
	Lysozyme	Promotes C-mediated cytolysis
	C-reactive protein	Acute phase response protein and opsonin
	Erythropoietin	Regulator of erythropoiesis
	Coagulation protein and inhibitors	Governing clotting mechanisms

Ed. Note: Details and characteristics of clinically important serum proteins and proteins in other biological fluids will be presented in "Synopsis of Proteins," Volume 3 in this series.

REFERENCES

1. Ritzmann SE, Daniels JC (eds): "Serum Protein Abnormalities, Diagnostic and Clinical Aspects," 2nd printing. New York: Alan R. Liss, Inc., 1982.
2. Dermer GB, Chapman JF, and Silverman LM: High-resolution two-dimensional electrophoresis of human body fluids proteins. Chapter 3, this volume.
3. Cullen GE, Van Slyke DD: Determination of the fibrin, globulin and albumin nitrogen of blood plasma. J Biol Chem 41:587, 1920.
4. Kabat EA and Mayer M: "Experimental Immunochemistry." Springfield, IL: C.C. Thomas, 1961, pp 476–483.
5. Howe PE: Use of sodium sulfate as a globulin precipitate in determination of proteins in blood. J Biol Chem 49:93, 1921.
6. Schultze HE, Heremans JF: "Molecular Biology of Human Proteins." Vol 1, Nature and Metabolism of Extracellular Proteins. Amsterdam: Elsevier, 1966.
7. Haurowitz F: "Chemistry and Biology of Proteins." New York: Academic Press, 1950.
8. Ritzmann SE, Wolf RE, Lawrence MC, et al: Sia euglobulin test-A re-evaluation. J Lab Clin Med 73:698, 1969.
9. Tiselius, A: A new apparatus for electrophoretic analysis of colloidal mixtures. Trans Faraday Soc 33:524, 1937.
10. König P: Employment of Electrophoresis in Chemical Experiments with Small Quantities. Acts and Works of the 3rd Congress of South American Chemists, Rio de Janeiro, 1937, Vol. 2, pp 334–336.
11. Durrum EL: Paper electrophoresis, In Block RJ, Durrum EL, Zweig G (eds): "Paper Chromatography and Paper Electrophoresis." Part II, 2nd ed. New York: Academic Press, 1958, pp 489–674.
12. Kohn J: A cellulose acetate supporting medium for zone electrophoresis. Clin Chim Acta 2:297, 1957.
13. Kohn J, Riches PG: A review of the development and application of cellulose acetate membrane electrophoresis. Chapter 1, this volume.
14. Sunderman FW: Micro-kjeldahl procedure for determination of serum protein nitrogen. In Sunderman FW, Sunderman FW Jr (eds): "Serum Proteins and Dysproteinemias." Philadelphia: Lippincott, 1964, pp 46–49.
15. Laurell CB: Composition and variation of the gel electrophoretic fractions of plasma, cerebrospinal fluid and urine. Scand J Clin Lab Invest 29 (Suppl 124):71–82, 1972.
16. Sun T: High-resolution agarose electrophoresis. Chapter 2, this volume.
17. Arnaud P, Wilson GB, Koistinen J, Fudenberg HH: Immunofixation after electrofocusing: Improved method for specific detection of serum proteins with determination of isoelectric points. I. Immunofixation point technique for detection of alpha-1 protease inhibitor method. J Immunol 16:221, 1977.
18. Raymond S, Weintraub L: Acrylamide gel as a supporting medium for zone electrophoresis. Science 130:711, 1959.
19. Ritchie RF, Smith R: (a). I. General principles and application to agarose gel electrophoresis. Clin Chem 22:497, 1976; (b). II. Application to typing of alpha-1 antitrypsin at acid pH. Clin Chem 22:1735, 1976; (c). III. Application to the study of monoclonal proteins. Clin Chem 22:1982, 1976.
20. Sun T: Immunofixation electrophoresis. Chapter 5, this volume.
21. Svedberg T, Pederson KP: "The Ultracentrifuge." Oxford: Clarendon, 1940.
22. Poulik MD: Immunoelectrophoresis. Introduction and historical aspects, In Ritzmann SE

(ed): "Protein Abnormalities." Vol IV. New York: Alan R. Liss, Inc., 1983.

23. Grabar P, Williams CA: Méthode permettánt l'étude conjugée des propriétés électrophorétiques immunochimiques d'un mélange de protéines. Application du sérum sanguin. Biochem Biophys Acta 10:193, 1953.

24. Scheidegger JJ: Une microméthode de l'immunoeléctrophorèse. Int Arch Allergy Appl Immunol 7:103, 1955.

25. Ressler N: Two-dimensional electrophoresis of serum protein antigens in an antibody containing buffer. Clin Chim Acta 5:795, 1960.

26. Clark MHG, Freeman T: Quantitative immunoelectrophoresis of human serum proteins. Clin Sci 35:403, 1968.

27. Fahey JL, McKelvey EM: Quantitative determination of serum immunoglobulins in antibody-agar plates. J Immunol 94:84, 1965.

28. Mancini G, Carbonara AO, Heremans JF: Immunochemical quantitation of antigens by single radial immunodiffusion. Immunochemistry 2:235, 1965.

29. Ritzmann SE: Radial Immunodiffusion—Revisited. ASCP Lab Med, Vol 9, Part 1, 7:23–33, 1978; Part 2, 8:27–40, 1978.

30. Laurell CB: Quantitative estimation of proteins by electrophoresis in agarose gel containing antibodies. Anal Biochem 15:45, 1966.

31. Hartley TF, Merrill DA, Claman HN: Quantitation of immunoglobulins in cerebrospinal fluid. Arch Neurol 15:472, 1966.

32. Kato K, Hamaguchi Y, Okawa S, et al: Enzymeimmunoassay in rapid progress. Lancet I:40, 1977.

33. Berson SA, Yalow RS: Immunoassay of protein hormones. In Pincus G, et al. (eds): "The Hormones: Physiology, Chemistry and Application." Vol 4. New York: Academic Press, 1964, pp 1–557.

34. Nakamura RM, Dito WR, Tucker ES III (eds): "Immunoassays in the Clinical Laboratory." New York: Alan R. Liss, Inc., 1979, pp 1–366.

35. Nakamura, RM, Dito, WR, Tucker ES III (eds): "Immunoassays. Clinical Laboratory Techniques for the 1980s." New York: Alan R. Liss, Inc., 1980, pp 1–464.

36. Ritchie RF (eds): "Automated Immunoanalysis." New York and Basel: Marcel Dekker, Inc., Part 1, pp 1–333, 1978; Part 2, pp 335–620, 1978.

37. Ritzmann SE, Aguanno JJ, Finney MA, Hughes RC: Quantitation of normal and abnormal serum IgG, A, and M by radial immunodiffusion, nephelometry and turbidimetry. Chapter 7, this volume.

38. Dito WR: Quantitation of serum proteins by centrifugal fast analyzer. Chapter 6, this volume.

39. Ritchie RF: Automated immunoprecipitation analysis of serum proteins. In Putnam FW (ed): "The Plasma Proteins. Structure, Function and Genetic Control." 2nd ed, Vol II. New York: Academic Press, 1975, pp 375–425.

40. Ritzmann SE, Aguanno JJ: The Immunoglobulins in Health and Disease. Monograph III. Wilmington, DE: du Pont de Nemours, 1981, pp 1–21.

41. Seligmann M, et al: IUIS/WHO working group. Use and abuse of laboratory tests in clinical immunology. Critical considerations of eight widely used diagnostic procedures. Clin Exp Immunol 46:662–674, 1981.

42. Williams FG Jr: Electrophoresis of serum proteins. B. Microzone electrophoresis of serum proteins. In Sunderman FW, Sunderman FW Jr (eds): "Serum Proteins and the Dysproteinemias." Philadelphia: Lippincott, 1964, pp 125–130.

43. Sunderman FW Jr: Recent advances in clinical interpretation of electrophoretic fraction-

ations of the serum proteins. In Sunderman FW, Sunderman FW Jr (eds): "Serum Proteins and the Dysproteinemias." Philadelphia: Lippincott, 1964, pp 323–395.

44. Cremer H, Tiselius A: Elektrophorese von Eiweiss in Filtrierpapier. Biochem Z 320:273, 1950.
45. Grassman W, Hannig K: Ein einfaches Verfahren zur Analyse der Serumproteine und anderer Proteingemische. Naturwissenschaften 37:496–497, 1950.
46. McDonald HH: Development of paper electrophoresis. Clin Chem 27:781, 1981.
47. Rosenfeld L: Origins of protein electrophoresis on paper. Clin Chem 27:1948–1949, 1981.
48. Anderson NG, Anderson NL: Molecular anatomy. Behring Inst Mitt 63:169–210, 1979.
49. Killingsworth LM: Clinical interpretation of protein patterns in cerebrospinal fluid, urine and other biological fluids. In Race GJ (ed): "Laboratory Medicine." Vol 4. Hagerstown, MD: Harper and Row, 1980, pp 1–14.
50. Alper CA, Johnson AM: Immunofixation electrophoresis: A technique for the study of protein polymorphism. Vox Sang 17:445, 1969.
51. Special Issue: Two-dimensional gel electrophoresis. Clin Chem Part II 28:737–1092, 1982.
52. Rose NR, Friedman H (eds): "Manual of Clinical Immunology." 2nd ed. Washington, DC: Amer Soc Microbiol, 1980, pp 1–1105.
53. Cawley LP, Minard BJ, Tourtellote WW: Immunofixation electrophoretic techniques applied to identification of proteins in serum and cerebrospinal fluid. Clin Chem 22:1262, 1976.
54. Svedberg T, Rinde H: The ultracentrifuge, a new instrument for the determination of size and distribution of size particle in amicroscopic colloids. J Am Chem Soc 46:2677, 1924.
55. Oudin J: Specific precipitation in gels and its application to immunological analysis. Methods Med Res 5:335–378, 1942.
56. Ouchterlony, Ö: Antigen-antibody reactions in gels and the practical application of this phenomenon in the laboratory diagnosis of diphtheria. Stockholm: Thesis, 1949.
57. Ouchterlony Ö: Diffusion-in-gel methods for immunological analysis. Progr Allery 5:1, 1958.
58. Killingsworth LM, Tillia MM, Killingsworth CE: Two-dimensional immunoelectrophoretic analysis of body fluid proteins. Chapter 4, this volume.
59. Koch TR, Adolf PK, Zimmerman DH, et al: Rapid quantitation of serum immunoglobulins with a miniature centrifugal analyzer. Clin Chem 28:502–504, 1982.
60. Jonker GH III: Optical properties of colloidal solutions. In Kruyt HR (ed): "Colloid Sciences." Vol I Amsterdam: Elsevier, 1952, p 90.
61. Pesce, MA, Bodourian SH: Nephelometric measurement of ceruloplasmin with a centrifugal analyzer. Clin Chem 28:516–519, 1982.
62. Immunochemical techniques. In: "Methods in Enzymology." New York: Academic Press. Part A, Vol 70: Vunakis H van, Langone JJ (eds), 1980, pp 1–525. Part B. Vol 73: Langone JJ, Vunakis H van (eds), 1981, pp 1–739. Part C. Vol 74: Langone JJ, Vunakis H van (eds), 1981, pp 1–729.
63. Natelson S, Pesce AJ, Dietz AA (eds): "Clinical Immunochemistry, Chemical and Cellular Bases and Applications in Disease." Washington, DC: Amer Assn Clin Chem, 1978, pp 1–505.
64. Maggio ET (ed): "Enzyme-Immunoassay." Boca Raton, FL: CRC Press, Inc., 1980, pp 1–295.
65. Engvall E, Pesce AJ (eds): "Quantitative Enzyme Immunoassay." Scand J Immunol 8 (Suppl 7):129, 1978.
66. Ornstein, L: Disc electrophoresis. I. Background and theory. Ann NY Acad Sci 121:321–349, 1964.

67. Kingsley GR: The determination of serum total protein, albumin and globulin by the biuret reaction. J Biol Chem 131:197, 1939.
68. Kingsley GR, Getchell G: The determination of microgram quantities of protein in biological fluid. J Biol Chem 225:545, 1957.
69. Reiss E: Der Brechungskoeffizient des Blutserums als Indikator für den Eiweissgehalt. Strassbourg: Inaugural Dissertation, 1902.
70. Naumann HN: Determination of total serum proteins by refractometry. In Sunderman FW, Sunderman FW Jr, (eds): "Serum Proteins and the Dysproteinemias." Philadelphia: Lippincott, 1964, pp 86–101.
71. Gocke JJ, Howe C: Rapid detection of Australia antigen by counter immunoelectrophoresis. J Immunol 104:1031, 1970.
72. Cohn EJ, Strong LE, Hughes WL, et al: Preparation and properties of serum and plasma proteins. IV. A system for the separation into fractions of the protein and lipoprotein components of biological tissues and fluids. J Am Chem Soc 68:459–475, 1946.
73. Pesendorfer F, Krassnitzky O, Wewelka F: Immunoelektrophoretischer Nachweis von "Hepatitis-Associated Antigen" (AU/SH Antigen). Klin Wochenschr 48:58, 1970.
74. Poulik MD: Filter paper electrophoresis of purified diphtheria toxoid. Can J Med Sci 30:417–419, 1952.
75. Oudin J: IIIB. Specific precipitation in gels and its application to immunochemical analyses. In Corcoran AC (ed): "Methods in Medical Research," Vol 5. Chicago: Year Book Med Publ, 1952, pp 335–378.
76. Schultze HE, Schwick G: The synthesis of antibodies and proteins. Clin Chim Acta 4:610–626, 1959.
77. Yalow RS, Berson SA: Assay of plasma insulin in human subjects by immunological methods. Nature 184:1648–1649, 1959.
78. Yalow RS, Berson SA: Immunoassay of endogenous plasma insulin. J Clin Invest 39:1157–1175, 1960.
79. O'Farrell PH: High resolution two-dimensional electrophoresis of proteins. J Biol Chem 250:4007–4021, 1975.
80. Kolin A: Isoelectric spectra and mobility spectra: A new approach to electrophoretic separation. Proc Natl Acad Sci (USA) 41:101, 1955.
81. Ishikawa E, Kato K: Ultrasensitive enzyme immunoassay. Scand J Immunol 8 (Suppl 7):43–55, 1978.
82. Engvall E, Perlman P: Enzyme-linked immunosorbent assay (ELISA). Quantitative assay of immunoglobulin G. Immunochemistry 8:871, 1971.
83. Van Weemen BK, Schuurs AHWM: Immunoassay using antigen-enzyme conjugate. FEBS Lett 15:232, 1971.
84. Anderson NL, Anderson NG: High resolution two-dimensional electrophoresis of human plasma proteins. Proc Natl Acad Sci (USA) 74:5421–5425, 1977.
85. Killingsworth LM, Savory J: Manual nephelometric methods for immunochemical determination of immunoglobulins IgG, IgA and IgM in human serum. Clin Chem 18:335, 1972.
86. Buffone, GJ, Cross RE, Savory J: A novel modification of a parallel fast analyzer for light scattering measurements: Kinetic measurement of IgG by laser induced near forward light scattering with an Aminco Rotochem. Clin Chem. 20:893, 1974.
87. Svensson H: Isoelectric fractionation analysis and characterization of ampholytes in natural pH gradients. I. The differential equation of solute concentrations at a steady state and its solution for simple cases. Acta Chem Scand 15:325–341, 1961.

DIAGNOSTIC METHODOLOGY AND INTERPRETATION

Protein Electrophoresis

Physiology of Immunoglobulins: Diagnostic and
Clinical Aspects, pages 15-27
© 1982 Alan R. Liss, Inc., 150 Fifth Avenue, New York, NY 10011

1

A Review of the Development and Application of Cellulose Acetate Membrane Electrophoresis

Joachim Kohn, MD, and Pamela G. Riches, PhD

INTRODUCTION

The introduction of cellulose acetate membrane (CAM) electrophoresis by Kohn in 1956 [19] was a good example of serendipity. A chance remark by a commercial traveler that CAM bacteriological filters could be made transparent by the use of a suitable clearing agent started a train of thought which led to the development of CAM, which in most respects was superior to the commonly used filter paper as a substrate for zone electrophoresis. CAM is now widely used in clinical laboratories for the examination of proteins of biological fluids, particularly the pattern of human serum proteins [11,12,23,25,36].

CAM electrophoresis separates the proteins of normal serum into seven zones (prealbumin, albumin, α_1-globulin, α_2-globulin, β_1-globulin, β_2-globulin and γ-globulin) as is shown in Figure 1.

The supporting medium can affect the conditions of zone electrophoresis and hence influence separations. The charge effect of the support medium causes interactions with macromolecules, and this together with variations in the degree of electroendosmosis causes differences in comparative patterns obtained. CAM shows the property of high electroendosmosis. Electroendosmosis is set up by the net negative charge on the ions of the supporting medium. In practical terms, the high electroendosmosis of CAM means that samples may be applied in the center of the membrane, and the resulting separation, which should ideally be 3.5–4.0 cm, will show an appreciable spreading of the clinically important γ-globulin zone. This can be clearly seen in Figure 1.

Ed. note: Dr. J. Kohn is the recognized pioneer of the cellulose acetate electrophoresis methodology.

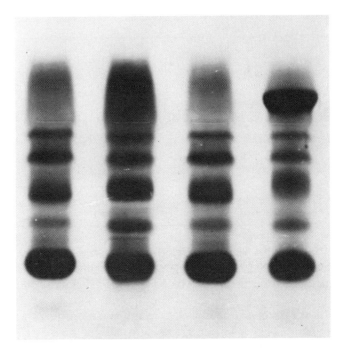

Fig. 1. Electrophoretic pattern of serum proteins on CAM using multiple applicator. Note the presence of the prealbumin fraction.

PHYSICAL AND CHEMICAL CHARACTERISTICS OF CAM

CAM is microporous (0.3–3.0 μ), homogeneous and contains few chemical contaminants. The content of heavy trace metals is very low. The acetylation of the cellulose of the CAM renders the material less hydrophilic and has almost completely eliminated the adsorptive properties of cellulose.

CAM is now available under a variety of different trade names, e.g., Oxoid (UK), Millipore (USA), Sartorius (Germany), Schleicher and Schüll (Germany), Cellogel (Italy), Separex (Japan), Sepraphor (USA), Titan Mylar backed (USA) and Helena (USA). The differences between the various brands are relatively small and are mainly in structure, pore size, and degree of acetylation.

When first introduced, CAM was almost exclusively available in the form of strips of varying length and width. It soon became apparent that sheets of CAM were to be preferred as these allowed multiple sample applications with obvious advantages [23]. With the introduction of multiple applicators [20] and electrophoresis equipment specifically for use with CAM, the material became firmly established for routine electrophoresis. More recently, CAM supported by rigid, flexible backing material, e.g., Mylar film, has been introduced. This modification makes the material rather costly, and it has not gained universal acclaim. However, the most modern innovation of automated equipment for CAM electrophoresis is based on the Mylar-backed material.

A special manufacturing process is used to produce Cellogel, the "gelatinized" (only by name) cellulose acetate as it has a gel-like consistency. This substrate, introduced in Italy [9], enjoys a practically unrivaled popularity in the country of its origin and in Latin America. It has certain advantages. By its nature it is less prone to drying during the manipulative stages, and it is thicker than CAM and hence less likely to suffer from heat distortion effects; it is also available in "slab" form (up to 10-mm thickness) and can be used for preparative purposes. The main drawbacks are its rather high cost and necessary storage in methanol.

APPARATUS FOR CAM ELECTROPHORESIS

A great variety of chambers for CAM electrophoresis have been recommended, and new modifications with special features are being continuously introduced on the market. The first significant departure from the horizontal type of chambers designed for filter-paper electrophoresis was the reversal of the position of the electrode compartment in relation to the buffer compartment [22], which is illustrated in Figure 2.

A chamber suitable for electrophoresis using a thin, microporous supporting medium such as CAM should incorporate features which will prevent or at least considerably reduce excessive and uneven evaporation resulting in drying up of the CAM. The classical, conventional horizontal chamber for filter-paper or gel electrophoresis had the buffer and electrode compartments separated by glass or plastic "spacer planes" over which the strips were stretched. This led to temperature differences between the relatively cooler areas around the buffer-filled compartments and those above the dry separating spacer plane. This in turn led to the impairment of the humidifying capacity of the chamber and to convection currents with their distorting effect on the separation pattern.

The main feature of the new design was that the buffer compartments occupied the whole width and length of the chamber without any dividing planes, providing a continuous fluid surface under the supporting medium.

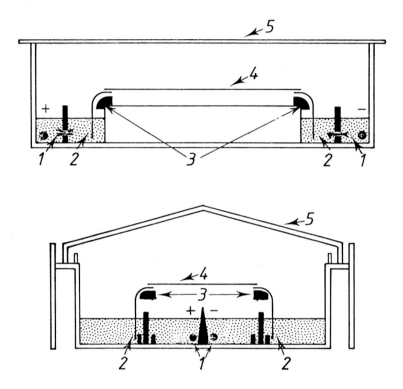

Fig. 2.   Diagram illustrating the essential features of the old-style (top) and new-style (bottom) tanks: 1) electrode compartment; 2) buffer compartment; 3) adjustable bridge pieces; 4) CAM; 5) tank cover.

The second innovation was the miniaturization of the chamber made feasible by the reduction in size—due to the above-mentioned positioning of the electrode and buffer compartments—and the much shorter separation patterns resulting from the superior discriminating power of the CAM. It also allowed a much larger number of samples to be processed at the same time with a concomitant economy of time and space.

However, miniaturization in some cases went too far, with the result that the separation patterns obtained were too short with the inherent risk of overlapping of fractions and making interpretation and/or reliable scanning much more difficult. A dense γ-globulin fraction could mask the presence of a monoclonal band, or alternatively, "crowding" and "condensation" may cause a polyclonal pattern to appear monoclonal. Sacrificing adequate resolution for a spurious benefit of time saving did not contribute to the performance of correct and reliable laboratory procedures.

STAINING OF CAM

Many protein stains have been successfully used with CAM [13]. The most commonly used in routine laboratories are Ponceau S, Amido Schwarz (amido black), Nigrosin, and Coomassie blue (now more commonly available as Page blue). It should be pointed out that the highest resolution of CAM electrophoresis, comparable to that obtained on agarose, can be achieved by applying diluted serum samples followed by a sensitive staining technique, e.g., Nigrosin [23]. In general, aqueous stains are preferred to alcoholic stains, which may cause some shrinkage of the membrane.

EVALUATION OF CAM ELECTROPHORESIS PATTERNS

CAM electrophoresis has now been in use in many laboratories for 25 years, and the experience gained over these years indicates that visual inspection of stained patterns by the experienced worker is more valuable than scanning densitometry [23], which may convey a false sense of accuracy.

The interpretation of numerical values is further complicated by the fact that all the electrophoretic zones with the exception of albumin represent a mixture of unrelated proteins whose concentrations may vary independently. The development of immunochemical methods such as radial immunodiffusion, electroimmunodiffusion, and more recently, nephelometric and turbidimetric methods for determination of specific proteins has radically changed the problem of quantitation of serum protein fractions. Quantitative electrophoresis, except for estimation of paraproteins and hemoglobins, offers no real information and will hopefully be replaced by analysis of a judiciously selected panel of specific proteins. Attention should also be drawn to the relatively little-known and little-used CAM solution technique. The fractions are cut out and dissolved in a suitable solvent—e.g., 10% ethanol, 90% chloroform. The technique is rapid, simple, and reproducible. An essential point not widely recognized is that the inspection of electropherograms should be carried out on uncleared, dry cellulose acetate against a strong source of light. Inspection using incident light is far less satisfactory, and the high sensitivity of the technique is grossly impaired.

There can be little doubt that the interpretation of CAM electrophoresis by the skilled laboratory worker is a valuable aid in many aspects of clinical diagnosis. One can do no better in this respect than to quote C-B Laurel [28], one of our greatest authorities in the field of plasma protein analysis:

> The clinical chemist may offer not only figures but with the aid of his increasing knowledge of the regulation of homeostasis of the individual proteins, a critical pathophysiologic interpretation of the results. The clinical chemist comes into contact with many more odd and crucial plasma protein abnormalities than the individual clinician and, therefore, has a better opportunity of gathering experience and interpreting findings.

APPLICATIONS OF CAM

The applications of CAM electrophoresis to serum proteins and to biological fluids other than serum are extensive. The brief survey that follows illustrates the potentially wide scope and usefulness of CAM electrophoresis.

Glycoproteins

Demonstration of serum glycoprotein patterns has been greatly improved by the use of CAM as supporting medium. The periodic acid-Schiff (PAS) reaction formed the base of the glycoprotein staining procedures [3,18].

Lipoproteins

Lipoprotein electrophoresis and quantitative estimation of the individual fractions on CAM has been vastly superior to the previous universally used filter-paper technique, and it gained in popularity due to its simplicity, rivaling that of gel electrophoresis [5,8]. Various staining methods such as Sudan black and Oil red O have been recommended and widely used. A different principle has been utilized in the ozone-Schiff technique, in which the separated lipoproteins after electrophoresis are exposed to the action of ozone followed by immersion in the Schiff reagent [21]. Ozone splits the double bonds and makes aldehyde groups available to the Schiff reagent. In a number of laboratories, this technique has been used successfully, particularly in Holland and Japan.

Prealbumin

A correct separation of serum on CAM permits visual assessment of reduction or absence of the prealbumin fraction [17].

Urinary Proteins

CAM electrophoresis has been found eminently suitable for the separation, detection, and identification of urinary proteins [23,29], particularly for the investigations in cases of suspected lymphoproliferative diseases such as myeloma and macroglobulinemia. In conjunction with immunodiffusion techniques, the monoclonal immunoglobulins and the monoclonal free light chains (the Bence Jones proteins) can be easily detected and identified.

Another useful application of CAM electrophoresis for the analysis of urinary proteins is in following the response to treatment in nephrotic syndrome. As proteinuria is a characteristic feature of the nephrotic syndrome, there is no need for urine concentration; a multiple or even single sample application, depending on the protein level, will usually be perfectly adequate to obtain a satisfactory and prognostically valuable separation pattern (Fig. 3). CAM electrophoresis could supplement or even replace the more com-

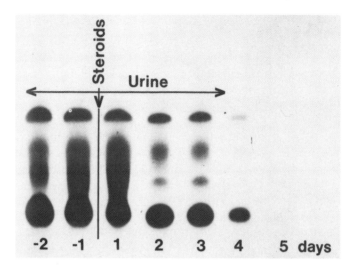

Fig. 3. Electrophoretic patterns of nonconcentrated urine samples on two pretreatment and five posttreatment days. Note the gradual disappearance of protein bands demonstrating response to treatment.

plicated clearance studies. The presence of β_2-microglobulin in urine can, with some experience, be detected by CAM electrophoresis and eventually confirmed, if required, by additional immunological techniques, e.g. immunofixation, on the same substrate.

Cerebrospinal Fluid (CSF) Proteins

Electrophoresis of CSF can be successfully performed on cellulose acetate, even without concentration. Repeated applications on the same site coupled with the use of a sensitive stain like Nigrosin or Coomassie blue may be able to reveal the abnormal patterns indicative of central nervous system (CNS) pathology [6,10,14,33].

Other Fluids

Proteins of ascitic, pleural, and synovial fluids, as well as those of saliva, tears [1], seminal fluid [34], and labyrinthine fluid [24], have been satisfactorily separated on CAM. In some instances prior concentration of these fluids is required before electrophoresis.

Hemoglobinopathies

One of the first applications of CAM electrophoresis was in the field of hemoglobinopathies [23,31]. The neatness and high discrimination power of

CAM resulted in much better separation of the hemoglobin variants than that obtained by filter-paper electrophoresis. The procedure was essentially the same as that used for serum proteins, discontinuous buffer systems being reported as more satisfactory for hemoglobin separation. The CAM has been particularly useful for large-scale population screening surveys.

Haptoglobin

On CAM electrophoresis, free hemoglobin in serum has a β-mobility, whereas the hemoglobin-haptoglobin complex migrates with α_2-mobility. By increasing the amounts of hemoglobin added to the serum sample a saturation point is reached when the free hemoglobin band moving with β-mobility can be demonstrated. The lowest concentration of added hemoglobin at which a free hemoglobin band can be detected is taken as the hemoglobin-binding capacity of the serum tested [16,37]. This method has now been superseded by immunological assays. CAM has also been used for haptoglobin typing [4].

Isotope-Labeled Substances

The absence of adsorption makes CAM eminently suitable as a supporting medium for isotope-labeled proteins. The detection and quantitation of the individual fraction containing the labeled material can be performed by cutting out the fractions, followed by measuring their radioactivity or by special scanners. Autoradiography, thanks to the homogeneity and very thin layer of CAM, is particularly satisfactory [23].

Coagulation Factors

CAM electrophoresis has been reported to be a useful and sensitive technique for the separation and detection of coagulation proteins in the plasma [32].

Forensic Medicine

CAM electrophoresis plays a major part in the field of forensic medicine, particularly in the identification of blood stains and in paternity cases [15].

Research Applications

CAM electrophoresis has been widely used in research. Some of its uses are 1) separation and identification of biologically active substances in biological fluids; 2) protein patterns in tumor tissue extracts; and 3) amino acid separations.

CAM electrophoresis is well suited for isoenzyme separation. The technique is simple, rapid, and economical and has been used with various modifications in routine and research laboratories for the separation of lactic dehydrogenase, alkaline phosphatase, amylase, leucine aminopeptidase, trypsin and in forensic medicine for the identification of isoenzymes of the red blood cell [23]. CAM may be used for isoelectric focusing, but the superiority of other support media makes its use very limited.

Immunodiffusion Techniques of CAM

CAM may be used for double immunodiffusion and radial immunodiffusion techniques [23].

Immunoelectrophoretic Techniques of CAM

CAM may also provide a support medium for a number of immunoelectrophoretic techniques [23,35]. It may be used alone, e.g., immunoelectrophoresis, or in combination with agar gel, e.g., transfer immunoelectrophoresis [22,23].

Counter-current electrophoresis is most successful on CAM [23,26]. It is very sensitive and has found many applications in identification of antigens or antibodies. It has been most widely used in serum protein analysis for the detection of α-fetoprotein and Australia antigen.

Cellogel provides a successful support medium for electroimmunodiffusion and two-dimensional immunoelectrophoresis.

A more recent application of CAM has been as the support medium for immunofixation [7,27,30]. This method combines the speed and simplicity of electrophoresis with a rapid antigenic identification of individual proteins in a complex mixture. A parallel stained pattern provides the localization of the antigen (Fig. 4).

The term "immunofixation" electrophoresis was first used by Alper and Johnson in 1969 [2]. In this technique the proteins separated by electrophoresis on agarose gel were exposed to specific antisera.

An immunofixation method carried out entirely on CAM for locating and identifying individual proteins in biological fluids has all the advantages of the agarose system in terms of sensitivity, exact location of minor monoclonal bands, and high resolution, with the added advantage of extreme speed and simplicity.

Immunofixation on CAM has proved invaluable in several areas where previously there were difficulties in localization and/or identification. In particular:

1) Identification of low concentrations of a paraprotein (in the region of 1 g/L) particularly in the presence of normal levels of immunoglobulins.
2) Localization of paraproteins masked by the α_2- and β-fractions.
3) Detection and identification of Bence Jones proteins in serum.
4) Identification of more than one paraprotein in serum.
5) Light-chain typing of IgM paraproteins, which may be a problem by other methods.

Immunofixation may also be used for the detection of conversion factors produced by activation of complement components [38]. The immunofixation pattern of native and converted C3 is shown in Figure 5.

The technique of immunofixation has considerable advantages over immunoelectrophoresis, particularly in the clinical field. In the UK it is gradually replacing immunoelectrophoresis.

CONCLUSION

The success of CAM may be attributed to its several advantages, which are as follows:

1. Adsorption is minimal.
2. Clear separation of all fractions with considerable "spreading" of the important γ-globulin zone.
3. Rapid separation (2 hours to obtain a completely stained and dried strip).
4. Sensitivity. With suitable staining, e.g. Nigrosin, as little as 1 μg of protein can be detected.

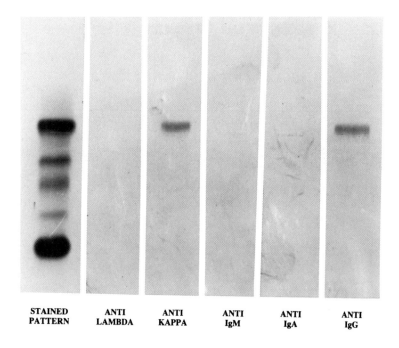

| STAINED | ANTI | ANTI | ANTI | ANTI | ANTI |
| PATTERN | LAMBDA | KAPPA | IgM | IgA | IgG |

Fig. 4. CAM immunofixation showing the identification pattern of an IgG paraprotein. Serum diluted 1:2 for stained pattern and 1:150 for the immunofixation with specific antibody.

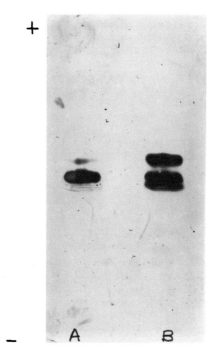

Fig. 5.   Immunofixation of serum diluted 1:10 to show C3 (A) and C3 with conversion product (B).

The technique is robust and rarely fails completely. When there are unsatisfactory results, they may be attributed to one or more of the following factors:

1. Incorrect buffer due to ionic strength, pH, excessive reuse, or evaporation.
2. Uneven running conditions—too-high current, uneven distribution across strip, or variations during run.
3. Too large or diffuse sample application (may be due to excessive moisture on surface of strip or overloading of applicators).
4. Drying of CAM, particularly when applying samples.

   There can be no doubt that since the first introduction of CAM electrophoresis, it has become a valuable, firmly established, and widely used technique in many laboratories. The usefulness of CAM as a support medium for zone electrophoresis has been emphasized and illustrated by the preceding brief survey of its development and many applications.

REFERENCES

1. Allerhand J, Karelitz S, Penbharkkul S, Ramos A, Isenberg HD: Electrophoresis and immunoelectrophoresis of neonatal tears. J of Pediatr 62:85, 1963.
2. Alper CA, Johnson AM: Immunofixation electrophoresis: A technique for the study of protein polymorphism. Vox Sang 17:445, 1969.
3. Arai K, Wallace HW: Electrophoretic determination of glycoproteins. An improved method with cleared cellulose acetate membranes. Anal Biochem 31:71, 1969.
4. Blackwell RQ, Lin CS: Haptoglobin type determination by cellulose acetate zone electrophoresis. Clin Chim Acta 8:868, 1963.
5. Beckering RE, Jr, Ellefson RD: A rapid method for lipoprotein electrophoresis using cellulose acetate as a support medium. Am J Clin Pathol 53:84, 1970.
6. Carrieri P: CSF electrophoresis: An adaptation cellogel RS for identification of protein banding. Boll Soc Ital Biol Sper 55:2341, 1979.
7. Chang C-H, Inglis NR: Convenient immunofixation electrophoresis on cellulose acetate membrane. Clin Chim Acta 65:91, 1975.
8. Chin HP, Blankenhorn W: Separation and quantitative analysis of serum lipoproteins by means of electrophoresis on cellulose acetate. Clin Chim Acta 20:305, 1968.
9. Del Campo GB: New simple technique for the multifractionation of serum proteins (18–21 fractions) on cellogel RS cellulose acetate strips. Clin Chim Acta 22:475, 1968.
10. Ebers GC: CSF electrophoresis in one thousand patients. Can J Neurol Sci 7:275, 1980.
11. Fischl J, Gordon C: Ultramicro-electrophoresis. Clin Chem 12:287, 1966.
12. Friedman HS: A standard procedure for serum protein electrophoresis on cellulose acetate membrane strips. Clin Chim Acta 6:775, 1961.
13. Gadd KG: Staining of proteins on cellulose acetate. Nature 212:628, 1966.
14. Glasner H: Microzone protein electrophoresis in non-concentrated CSF. Klin Wochenschr 55:4, 1977.
15. Grunbaum BW: Rapid phenotyping of group specific components by immunofixation on cellulose acetate. J Forensic Sci 22:586, 1977.
16. Hall R: A simple and rapid method for the estimation of haptoglobin in serum. J Med Lab Technol 21:64, 1964.
17. Harris RI, Kohn J: The pre-albumin fraction: A useful parameter in the interpretation of routine protein electrophoresis. J Clin Pathol 27:986, 1974.
18. Klainer AS, Beisel WR, Atkins WK: Determination of serum glycoproteins on cleared cellulose acetate strips. Amer J Clin Pathol 50:137, 1968.
19. Kohn J: A new supporting medium for zone electrophoresis. J Biochem 65:9, 1956.
20. Kohn J: Multisample applicator for zone electrophoresis. Clin Chim Acta 18:65, 1967.
21. Kohn J: A lipoprotein staining method for zone electrophoresis. Nature 189:312, 1961.
22. Kohn J: Small scale membrane filter electrophoresis and immunoelectrophoresis. Clin Chim Acta 3:450, 1958.
23. Kohn J: In Smith I (ed): "Chromatographic and Electrophoretic Techniques, Vol 2." (4 Ed) London: William Heinemann Medical Books Ltd, pp 90–137, 1976.
24. Kohn J: Electrophoretic and immunological studies on some body fluids in normal and pathological conditions and a preliminary communication on the separation of proteins of the labyrinthine fluids. Protides Biol Fluids Proc of the 7th Colloq Bruges, 1959.
25. Kohn J: Cellulose acetate electrophoresis, In Race G (ed): "Laboratory Medicine, Vol 1." Clinical Chemistry 12B York Pennsylvania: The Maple Press Company, 1976.
26. Kohn J, Kahan M: Countercurrent immunoelectrophoresis on cellulose acetate. J Immunol Methods 11:303, 1976.
27. Kohn J, Riches PG: A cellulose acetate immunofixation technique. J Immunol Methods 20:325, 1978.

28. Laurell C-B: Electrophoresis, specific protein assays, or both, in measurement of plasma proteins? Clin Chem 19:99, 1973.
29. Lombardo T, et al: Use of a particular cellulose acetate supporting agent on the electrophoretic evaluation urinary proteins. Boll Soc Ital Biol Sper 121:593, 1979.
30. Martin W, Voss C: Gc-immunofixation auf cellogel-Folien. Ärtzl Lab 23:337, 1977.
31. Marengo-Rowe AJ: Rapid electrophoresis and quantitation of haemoglobins on cellulose acetate. J Clin Pathol 19:790, 1966.
32. Meyer D, et al: Migration electrophoretique des facteurs de coagulation sur acetate de cellulose. Nouv Rev Fr d'Haemat 9:611, 1967.
33. Paty DW, et al: CSF electrophoresis: An adaptation of using cellulose acetate for the identification of oligoclonal banding. Can J Neurol Sci 5:297, 1978.
34. Quinlivan WLG: Analysis of the proteins in human seminal plasma. Arch Biochem Biophys 127:680, 1968.
35. Rao KM, et al: A rapid micro radial electrophoretic method of protein separation on cellulose acetate membranes. Experientia 35:569, 1979.
36. Rice RE, Ondrick FW: Electrophoresis of serum proteins on cellulose acetate. Am J Clin Pathol 41:321, 1964.
37. Valeri CR, Bond JC, Forlwer K, Sobucki J: Quantitation of serum haemoglobin-binding capacity using cellulose acetate membrane electrophoresis. Clin Chem 11:582, 1965.
38. Whicher JT, Higginson J, Riches PG, Radford S: Clinical applications of immunofixation: Detection and quantitation of complement activation. J Clin Pathol 33:781, 1980.

Physiology of Immunoglobulins: Diagnostic and
Clinical Aspects, pages 29–63
© 1982 Alan R. Liss, Inc., 150 Fifth Avenue, New York, NY 10011

2

High-Resolution Agarose Electrophoresis

Tsieh Sun, MD

THE EVOLUTION OF ELECTROPHORESIS

As more plasma proteins are being characterized and their clinical significance is being elucidated, it is only natural that a higher resolution of protein bands in the electrophoretogram is continuously demanded. To achieve this goal, improvements have been made along three lines in the last four decades.

Improvement in Support Medium

This is probably the most important factor in determining the resolution of protein bands. Approximately 13 different materials have been utilized for electrophoretic support media; however, only three media, namely filter paper, cellulose acetate, and agarose, have been extensively employed in clinical laboratories. Polyacrylamide and starch gels, acting as molecular sieves, can separate large numbers of protein bands, but the failure to identify the bands limits the clinical application of these media. Therefore, polyacrylamide and starch gels are being confined to preparative electrophoresis or to the identification of limited numbers of protein fractions of the same functional group, such as isoenzymes, hemoglobins, and lipoproteins.

In recent years, *agarose gel* has gradually gained in popularity [14, 15, 24, 35, 39]. It possesses many advantages: High and uniform porosity of the gel enables the molecules of the same protein (or proteins with the same isoelectric point) to move at an equal speed without obstruction, thus avoiding zone broadening and achieving high resolution. Agarose gel has no chromatographic effects, such as adsorption and ion exchange, and no chemical reactions with plasma proteins. Its complete transparency due to a high water content (98%) avoids distortion in the tracing and the resultant erroneous estimation of protein percentages that can be seen in other opaque media, the so-called hyperchromic effect [47]. With low endosmosis, agarose gel minimizes the influence of the buffer flow upon the electrophoretic mobility of individual proteins.

Application of Higher Voltage

Another important factor affecting the separation of protein fractions is the voltage applied during electrophoresis [35], the higher the voltage, the better the resolution. Although the heat generated during electrophoresis is partially dissipated by the evaporation of part of the large water content from the agarose gel, both the gel and plasma proteins are still subject to heat damage when high voltage is applied. Therefore, a cooling system is needed to absorb the excessive heat. This can be accomplished by using a thermoelectric refrigerator, a water-cooled system, or heat-absorbing crystals. Lithium nitrate, for instance, has a very low melting point. When its crystal form is sealed in an electrophoresis apparatus, a large amount of heat can be absorbed by the crystals as they melt into a liquid state. When the temperature drops after electrophoresis, the liquid lithium nitrate recrystallizes and is ready for use.

Modification of Electrophoresis Buffer

Barbiturate buffers at pH 8.6 are still most commonly used, but addition of calcium lactate to the buffers adds an important contribution to the resolution of the β-globulin band into transferrin, β-lipoprotein, and C_3 complement [14,24]. Calcium ions also enhance the staining of globulins and affect the electrophoretic mobility of the C-reactive protein [14,19,24].

The so-called *high-resolution electrophoresis (HRE)* is the *combination of the use of agarose medium,* the *application of high voltage with adequate temperature control,* and the *modification of electrophoresis buffer.* The advantages of HRE do not lie only in the improved identification of more protein fractions but also in the enhanced sensitivity of detecting abnormal bands, such as monoclonal or oligoclonal bands, C-reactive proteins, α-fetoprotein, and others. An additional attractive feature of HRE is its ability to identify the genetic variants of albumin, α_1-antitrypsin, haptoglobin, transferrin, and C_3 complement [14,24,39]. It is probably safe to state that HRE is one of the most informative tests in the clinical laboratory today.

SPECIMEN REQUIREMENTS

For the conventional five-fraction electrophoresis, serum specimens can be stored at 4°C for as long as a week without obvious alteration in electrophoretic patterns, with the possible exception of α_1-antitrypsin, which appears decreased after lengthy storage periods. HRE, however, is very sensitive to the "aging" effects of serum; thus, in general, serum specimens kept at 4°C should be tested not later than three days after specimen collection. If the analysis has to be delayed until the fourth day, plasma specimens with ethylenediaminetetraacetate (EDTA) as an anticoagulant should be used, as EDTA inactivates proteases and stabilizes C_3 complement and lipoprotein bands. The aging of serum usually causes a blurred electrophoretic pattern with a pale background, easily mistaken for generalized hypoproteinemia (Fig. 1C,D), and more profound effects are seen in C_3 complement and β-lipoprotein [14,24]. Both fractions can partially or completely disintegrate with frequent appearances of their split products, C_3c or fast-moving lipoprotein, which overlap or anodally move toward the transferrin band (Fig. 1A,B). In addition to aging, marked degrees of hyperbilirubinemia (Fig. 1E,F) and *hypertriglyceridemia* (Fig. 1G,H,I), but not hypercholesterolemia, may also cause a blurred pattern that renders the interpretation difficult or invalid. Hemolysis generally does not affect the patterns, but in severe cases, a hemoglobin band can be seen in the $α_2$-β-interzone.

If HRE can be performed within three days, serum is preferred to plasma. This is because most chemical and serological tests are done on serum, and additional plasma specimen collection can be avoided. Also a strong fibrinogen band present in plasma can mimic or overlap a paraprotein band, which is quite frequently located near the fibrinogen position. Furthermore, the superimposition of fibrinogen over the γ-zone makes it difficult to calculate the percentages when scanning is performed.

ELECTROPHORESIS PROCEDURES

There are several electrophoresis apparatuses with a cooling system available commercially (e.g., Bio-Rad, LKB, MRA Corp., Bioware Products, Worthington Diagnostics). As the Panagel™ system of Worthington Diagnostics is being used in our laboratory, the procedures described below are based mainly on this system.

Sample Application

The amount of specimen required is 10 μL of serum or plasma or equal amounts of concentrated cerebrospinal fluid (CSF) or urine with a protein content of approximately 1 g/dL. The samples are applied through the slits of a plastic sheet that covers the prebuffered agarose gel slide. Prior to application, the application site should be dried by blotting with a strip of Whatman No. 1 filter paper. The time interval between sample application is about 15–30 seconds, depending on the skill of the technician. However, it is critical that excess sample be removed with filter paper seven minutes after application and that electrophoresis be started as soon as possible.

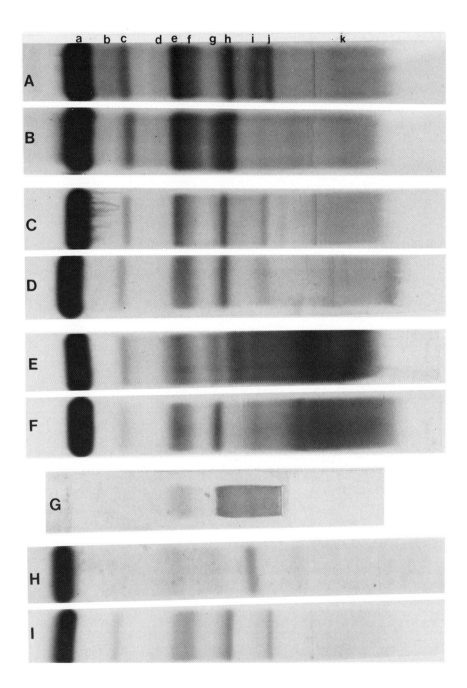

Electrophoresis

The slide is placed, gel side up, onto the curved surface of the cooling block, and the cooling block is then placed into the buffer cell. When the voltage is set at 200 V, the milliameter should read about 80 mA if an 8-sample slide is used, or 160 mA for a 16-sample slide. The electrophoresis time is 45 minutes or when the bromphenol blue stained albumin has migrated 5.5 cm. The cooling block of the Worthington System contains heat-absorbing crystals; therefore, no cool-water circulation is needed. However, after three electrophoretic runs the cooling block should be placed in the ice water to recrystallize the melted crystals prior to reuse.

Fixing, Drying, and Staining

Immediately after completion of electrophoresis, the slide is fixed in picric acid for ten minutes and rinsed twice in methanol solution. The slide is then press-dried and air-dried. For serum or plasma, the slide is stained with Amido black 10B and, for urine or CSF, with Coomassie brilliant blue. After staining, the slide is rinsed in running tap water and destained with 5% acetic acid solution. After air-drying, the slide is ready for inspection or scanning.

ELECTROPHORESIS REPORT FORMAT

Thirteen protein fractions can be identified by HRE (Fig. 2A,B; Table I). Prealbumin, albumin, α_1-antitrypsin, transferrin, β-lipoprotein, C_3 complement, and fibrinogen are usually present as discrete bands. β-Lipoprotein is

---

Fig. 1.   Factors affecting electrophoretic patterns. A–D: Serum electrophoresis affected by the aging effects. (A) An electrophoretic pattern performed on the day of specimen collection. (a) albumin, (b) α-lipoprotein, (c) α_1-antitrypsin, (d) antichmotrypsin group, (e) α_2-macroglobulin, (f) haptoglobin, (g) hemopexin, (h) transferrin, (i) β-lipoprotein, (j) C_3 complement, (k) immunoglobulins. (B) The same specimen as (A) was run three days later showing total disappearance of C_3 complement and a fast-moving lipoprotein, partly overlapping with transferrin. (C) A specimen was electrophoresed two days after collection showing a pale background mimicking generalized hypoproteinemia, the β-lipoprotein band has disintegrated. (D) The same specimen as (C) was electrophoresed three days after collection, showing marked decrease in C_3 complement and blurring of α_1-antitrypsin. α_2-Macroglobulin and haptoglobin are no longer distinguishable. E,F: A case of alcoholic cirrhosis with cholestasis. (E) A specimen with a bilirubin of 10.8 mg/dL and serum glutamic-oxaloacetic transaminase (SGOT) 156U/L showing blurring of all the fractions except albumin. (F) A specimen from the same patient when bilirubin decreased to 3.4 mg/dL and SGOT 52 U/L All the fractions are better defined, especially the transferrin. G,H,I: A case of type V hyperlipidemia. (G) Lipoprotein electrophoresis pattern. The specimen contains greater than 5,000 mg/dL of triglyerides and 353 mg/dL of cholesterol. (H) Protein electrophoresis of the same specimen showing only the albumin and transferrin bands. (I) A specimen from the same patient when triglyceride dropped to 1752 mg/dL. More fractions are recognizable than before.

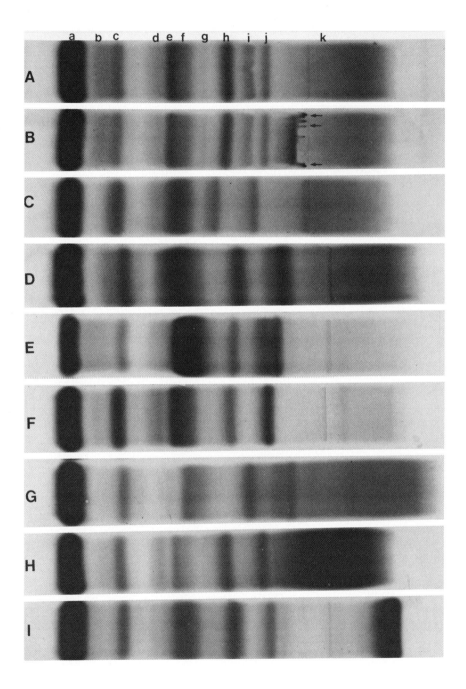

characterized by its irregular edge and tortuous configuration. α_2-Macroglobulin and haptoglobin almost always fuse into one band, but the intensity of staining makes the distinction: The former stains darker and the latter lighter.

The γ-globulins or immunoglobulins stain homogeneously, covering a broad area. Normally, IgM, as a macroglobulin, remains near the application site; IgA is present anodally to the application site, extending to the α_2-β-interzone; and IgG covers the area from the cathodal end of γ- to the α_2-β-interzone. IgD and IgE are normally present at undetectable levels; however, in case of monoclonal gammopathy, IgD and IgE can be detected as discrete bands; and the location of IgA- and IgM-monoclonal bands is not always confined to their normal positions.

TABLE I. Percentages of Protein Fractions Detected by High-Resolution Electrophoresis and Their Correlation With the Classical Five Fractions

		Percentage[a]	
Five-zone	High-resolution	Helena	Gelman
Albumin	Albumin	43.2 ± 3.9	62.6 ± 3.1
α_1-globulin	α-lipoprotein	3.0 ± 0.6	1.8 ± 0.4
	α_1-antitrypsin	3.3 ± 0.7	2.5 ± 0.6
α_2-globulin	Antichymotrypsin group	12.0 ± 2.8	8.0 ± 2.0
	α_2-macroglobulin		
	Haptoglobin		
β-globulin	Hemopexin	2.3 ± 0.5	1.2 ± 0.4
	Transferrin	6.6 ± 0.9	4.7 ± 0.7
	β-lipoprotein	2.7 ± 0.7	1.5 ± 0.5
	C_3 complement	4.2 ± 1.1	3.0 ± 0.6
γ-globulin	γ-globulin	22.9 ± 3.6	14.9 ± 3.1

[a]Twenty-two normal control specimens were scanned by densitometers manufactured by Helena and Gelman, respectively.

Fig. 2. Serum electrophoresis patterns in normal and disease status. (A) Normal serum. Abbreviations are the same as those used in Figure 1. (B) Normal plasma: The additional fraction anodal to the application site is fibrinogen, which shows the characteristic fibrin debris deposition (arrows). (c) Immediate response pattern. (D) Delayed response pattern. (E) Nephrotic syndrome. (F) Protein-losing enteropathy. (G) Hepatic cirrhosis. (H) Autoimmune hemolytic anemia: A case of Coombs' positive hemolytic anemia with splenomegaly. Haptoglobin was less than 50 mg/dL, IgG 4644 mg/dL, IgA 558 mg/dL, IgM 25 mg/dL, hemoglobin 10.5 g/dL, hct 30.8%, reticulocyte count 10%, and C_3 complement was at low normal level. (I) Monoclonal gammopathy: A case of IgG multiple myeloma.

The remaining electrophoretic zones are each dominated by one protein fraction, but they are also comprised of minor fractions [14,17,24,35]. When the minor fractions are increased, the dominant fraction will be masked, thus possibly leading to misinterpretation. For instance, the α-lipoprotein zone can be masked by α_1-acid glycoprotein during inflammatory processes or by α-fetoprotein in case of hepatoma. The antichymotrypsin zone is composed of antichymotrypsin, the group-specific components (Gc), and inter-α-trypsin inhibitor. This zone is also overlapped by haptoglobin in case of haptoglobin type 1-1 or type 1-2. The hemopexin zone is superimposed by cold insoluble globulin. In an aging serum specimen, the split products of C_3 complement and β-lipoprotein will also migrate to this area. In addition, the heterozygous phenotypes of albumin, α_1-antitrypsin, transferrin, and C_3 complement may project an extra band to their adjacent zones.

In view of these complexities, it is obvious that the considerable degree of expertise of a proteinologist is required to correctly interpret the HRE patterns in the clinical laboratory. Suffice it to say that the interpretation should always be done in conjunction with the clinical conditions. Merely mentioning which fraction is changed is hardly adequate, as it is not any better than reporting the percentage of fractionation without comments. Inexperience of clinical pathologists or clinical chemists and batch-to-batch variation of commercial products frequently lead to misinterpretations of some fractions as elevated or decreased, when the staining intensity changes. Using a normal serum control is helpful, but this normal control has to be changed every three days or the aging effects render it unsuitable for use. The electrophoretic pattern of a particular serum will remain the same only if the specimen is stored at $-70°C$ [14], which is usually not feasible in an ordinary clinical laboratory. Furthermore, mild to moderate changes in some fractions cannot be detected by direct inspection. Laurell states that hypoalbuminemia cannot be perceived with certainty unless the concentration of albumin is reduced by at least 30% [24].

Densitometric scanning of electrophoretic patterns is useful for the detection of changes in fractions which cannot be recognized by direct visualization because of the abovementioned reasons [45]. Quantitative or kinetic monitoring of protein electrophoretic patterns in a given patient is another important indication for scanning. As the quantitative measurement of immunoglobulins by techniques other than densitometry usually does not distinguish monoclonal M-proteins from normal immunoglobulins of the same class, calculation of the quantity of the M-proteins by multiplying their percentages by the total proteins is still a relatively accurate method [7].

There are, however, many factors affecting the results of densitometric scanning. These factors include the dye used for staining, the densitometer, the wavelength used, the agarose slides, the duration for electrophoresis, fixation, staining, and decolorization [47]. All these factors should be standardized when kinetic studies are desired. For the staining of agarose gel, Amido black is superior to Ponceau S in terms of definition of the protein fractions. When electrophoresis is performed on body fluids other than serum, such as cerebrospinal fluid and urine, Coomassie brilliant blue is preferred, because it is two to three times more sensitive in protein staining than Amido black [14]. With Amido black stained slides, the Helena densitometer may yield spuriously low percentages of albumin fractions, whereas the Gelman densitometer may produce a falsely low percentage of γ-fractions.

INTERPRETATION OF ELECTROPHORETIC PATTERNS

The usefulness of recognizing electrophoretic findings is determined by their specificity, which, in turn, depends on the number of diseases that may show this particular change. For instance, the absence or decrease of α_1-antitrypsin usually indicates a specific state—α_1-antitrypsin deficiency; thus, this finding is clinically useful. Increase in α_1-antitrypsin, on the other hand, can be seen in many acute and subacute disorders; therefore, this finding alone is not specific and not as useful. While the changes in a single fraction may not be specific, the combination of changes of several fractions can become meaningful. This is called a "specific pattern." For example, hypoalbuminemia is frequently seen in many clinically abnormal situations; however, when there is coexistence of hypogammaglobulinemia, hyper-α_2-macroglobulinemia, and hyper-β-lipoproteinemia, the pattern becomes almost specific for nephrotic syndrome. Electrophoretic patterns have provided a great deal of useful information [1,4,5,17,20,22,24,30,39,40,41]. Unfortunately, pattern reading is frequently abused and the electrophoretic pattern has often been mistreated and overinterpreted. If serum protein changes in diseases are computerized, probably each disease will be showing a predominant pattern, but this pattern is neither specific nor diagnostic. Examples from the literature of nonspecific and nondiagnostic patterns include myocardial infarction, rheumatic disease, systemic lupus erythematosus, pregnancy, sarcoidosis, collagen disease, Hodgkin's disease, essential hypertension, congestive heart failure, myxedema, thyrotoxicosis, diabetes mellitus, and many others [20,40]. However, by critical scrutiny, there is only a limited number of patterns that can be considered specific because of their high predictive values (Table II) [39].

SERUM PATTERNS
Immediate Response Pattern (Fig. 2C)

This pattern is not disease-specific but rather stage-specific [4,39,44]. It denotes that the disease is at an acute stage, and is usually due to inflammation or injury. The basic components of this pattern are elevation of acute phase

TABLE II. Composition of Seven Common Electrophoretic Patterns

Pattern	Alb	AAT	AM	Hp	Tf	BL	C_3	Fb	γ
Immediate response	↓	↑	N[a]	↑	↓	N	↑	↑	N
Delayed response	↓	↑	N	↑	↓	N	↑	↑	↑
Nephrotic syndrome	↓	N	↑	N	N	↑	N	↑	↓
Protein-losing enteropathy	↓	N	N or ↑	N	N	N	N	↑	↓
Hepatic cirrhosis	↓	N	N	N	N	N	N	N	↑[b]
Autoimmune hemolytic anemia	↓	N	N	↓	N	N	↓ or N	N	↑
Monoclonal gammopathy	↓	N	N	N	N	N	N	N	↑[c]

Alb = albumin, AAT = α_1-antitrypsin, AM = α_2-macroglobulin, Hp = haptoglobin, Tf = transferrin, BL = β-lipoprotein, C_3 = C_3 complement, Fb = fibrinogen, γ = γ-globulin.
[a]N = Normal.
[b]Polyclonal gammopathy with β-γ bridging.
[c]Increase in monoclonal protein only. Normal immunoglobulins may be decreased (background suppression).

reactants and decrease of some carrier proteins that sometimes are called the negative acute phase reactants (e.g., transferrin). The acute phase reactants which are demonstrable in HRE include α_1-antitrypsin, haptoglobin, C_3, and C-reactive protein. The changes of C_3, however, are less frequently encountered because its increase does not occur until late in the disease (e.g., a week after the onset of an acute episode) while changes of other acute phase reactants have occurred during the incipient stages of the disease. The elevation of C-reactive protein is not demonstrable until it reaches the peak level when a discrete band is present at the cathodal end of the γ-zone. As to the changes in carrier proteins, only when there is hypoalbuminemia, and sometimes also hypotransferrinemia, are they demonstrable. The decrease in α- and β-lipoproteins cannot be reliably measured by HRE.

Delayed Response Pattern (Fig. 2D)

This pattern is again stage-specific. It appears after the immediate response pattern, when the acute reaction is still in progression, and, simultaneously, the immune response joins in [4,39,44]. This pattern shows, in addition to the changes seen in the immediate response pattern, an elevation of immunoglobulins. This is usually found in subacute or chronic infectious diseases, especially in fungal, parasitic, or mycobacterial infections.

Nephrotic Syndrome (Fig. 2E)

This pattern is caused by the loss of proteins into the urine and reflects, therefore, a decrease in both albumin and γ-globulin. As long as the glomerular filtration maintains certain selectivity, macromolecules such as α_2-

macroglobulin and fibrinogen will be retained or even elevated in the blood [1,5,17,22,30,39,40]. The elevation is probably due to overproduction of these proteins by the liver via compensatory mechanisms. The increase of β-lipoprotein in this pattern reflects hypercholesterolemia, which is characteristically seen in nephrotic syndrome, and distinguishes this pattern from that of protein-losing enteropathy.

Protein-Losing Enteropathy (Fig. 2F)

This pattern is caused by the disturbance of absorptive function of the digestive tract, usually seen in patients with malignancies and chronic ailments as well as in cases with genuine malabsorption syndrome such as tropical sprue. It differs from the nephrotic pattern in that it presents a "bulk loss" of proteins irrespective of their molecular weights; there is no hyperbetalipoproteinemia, and hypoalbuminemia and hypogammaglobulinemia are not as prominent [4,14,39]. Elevation of α_2-macroglobulin may or may not be present.

Hepatic Cirrhosis (Fig. 2G)

This pattern is characterized by hypoalbuminemia and polyclonal gammopathy [1,4,5,14,17,39]. The specific feature of this pattern is the so-called β-γ-bridging. Normally, a pale area is present in between the β- and γ-zones. In hepatic cirrhosis, especially alcoholic cirrhosis, there often occurs a marked elevation of IgA that fills up the gap in between these two zones. The increase in acute phase reactants distinguishes the active cirrhosis from the inactive form.

Autoimmune Hemolytic Anemia (Fig. 2H)

This disorder is manifested by a decrease in haptoglobin and C_3 and an increase in γ-globulin in a polyclonal form. Hypohaptoglobinemia is due to increased consumption of haptoglobin in a complex form with liberated hemoglobin. Hypergammaglobulinemia is caused by the synthesis of autoimmune antibodies. As the antigen-antibody complexes are formed, complement components are consumed. However, the decrease in C_3 may not be obvious [14], while the more prominent decrease in C_4 complement is not demonstrable by HRE.

Monoclonal Gammopathy (Fig. 2I)

Detection of a monoclonal band (or M-protein, paraprotein band) is the most unique function of electrophoresis that still cannot be replaced by any of the quantitative techniques [10,21,29,39]. In this respect, HRE is often more sensitive than cellulose acetate electrophoresis in detecting early myeloma cases (Fig. 3). Although M-proteins can be seen anywhere from the

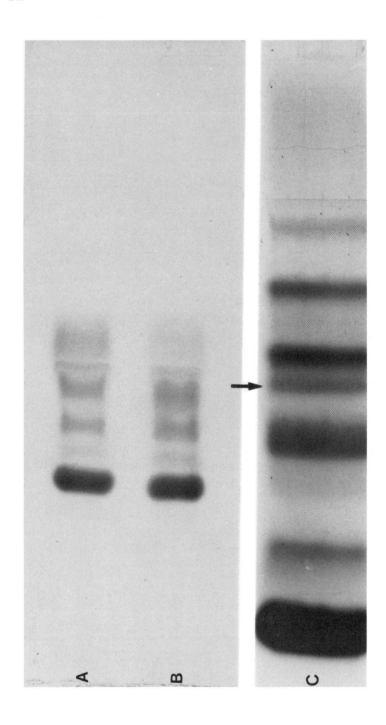

cathodal end of γ-zone to the α_1-zone, "ectopic" migration is but rarely seen, mostly in Bence Jones protein [10,21,28–30,39]. IgA is typically confined to the β-γ-interzone, and both IgG and IgM are usually encountered in the γ-zone. In malignant monoclonal gammopathy, the uninvolved immunoglobulins are usually decreased, a condition that is called "background suppression." In this pattern, hypoalbuminemia is almost invariably encountered (Fig. 3).

One of the unique features of HRE is its ability to demonstrate various configurations of different classes of M-proteins, thus providing a preliminary identification (Fig. 4) [39]. The IgG band usually shows smooth edges with slightly bulging ends. The IgM band is usually narrower than the IgG band and has sawtoothed edges and flattened ends. Background suppression in macroglobulinemia involves not only the γ-zone but also all the other fractions. This generalized hypoproteinemia background is often related to the therapeutic procedure, namely, plasmapheresis. The IgA band is usually much broader than the IgG and IgM bands due to its tendency to polymerize. It is also characterized by blurred edges and bulging ends and is usually tapered toward the anodal end, forming a trapezoid configuration. The configuration of light chain bands is similar to that of IgG, except that it is narrower. While these general configurations are valid on a statistical basis, in an individual serum sample they are not always diagnostic.

Immune complexes, especially for those with a monoclonal antibody component and those in the form of cryoglobulins, can be detected as a discrete band in the γ- or β-γ-zone. This band usually has blurred edges and flattened ends (Fig. 4G). Acidification of serum to pH 3.0 may dissociate the immune complexes [18].

CHANGES IN INDIVIDUAL FRACTIONS

The evaluation of individual fractions is based on their heterogeneity, electrophoretic mobility, and concentration. Heterogeneity reflects hereditary changes which can be seen as double bands in albumin, α_1-antitrypsin, haptoglobin, transferrin, and C_3 complement (Fig. 5). The changes in elec-

---

Fig. 3. A 57-year-old female with λ-L-chain myeloma proved by bone marrow and radiological examinations. (A) and (B) are cellulose acetate electrophoresis of normal control and of the patient's specimen, respectively. The latter shows hypogammaglobulinemia, but no monoclonal protein band is identified. (C) Agarose electrophoresis of the same specimen: A monoclonal band is shown in the α_2-β-interzone (arrow) with marked background suppression in the γ-zone. The monoclonal band was identified as monoclonal λ-light chain by immunofixation and immunoelectrophoresis. There was generalized hypoimmunoglobulinemia (IgG 319 mg/dL, IgA 24 mg/dL, IgM 34 mg/dL).

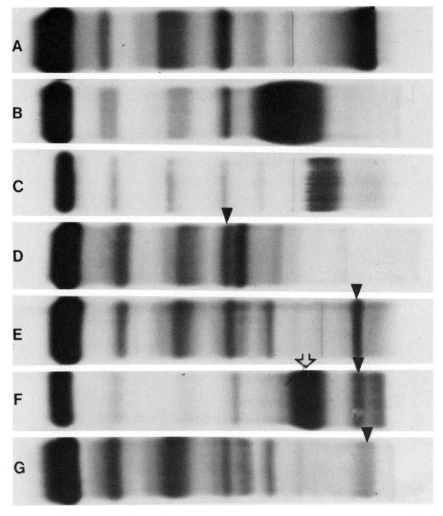

Fig. 4. Configuration and location of paraprotein M-bands. (A) IgG. monoclonal gammopathy. (B) IgA monoclonal gammopathy. (C) IgM monoclonal gammopathy. (D) IgD monoclonal gammopathy showing atypical location (arrow head) of the monoclonal band. This atypical location is the major reason for the frequent failure of cellulose acetate electrophoresis to detect IgD myeloma. (E) λ-Light chain myeloma. The arrow head indicates the M-protein band. (F) IgA-IgG biclonal gammopathy. The broad band is IgA-λ (hollow arrow) and the narrow one IgG-λ (arrow head). The cathodal end shows the remaining part of normal immunoglobulins. (G) Immune complex: A case of nephrotic syndrome with immune complex deposit on the basement membrane of the glomeruli. Rheumatoid factor titer was 1:320 by latex fixation. IgM-κ was identified in the cryoglobulin by immunoelectrophoresis. An additional IgG component was found in the immune complex by immunofixation, probably as the autologous antigen. The arrow head points at a poorly defined monoclonal band, representing the immune complex.

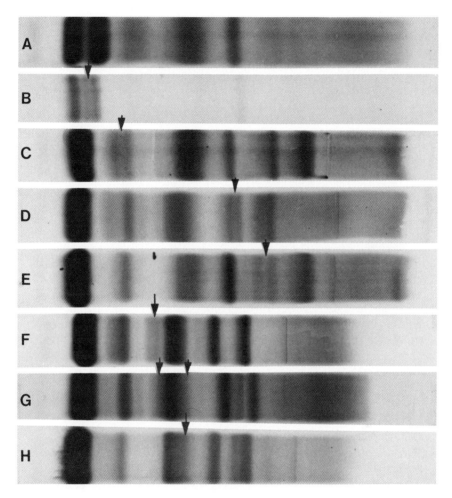

Fig. 5. Genetic variants of protein fractions. (A) Bisalbuminemia. (B) Bisalbuminuria: the slow albumin band further splits into two bands (arrow). (C) Heterozygous α_1-antitrypsin phenotype, showing double α_1-antitrypsin bands (arrow). (D) Double transferrin bands (arrows). (E) Double C_3 complement bands (arrow). (F) Haptoglobin phenotype Hp 1–1; the arrow indicates the location of the haptoglobin band. (G) Haptoglobin phenotype Hp 1–2; the arrows indicate the location of the haptoglobin bands. (H) Haptoglobin phenotype Hp 2–2; the arrow indicates the location of the haptoglobin band.

trophoretic mobility can be due to the following factors: (1) heredity; (2) binding of the individual fraction to a certain chemical substance, such as penicillin-albumin complex; and (3) disintegration of a protein fraction, such as lipoprotein and C_3 complement. The most common and significant findings in electrophoresis are the changes of individual protein fractions in their concentrations [30,33]. This will be discussed further in detail.

Prealbumin

Hypoprealbuminemia is supposed to be seen in inflammatory reactions, malnutrition, or conditions where functioning liver cell mass is decreased [14,24]. Increase in prealbumin is encountered in alcoholism. The problem is that prealbumin is only consistently seen in CSF but rarely discernible in serum or urine; thus its clinical significance is difficult to evaluate.

Albumin

Hypoalbuminemia is the only clinically important finding for this fraction. However, its presence is not specific as it can be seen in many situations, such as diseases of the liver, the gastrointestinal tract, and kidney; and malnutrition, malignancy, or any chronic ailments, including infections, that prevent either the synthesis or the absorption of albumin [1,5,22,29,33,40]. A broad albumin band with a diffuse anodal edge (see also Pseudobisalbuminemias) usually indicates the presence of increased bilirubin levels or certain drugs (e.g., penicillin and aspirin), which conjugate with albumin fraction (Fig. 6B) [14,24,39]. A double albumin band denotes bisalbuminemia (Fig. 5A), which is not disease-associated but is the only known cause of genuine "hyperalbuminemia" [11,42].

Alpha-Lipoprotein (AL)

AL occupies the albumin-α_1-antitrypsin interzone. It is not a discrete band; therefore, the estimation of its concentration by HRE is not reliable. Only a marked decrease in AL can be appreciated from an electrophoretogram, which may represent the existence of liver diseases [14,24]. Increase in density in this zone is more likely due to elevation of α_1-glycoprotein, an acute phase reactant, rather than AL. α_1-Fetoprotein can be present as a discrete band in this zone when it is markedly increased in hepatoma or other related tumors [14,24]. However, heterozygous α_1-antitrypsin, bisalbuminemia, and even Bence Jones proteinemia should be excluded before identifying a band as α-fetoprotein.

Alpha-1-Antitrypsin (AAT)

In HRE, AAT is present as a discrete band without any superimposed component; thus it is far more accurate in estimating this fraction than the

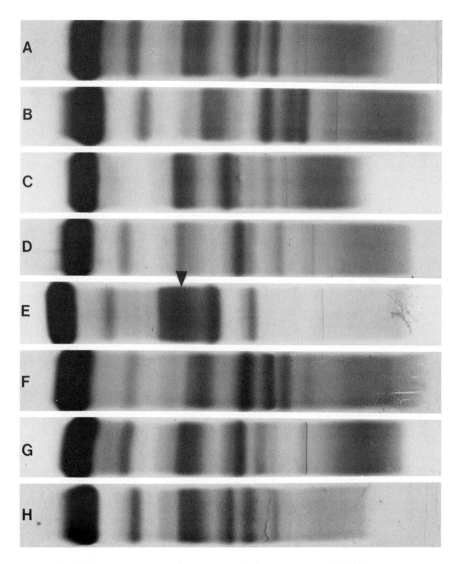

Fig. 6. Changes in individual fractions. (A) Normal serum. (B) Hyperbilirubinemia, showing bilirubin-conjugated albumin. (C) Homozygous α_1-antitrypsin deficiency, showing absence of α_1-antitrypsin. The phenotype of this case was PiZ. (D) Hypohaptoglobinemia in a case of hemolytic anemia. (E) Haptoglobin-hemoglobin complex in a case of hemolytic disease. Note the α_2-β-interzone is entirely occupied by the complex (arrow head). The pattern also shows severe hypogammaglobulinemia. (F) Hyperbetalipoproteinemia, showing prominent β-lipoprotein band. (G) Hypocomplementemia, showing markedly decreased C_3 complement. (H) Hypogammaglobulinemia.

five-fraction system. As an acute phase reactant, its elevation is frequently seen and is therefore nonspecific. Its decrease, however, is highly significant clinically. Absence of AAT band is seen in PiZ of PiS phenotypes (Fig. 6C). Heterozygous AAT deficiency may show decreased staining intensity or may appear as a double band (Fig. 5C). Most AAT deficiencies are of hereditary origin [27,36,37], although it can be present in respiratory distress syndrome [9]. In multiple myeloma, M-proteins such as IgA or Bence Jones protein may be bound to AAT, causing a relative deficiency when measured by radial immunodiffusion technique [36].

Antichymotrypsin

This fraction is present at the α_1-α_2-interzone, which is also occupied by inter-α-trypsin inhibitor, the group-specific components, and the fast haptoglobin in the case of phenotype 1–1 and 2–1 [24,35]. Therefore, it is difficult to estimate the individual fractions in this zone.

Alpha-2-Macroglobulin (AM)

The elevation of AM is most striking in nephrotic syndrome and to a lesser degree may also be seen in protein-losing enteropathy, pregnancy, and administration of estrogen preparations [17,22,24,33,39]. The decrease in AM is nonspecific and usually not detectable in electrophoresis because of its overlapping position with haptoglobin.

Haptoglobin (Hp)

The ability to identify Hp phenotypes is one of the special features of HRE [24]. The fast Hp represents phenotype 1 and the slow one, phenotype 2. If Hp can be seen only on the anodal side of AM, the phenotype is denoted Hp 1–1 (Fig. 5F); when seen only on the cathodal side of AM, Hp 2–2 (Fig. 5H); the phenotype Hp 2–1 is present when Hp is seen on both sides of AM (Fig. 5G). The decrease of Hp concentrations is rather specific, as it indicates intravascular hemolysis (Fig. 6D). Occasionally Hp-hemoglobin complexes can be demonstrated in the α_2-zone or α_2-β-interzone as a dense protein band (Fig. 6E) [14,24,39]. *In vitro* hemolysis and formation of Hp-Hb complexes often results in a cathodal shift and increase of the Hp fraction. As an acute phase reactant, elevation of Hp is frequently seen and is thus nonspecific.

Hemopexin (Hx)

During hemolysis, the free heme binds with Hx, forming a complex for possible further disposal by the hepatocyte. The determination of Hx is therefore very useful for the evaluation of hemolysis when haptoglobin is exhausted. The Hx zone in HRE is, however, poorly defined, and is overlapped by cold insoluble protein [14,24]. The information provided by HRE from this zone is therefore not helpful.

Transferrin (Tf) (Fig. 7)

As a negative acute phase reactant, the decrease in Tf is frequently seen in inflammation, injury, and malnutrition. The increase in Tf is, however, more specific as it is only encountered in iron deficiency, pregnancy, ingestion of estrogen preparations, and possibly hepatitis [14,24]. In aged specimens, Tf can be overlapped by degradation products of β-lipoprotein or C3 complement, yielding falsely high results.

Beta-Lipoprotein (BL)

Hyperbetalipoproteinemia causes slower mobility and darker staining of BL (Fig. 6F). Disintegration of BL and increase nonesterified fatty acid content induce fast mobility [14,24]. It should be borne in mind, however, that IgA overlaps with BL and may affect the intensity of the latter. Heparin therapy may result in anodal extension of lipoprotein moieties (see Pseudobisalbuminemias).

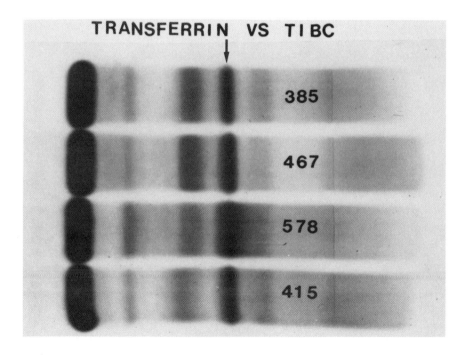

Fig. 7. Comparison of the density of transferrin bands (arrow) with the total iron binding capacity in μg/dL, showing proportional changes.

C₃ Complement (C₃)

C₃ is very labile and it readily disintegrates. Its conversion product C_3c has a fast β_1-mobility. However, it is difficult to distinguish its *in vitro* activation from *in vivo* activation based on electrophoretic pattern alone [14,24]. A more reliable technique for the detection of the C_3 conversion product is counterimmunoelectrophoresis [2]. To rule out *in vitro* activation, in cases where C_3 determination is especially important, fresh serum or, preferably EDTA plasma should be used. Decrease in staining intensity also indicates activation (*in vivo* or *in vitro*) or congenital deficiency (Fig. 6B). Complement activation associated with autoimmune diseases or immune complex disorders, such as lupus erythematosus and poststreptococcal glomerulonephritis, usually occurs via the classic pathway [46]. Infections such as bacterial endocarditis and gram-negative sepsis, on the other hand, activate the complement system mainly through the alternative pathway [46]. Regardless of the pathway involved, C_3 is inevitably decreased. Elevation of C_3 is seen five to seven days after injury or inflammation, as an acute phase reaction.

Fibrinogen (Fb)

Fb is also an acute phase reactant and its elevation is frequently seen in acute disorders [44]. Decrease in Fb denotes fibrinolysis or a congenital anomaly [14,24]. However, as mentioned under Specimen Requirements, the disadvantages of using plasma specimens outweigh the information obtained by the presence of an Fb band. The most important disadvantage, however, is that this band frequently mimics or masks a monoclonal band. As a result, immunoelectrophoresis is often unnecessarily performed in order to identify the "monoclonal protein." A fibrinogen band can be occasionally seen in serum specimens, if the patient is receiving heparin therapy or if the serum is separated from red cells before clotting is completed.

Gamma-Globulin or Immunoglobulin (Ig)

HRE is an excellent tool for the study of gammopathies and is superior to any other type of electrophoresis in this respect [14,24,39]. Based on the electrophoretic findings, gammopathies can be divided into three groups: monoclonal, polyclonal, and oligoclonal (Fig. 8).

Monoclonal gammopathy, as discussed previously, is manifested as a discrete band in a restricted area (Fig. 8A). *Polyclonal gammopathy,* on the other hand, shows a generalized diffuse elevation of staining intensity, covering a part of or the entire γ-zone (Fig. 8B). Polyclonal gammopathy usually involves all classes of Igs. However, it may also involve only a single class of Ig that is produced by different clones of plasma cells, as evidenced by

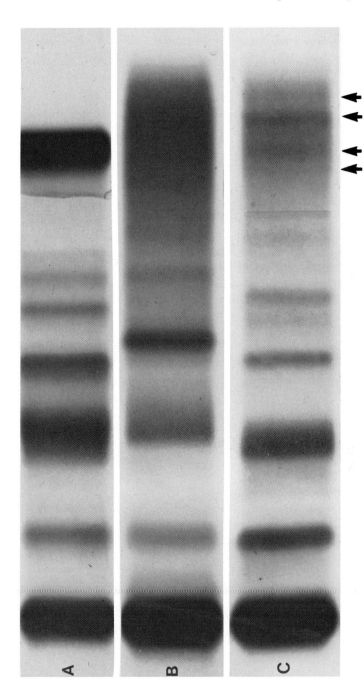

Fig. 8. Three types of gammopathy: (A) monoclonal, (B) polyclonal, and (C) oligoclonal gammopathy (arrows).

the elevation of both κ- and λ-light chains in a normal ratio, but only one heavy chain. In the latter situation, only IgG polyclonal gammopathy can be readily appreciated from an electrophoretogram. If IgA is markedly elevated, the β-γ-interzone may show increased staining intensity, but this phenomenon usually does not occur alone; frequently other classes of Ig are also increased. Selective IgM polyclonal gammopathy is hardly discernible on HRE as it overlaps entirely with IgG and its increase can be masked by the bulk of IgG. Marked polyclonal gammopathy is usually seen in autoimmune or collagen diseases, for example, lupus erythematosus and rheumatoid arthritis, and sometimes in hepatic diseases [29]. However, it is seldom found in infectious diseases in this country perhaps because they are mostly only transient and not severe. Parasitic diseases involving the reticuloendothelial system, such as kala-azar and leishmaniasis, can cause extreme hypergammaglobulinemia, but again they are rare in the United States.

Oligoclonal gammopathy denotes multiple rather narrow faint bands in the γ-zone, usually near the cathodal end (Fig. 8C). The ability to detect oligoclonal banding is one of the distinguishing features of HRE [16,39]. Its presence usually indicates an early immune response in infectious diseases, especially in viral infections, and represents the products of several small clones of plasma cells [24]. Oligoclonal gammopathy frequently is also associated with malignancy [24,39]. If this pattern is detected in a clinically nonmalignant case, it is probably worthwhile to check for an occult tumor. Oligoclonal bands are usually seen in the CSF of patients with demyelinating diseases but may be occasionally also demonstrated in the serum of those cases [16,23,26,34].

Hypogammaglobulinemia is one of the most frequent findings in electrophoresis (Fig. 6H). [39]. Secondary hypogammaglobulinemia, if due to nephrotic syndrome or protein-losing enteropathy, can be traced by pattern reading [29,39]. When the Ig is extremely low, however, a primary cause should be considered.

C-Reactive Protein (CRP)

HRE is the only electrophoresis system that can detect a discrete CRP band if present in appreciable amounts, because of its resolution power and also because the CRP is located in the terminal γ-zone without being superimposed by any other discrete band (see Fig. 11C, p. 58) [19,24,39]. In other systems, such as cellulose acetate electrophoresis, where the buffer does not contain calcium ion, CRP is present in the α_2- or β-zone, overlapping with other protein bands. The sensitivity of HRE for the detection of CRP is comparable to that of the Ouchterlony double diffusion technique. When a suspected CRP is present, Ouchterlony technique or other assays (e.g., nephelometry, latex agglutination) can be used for further confirmation. CRP is considered to be superior to the time-honored markers of acute phase phenomena, such as fever, leukocytosis, and the erythrocyte sedimentation rate for the evaluation of inflammation or for postoperative follow-up [33].

CSF ELECTROPHORESIS

The study of CSF electrophoresis is mostly confined to the γ-zone [8,14,24,39].

The most important finding is *oligoclonal banding,* which is characteristic of demyelinating disorders [16,23,26,34]. These bands represent local production of immunoglobulins by immunocytes in the central nervous system (CNS). In most of the large series, 90% of the patients with multiple sclerosis have oligoclonal gammopathy (Fig. 9D) [16,23,26,34]. On the other hand, this pattern is not only seen in multiple sclerosis, but also seen in infections, especially in viral infections of the CNS [16,23,26,34]. The banding in the latter group is, however, only transient, whereas in multiple sclerosis, it is usually persistent. These bands are mostly composed of IgG, especially IgG-1 subclass [6,34], although in some cases, IgA, IgM, and light chains can also be demonstrated [34,48]. It is of interest to note that the oligoclonal bands seen in subacute sclerosing panencephalitis (SSPE) contain antibodies against measles virus, suggesting a possible causative role of this virus in the development of SSPE [6,34].

A normal fraction, which is frequently confused with oligoclonal bands, is *γ-trace* [22]. It is usually present as a faint but discrete band at the cathodal end of γ-zone. As γ-trace is unrelated to immunoglobulins, immunofixation technique can distinguish it from oligoclonal gammopathy in which usually more than one band should be detectable.

Polyclonal gammopathy in CSF usually indicates inflammation of CNS with resultant increased permeability of the blood-CSF barrier. It can also be seen in brain tumors, polyneuropathies, and cerebral infarcts (Fig. 9A,B) [5,14,24,39].

Monoclonal gammopathy in CSF (Fig. 9C) is often due to multiple myeloma, thus the abnormal protein is usually of serum source [39], but it can also be locally produced in the CNS if there is myelomatous infiltration in the brain. Monoclonal bands are occasionally seen in epilepsy and syphilis [39]. When CSF electrophoresis is performed, it is advisable to also assay a serum sample from the same patient simultaneously to evaluate the origin of any change in the γ-zone. If both serum and CSF show a monoclonal band, for instance, the change is usually of serum origin.

The presence of a carbohydrate deficient *β_2-transferrin* in addition to the *β_1-transferrin* is characteristic for CSF and has been used for its identification [13]. The so-called *degenerative pattern* consists of an increase of β_2-glob-

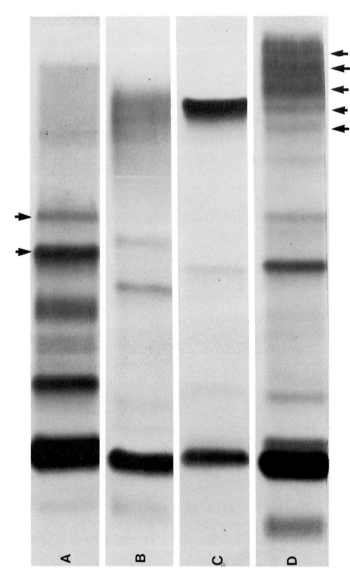

Fig. 9. Electrophoretic patterns of cerebrospinal fluid (CSF) (A) Marked increase in permeability of blood-CSF barrier showing almost all the serum protein components. Note slow and fast transferrin bands (arrows) are present. This is a case of acute idiopathic polyneuritis. The specimen contains total CSF protein of 970 mg/dL, γ-globulin 12%, albumin 660 mg/dL, IgG 90 mg/dL, and IgG/albumin ratio is 0.14. Serum IgG/albumin ratio is 0.17. (B) Polyclonal gammopathy: This is a case of bacterial meningitis. The specimen contains total protein of 55 mg/dL, γ-globulin 41%, albumin 18.8 mg/dL, IgG 23.2 mg/dL and IgG/albumin ratio 1.23. Serum IgG/albumin ratio is 1.39. (C) Monoclonal gammopathy: This is a case of IgG myeloma. The specimen contains total protein of 120 mg/dL, γ-globulin 43%, albumin 41mg/dL, IgG 82 mg/dL and IgG/albumin ratio 2.0. Serum IgG/albumin ratio is 4.2. (D) Oligoclonal gammopathy: This is a case of multiple sclerosis showing five narrow bands in the γ-zone (arrows). The specimen contains total protein of 37 mg/dL, γ-globulin 33%, albumin 17 mg/dL, IgG 12 mg/dL, and IgG/albumin ratio 0.71. The serum IgG/albumin ratio is 0.33.

ulin, which is mainly due to the elevation of the slow transferrin but can also be the result of changes in mobility of α_1-acid glycoprotein, α_1-antitrypsin, ceruloplasmin, haptoglobin, and hemopexin [5]. The degenerative pattern can be seen in cerebral atrophy, syringomyelia, amyotrophic lateral sclerosis, and recurrent anoxia [5]. A recent report correlates the presence of a rare genetic variant of transferrin (phenotype $B_{0-1}C$) with Marie-Sanger-Brown's ataxia [32]. The mechanism of the formation of the degenerative pattern is unknown; it can be either due to specific CNS protein synthesis, or protein alteration secondary to degenerative diseases.

URINE ELECTROPHORESIS

The most important function of urine electrophoresis is for the *screening of Bence Jones protein (BJP)*, which has been redefined as monoclonal free light chain to replace the original definition given by Bence Jones. The classical heat test shows approximately two-thirds false-negative [39] and one-fifth false-positive results [28], indicating that the physicochemical properties of this protein at different temperatures are not essential. It should be emphasized that dip-sticks for urine proteins are also not useful in detecting BJP, i.e., BJP may be present when the dip-stick indicates no protein in the urine. This phenomenon is due to the small number and low affinity of binding sites on BJP molecules for the indicator dye used in dip-sticks [3]. On the contrary, the HRE is a very reliable way for BJP screening.

BJP appears as one or more discrete bands in γ-, β- and, very rarely, α_2- or α_1-zones (Fig. 10H) [28,30,39]. The presence of large amounts of lysozyme, myoglobin, and hemoglobin (Fig. 10I,J) in urine may also mimic an M-protein band [21,29,31]. However, these findings are rare; in addition, the bands are usually fainter than the BJP band and are never multiple. On the other hand, false-negative results are even more uncommon, as they have never been encountered in our laboratory. If there is no monoclonal band detected in the electrophoretogram, BJP can usually be ruled out provided the urine specimen examined was sufficiently concentrated (e.g., $50\times$). Patterns of oligoclonal and polyclonal gammopathy are considered negative for BJP. Immunoelectrophoresis is a very helpful confirmative test for BJP, especially for typing, but false-positive results may be encountered. When renal permeability is increased or tubular reabsorption is decreased (or even in normal persons), polyclonal light chains may appear in the urine, especially when concentrated ≥ 100 times. However, the κ/λ ratio is about 2:1, and the light chains present in the urine are disintegrated by the action of bacteria or lysozyme; finally only free κ-light chain is left in the urine specimen. This result, when demonstrated by immunoelectrophoresis, can be misinterpreted as BJP, but if there is no monoclonal band present on the electro-

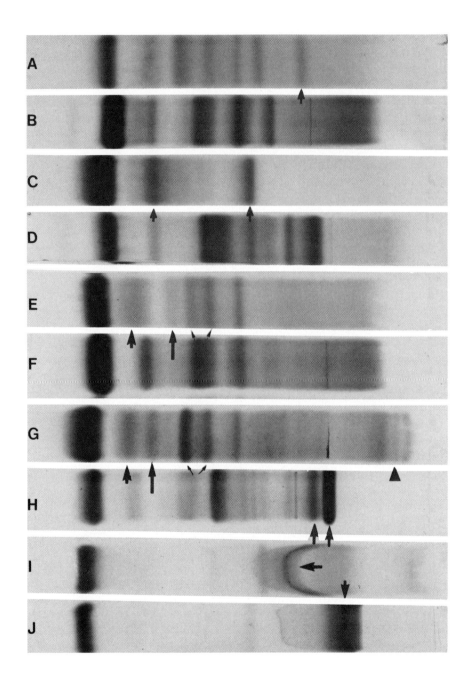

phoretogram, false positivity should be considered. Immunofixation electrophoresis [38] and Ouchterlony techniques [49] can further verify this situation. Bence Jones proteinuria can be classified as prerenal proteinuria because BJP as well as other low molecular weight proteins such as hemoglobin, myoglobin, and lysozyme may appear in the urine even if the kidneys are normal [5].

Recently, there has been an increasing interest in nephrology for the distinction between *glomerular and tubular proteinuria*. Here, electrophoresis can be helpful for the differential diagnosis except in the late uremic stage when glomeruli and tubules are both damaged. To evaluate the severity of kidney damage, however, quantitation of total urine protein is more revealing than electrophoresis. Tubular proteinuria is usually associated with protein loss of no more than 0.5 g/d; if the urine protein is higher than this quantity, glomerular or mixed proteinuria should be considered.

The distinction between glomerular and tubular proteinuria provides a clue to the possible etiology. Glomerular proteinuria is usually due to inflammation or increase in venous pressure, while tubular proteinuria may be caused by

Fig. 10. Electrophoretic patterns of urine. (A) Predominant nonselective glomerular proteinuria showing most of the plasma protein fractions. Note that the concentration of the immunoglobulins is proportional to that of albumin and that larger molecules like fibrinogen (arrow) are present in the urine. (B) Serum specimen from the same patient as (A). (C) Selective glomerular proteinuria showing predominantly albumin, α_1-antitrypsin (arrow) and transferrin (arrow). (D) Plasma specimen from the same patient as (C). (E) Selective glomerular proteinuria in acute inflammation showing albumin, α_1-acid glycoprotein (orosomucoid) (short arrow), Zn-α_2-glycoprotein (long arrow), α_2-microglobulin (double-banded, indicated by small arrow heads), and transferrin. The presence of orosomucoid and Zn-α_2-glycoprotein denotes the presence of inflammation, while the appearance of α_2-microglobulin indicates involvement of renal tubules. (F) Serum specimen from the same patient as (E). (G) Combination of glomerular nonselective proteinuria and tubular proteinuria showing the presence of albumin, α_1-antitrypsin (long arrow), orosomucoid (short arrow), α_2-microglobulin (double-banded, small arrows), transferrin and γ-trace (large arrow head). This is a case of end stage kidney with uremia. (H) Bence Jones proteinuria, showing a pair of monoclonal bands (arrows) with different staining intensity present near the application site at the γ-zone. The lighter-stained band is probably the split product of Bence Jones protein (BJP) and its presence is characteristic for BJP in agarose electrophoresis. The presence of several low molecular protein bands is due to competitive inhibition of tubular reabsorption of these proteins by BJP. (I,J) Hemoglobinuria: The hemoglobin is better illustrated as a "monoclonal" band (arrow) by Amido black stain (J), whereas in Coomassie brilliant blue stained slide (I), the diffuse portion of hemoglobin is stained as a curved arc (arrow). Hemoglobin band is more frequently seen in α_2-β- interzone than in γ-zone. This is a case of idiopathic autoimmune hemolytic anemia with a hemoglobin of 5.3 g/dL and hematocrit 16.3%. Reticulocyte count was 26%. Both direct and indirect Coombs' tests were positive. Chemistry profile showed total bilirubin 6.6 mg/dL, with direct bilirubin 6.0 mg/dL, lactic dehydrogenase 473 U/L, and haptoglobin less than 50 mg/dL. Hemoglobinuria was proved by a dip-stick test. During the second admission, splenectomy was performed. The patient's situation improved and all laboratory findings gradually returned to normal or near normal.

chemical poisoning, acute renal tubular failure, systemic lupus erythematosus, or hereditary disorders, such as Fanconi syndrome [5,17,30].

Glomerular proteinuria can be further divided into *nonselective and selective types*. In the nonselective type, the urine pattern can be very similar to that of the serum (Fig. 10A,B). In other words, most plasma proteins are filtered unchanged through the hyperpermeable glomeruli. A good indication of nonselective glomerular proteinuria is the elevated urine gamma/albumin ratio which will be very close to the serum ratio. The selective type is characterized by the presence of albumin, α_1-antitrypsin, and transferrin (Fig. 10C,D). In inflammatory conditions, α_1-acid glycoprotein and Zn-α_2-glycoprotein (a low molecular protein present in the α_1-α_2-interzone) also appear (Fig. 10E,F).

Tubular proteinuria is due to the inability of renal tubules to reabsorb the low molecular proteins (molecular weight below 20,000 dalton), which are then accumulated to detectable levels in urine [5,14,24,30]. As a result, α_2-microglobulin, β-microglobulin and γ-trace are present in the urine (Fig. 10G). For the identification of these protein bands, urine and serum specimens from the same patient should be electrophoresed side by side simultaneously. Urine α_2-microglobulin appears as a pair of protein bands at both sides of the serum α_2-macroglobulin when the urine and serum strips are compared (Fig. 10G). The urine β-microglobulin occupies the space of the serum β-lipoprotein, which is not filtered through the glomeruli because of its large size. The γ-trace in urine is present at the cathodal end of γ-globulin similar to its position on CSF electrophoresis.

The more accurate way of identifying these low molecular proteins is by sodium dodecyl-sulfate (SDS) polyacrylamide gel electrophoresis for the direct measurement of their molecular weights. However, this method is time-consuming since the required electrophoretic columns are not commercially available. A relatively convenient way to achieve this goal is simply *quantifying β-microglobulin,* as a representative protein, by radioimmunoassay. If there is an increase of β-microglobulin in a nonuremic patient, the diagnosis of tubular proteinuria is usually established.

SUPPLEMENTARY TESTS
Quantitative Tests

The issue of quantitation of individual protein fractions versus electrophoresis is of practical importance [25,45]. It is obvious that quantitation cannot at this time completely replace electrophoresis for some of its important functions, for instance, the demonstration of monoclonal and oligoclonal banding. On the contrary, it seems desirable that regardless of the method used for immunoglobulin quantitation, an electrophoresis should be done to screen for M-proteins. The presence of an M-protein may cause falsely high or low results in quantitation because of antigen excess, poly-merization of protein molecules, or coexistence of multiple protein moieties.

A routine performance of multiple protein quantitation is not only costly (thus not feasible in a clinical laboratory) but also not necessary [45]. Se-lective quantitation should be done only when indicated by electrophoretic findings and by clinical situations. For instance, if the γ-globulin in an electrophoretogram is normal, there is no need to quantify IgG, IgA, and IgM unless selective immunodeficiency or multiple myeloma is suspected clinically. On the other hand, when all the acute phase reactants are elevated in electrophoresis, the additional α_1-acid glycoprotein assay will not provide any new information.

Only total protein and albumin are quantified in our laboratory routinely. Total protein quantitation is also a satisfactory method for quality control, because it can be used for the comparison of the staining intensity of elec-trophoretic patterns, and it also serves as the basis for the calculation of the relative quantities of individual protein fractions. The measuring of albumin is also a means for quality assurance as comparison can be made with its calculated value. As mentioned before, the calculated value may not be accurate when certain densitometers are used. When the scanning reveals decreased levels of certain proteins, such as α_1-antitrypsin, haptoglobin, C_3 complement, and immunoglobulins, quantitation of the changed fraction should be performed to verify and substantiate the electrophoretic findings. Im-munoglobulins are also quantitated when increased.

Total protein should also be determined routinely on CSF and urine spec-imens. In addition, a routine IgG/albumin ratio should be done on CSF and, whenever feasible, compared with that of the serum [12,43]. When the ratio of the CSF is higher than that of the serum, local production of IgG in the central nervous system is indicated.

When financially feasible, serum specimens for electrophoresis should also be analyzed by a multichannel analyzer (SMAC), which provides val-uable information aiding in the interpretation of electrophoretic patterns. For instance, abnormal renal function tests will substantiate the nephrotic pattern, while abnormal liver function tests support the pattern of hepatic cirrhosis.

Qualitative Tests

The main purpose of the qualitative tests in this context is to distinguish paraproteins from pseudoparaproteins. While paraproteins may occasionally hide under a normal fraction, several protein bands can mimic paraproteins. The most common ones are the fibrinogen (Fig. 11B) and the C-reactive protein (Fig. 11C) [21,39]. The position of fibrinogen and the occasional presence of tiny fibrin debris near the band (Fig. 2B) are usually helpful in identifying this protein. The location, the width, and the low intensity of the CRP band often suggest its identity. The presence of an extra band in heterozygous

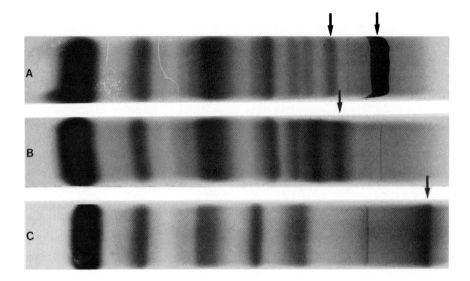

Fig. 11. Commonly encountered pseudoparaprotein bands. (A) A partially dried specimen stays at the application site forming a pseudoparaprotein band (arrow). A fibrinogen band is also present (arrow). (B) Fibrinogen band (arrow) in a serum specimen mimicking monoclonal band. (C) A distinct C-reactive protein (arrow) is seen at the cathodal end of the γ-zone.

phenotypes of transferrin, C_3 complement, albumin, and α_1-antitrypsin may also be mistaken as paraprotein [14,24]. The infrequent occurrence of bands of lysozyme, myoglobin, and hemoglobin may also cause some confusion [21,29,31]. Finally, if the specimen is partially desiccated after application (Fig. 11A) or an excessive specimen volume is applied, a thick band will appear at the application site, causing unnecessary diagnostic considerations. For the verification of the abovementioned situations the following tests should be used selectively [50].

Immunoelectrophoresis (IEP). This is the most frequently performed supplementary test in conjunction with electrophoresis for the confirmation, classification, and light chain typing in monoclonal gammopathy [10,21,29]. When a monoclonal band is located at cathodal end of the γ-zone, a reversed polarity IEP should be performed [39a]. It can also be used for the identification of other proteins that mimic paraproteins. However, it is a time-consuming and costly test. Therefore, its use is confined mainly to the study of immunoglobulin, whereas other proteins are identified by simpler techniques.

Immunofixation electrophoresis. Immunofixation appears to be gradually supplementing IEP in some laboratories. However, we are still more confident in diagnosing monoclonal gammopathies with IEP because of the presence of prominent changes in configuration, density and/or electrophoretic mobility of the precipitating arcs, and also because of the side-by-side comparison with normal controls in IEP.

The most important indication of immunofixation is probably the detection of abnormal, bound light chains which are not demonstrable by IEP either due to the umbrella effect of IgG (e.g., IgM macroglobulinemia) or due to precipitate inhibition (e.g., IgA myeloma) [6,38]. It is also easier to identify the composition of an oligoclonal band by immunofixation than by IEP, because the concentration of the antigens is not diluted by diffusion [6,38]. Therefore, immunofixation should be used for further investigation when IEP fails to verify the nature of a monoclonal band. Other indications for the use of immunofixation will be discussed in Chapter 5.

Ouchterlony immunodiffusion technique (OT). This is a convenient technique for the diagnosis of Bence Jones proteins if a reliable free light chain antiserum is available [31,49]. It can also be used to identify the nature of a non-γ-monoclonal band with C-reactive protein, lysozyme, and myoglobin antisera. In case of doubt, immunofixation should be used to verify the results by directly applying the monospecific antiserum to the monoclonal band.

Fibrinogen precipitation. It is always of diagnostic concern when a fibrinogen band is present in the serum or is markedly increased in plasma, as it mimics a M-protein band. Before proceeding to IEP, one can simply mix the specimen with an equal part of thrombin. The mixture is then centrifuged and the supernatant electrophoresed. If the pseudoparaprotein band is fibrinogen, it will disappear after this treatment (Fig. 12). Screening by Ouchterlony technique with antifibrinogen antiserum or by quantitating fibrinogen by fast nephelometry or turbidity methods [49] is also a practical approach.

Isoelectric focusing. This technique is excellent for the study of the genetic polymorphism of plasma proteins, especially when it is used in combination with immunofixation (see Chapter 5). If an extra band is present in the electrophoretogram due to a heterozygous phenotype of a certain protein, isoelectric focusing should verify its nature. This technique, however, is cumbersome and costly, and therefore not practical for routine phenotyping in a clinical laboratory. A more promising application of this technique is for the testing of CSF for oligoclonal banding [34]. This should be done in clinically highly suspected cases of multiple sclerosis, when electrophoresis fails to demonstrate the oligoclonal bands.

SUMMARY

The HRE provides information about 13 protein fractions, but only 10 of them can be reliably evaluated. These 10 fractions are prealbumin, albumin, α_1-antitrypsin, haptoglobin, α_2-macroglobulin, transferrin, β-lipoprotein, C_3

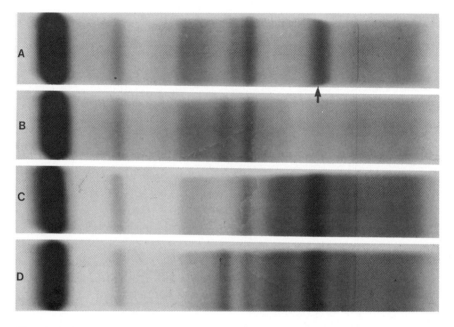

Fig. 12. Fibrinogen precipitation. (A) A plasma specimen diluted with equal part of normal saline, showing a fibrinogen band (arrow). (B) After adding equal part of thrombin, the fibrinogen band disappears. (C) A serum specimen showing a monoclonal band at the location of fibrinogen. (D) After thrombin treatment, the monoclonal band persists.

complement, fibrinogen and γ-globulins. In the zones of α-lipoprotein, antichymotrypsin, and hemopexin, there exist many superimposed components, making it very difficult to interpret their changes in a rational way.

The HRE not only demonstrates more protein fractions than conventional electrophoresis but also is the preferred system for the detection of monoclonal and oligoclonal bands; thus it is an invaluable tool for the diagnosis of monoclonal gammopathies as well as demyelinating disorders. It is very sensitive in the evaluation of the changes in α_1-antitrypsin, which assumes a discrete band without any superimposed components. The ability to identify the α-fetoprotein and C-reactive protein bands is another special feature of this system. Furthermore, HRE can be used to phenotype haptoglobin and to unveil the genetic variants of albumin, α_1-antitrypsin, transferrin, and C_3 complement. In urinalysis, HRE is very helpful in the detection of Bence Jones proteins and for the distinction between glomerular and tubular proteinuria.

Densitometric scanning of the electrophoretogram aids the interpreters with limited experience and it provides an objective comparison of different patterns obtained at different stages of a disease, e.g., before and after chemotherapy of myeloma patients. However, scanning can never replace the direct, thorough inspection of electrophoretic patterns by the experienced pathologist, chemist, or any other scientist specializing in this field.

Quantitative protein studies should be considered to be supplementary to, not a replacement for, electrophoresis. Total proteins and albumin should be quantitated routinely for sera and for CSF, but analysis of other fractions should be performed only when indicated by electrophoretic findings or clinical stiuations.

REFERENCES

1. Alper CA: Plasma protein measurements as a diagnostic aid. N Engl J Med 291:287, 1974.
2. Arroyave CM, Taylor DG, Gallup P, Nakamura RM: Screening test for complement activation by counterimmunoelectrophoresis. Am J Clin Pathol 69:440, 1978.
3. Bowie L, Smith S, Gochman N: Characteristics of binding between reagent-strip indicators and urinary proteins. Clin Chem 23:128, 1977.
4. Brackenridge CJ, Csillag ER: A quantitative electrophoretic survey of serum fractions in health and disease. Acta Med Scand 172 (suppl 383):1, 1962.
5. Cawley LP: "Electrophoresis and Immunoelectrophoresis." Boston: Little, Brown, 1969.
6. Cawley LP, Minard BJ, Tourtellotte WW, Ma BI, Challe C: Immunofixation electrophoretic techniques applied to identification of protein in serum and cerebrospinal fluid. Clin Chem 22:1262, 1976.
7. Daniels JC, Vyvial TM, Levin WC, Ritzmann SE: Methodologic differences in values for M-proteins in serum, as measured by three techniques. Clin Chem 21:243, 1975.
8. Epstein E, Zak B, Baginski ES, Civin WH: Interpretation of cerebrospinal fluid protein by gel electrophoresis. Ann Clin Lab Sci 6:27, 1976.
9. Evans HE, Mandl I, Keller S: Respiratory distress syndrome: Serum enzyme inhibitor levels and lung tissue elastin composition. In Mittman C (ed): "Pulmonary Emphysema and Proteolysis." New York: Academic Press, 1972, pp 91–98.
10. Franklin EC: Electrophoresis and immunoelectrophoresis in the evaluation of homogeneous immunoglobulin components. In Bach FH, Good RA (eds): "Clinical Immunobiology Vol. 3." New York: Academic Press, 1976, pp 21–36.
11. Frohlich J, Kozier J, Campbell DJ, Curnow JV, Tarnoky AL: Bisalbuminemia: A new molecular variant, albumin vancouver. Clin Chem 24:1912, 1978.
12. Ganrot K, Laurell CB: Measurement of IgG and albumin content of cerebrospinal fluid and its interpretation. Clin Chem 20:571, 1974.
13. Irjala K, Suonpaa J, Laurent B: Identification of CSF leakage by immunofixation. Arch Otolaryngol 105:447, 1979.
14. Jeppsson JO, Laurell CB, Franzen B: Agarose gel electrophoresis. Clin Chem 25:629, 1979.
15. Johansson BG: Agarose gel electrophoresis. Scand J Clin Lab Invest 29 (suppl 124):7, 1972.
16. Johnson KP, Arrigo SC, Nelson BJ: Agarose electrophoresis of cerebrospinal fluid in multiple sclerosis. Neurology 27:273, 1977.
17. Kawai T: "Clinical Aspects of the Plasma Proteins." Philadelphia and Toronto: JB Lippincott, 1973.

18. Kelly RH, Scholl MA, Harvey VS, Devenyi AG: Qualititative testing for circulating immune complexes by use of zone electrophoresis on agarose. Clin Chem 26:396, 1980.
19. Kindmark CO: Identification of C-reactive protein by agarose gel electrophoresis of human serum or plasma. Clin Chim Acta 35:491, 1971.
20. Killingsworth LM, Cooney SK, Tyllia MM: Protein analysis: The closer you look, the more you see. Diagn Med 3:46, 1980.
21. Kohn J: The laboratory investigation of paraproteinemia. Recent Adv Clin Pathol 6:363, 1973.
22. Larson PH: Serum proteins: Diagnostic significance of electrophoretic patterns. Hum Pathol 5:629, 1974.
23. Laterre EC, Callewaert A, Heremans JF, Sfaello Z: Electrophoretic morphology of gamma globulins in cerebrospinal fluid of multiple sclerosis and other diseases of the nervous system. Neurology 20:982, 1970.
24. Laurell CB: Composition and variation of the gel electrophoretic fractions of plasma, cerebrospinal fluid and urine. Scand J Clin Lab Invest 29 (suppl 124):71, 1972.
25. Laurell CB: Electrophoresis, specific protein assays, or both in measurement of plasma proteins. Clin Chem 19:99, 1973.
26. Link H, Muller R: Immunoglobulins in multiple sclerosis and infections of the nervous system. Arch Neurol 25:326, 1971.
27. Morse JO: Alpha-1-antitrypsin deficiency. N Engl J Med 299:1045, 1099, 1978.
28. Perry MC, Kyle RA: The clinical significance of Bence Jones proteinuria. Mayo Clin Proc 50:234, 1975.
29. Ritzmann SE: Immunoglobulin abnormalities. In Ritzmann SE, Daniels JC (eds): "Serum Protein Abnormalities, Diagnostic and Clinical Aspects," 2nd printing. New York: Alan R. Liss, Inc., 1982, pp 351–485.
30. Ritzmann SE, Daniels JC: Serum protein electrophoresis and total serum proteins. In Ritzmann SE, Daniels JC (eds): "Serum Protein Abnormalities, Diagnostic and Clinical Aspects," 2nd printing. New York: Alan R. Liss, Inc., pp 3–25.
31. Ritzmann SE, Nakamura RM: Ouchterlony double-diffusion technique. In Ritzmann SE, Daniels JC (eds): "Serum Protein Abnormalities, Diagnostic and Clinical Aspects," 2nd printing. New York: Alan R. Liss, Inc., pp, 85–93.
32. Stibler H: Direct immunofixation after isoelectric focusing: An improved method for identification of cerebrospinal fluid and serum protein. J Neurol Sci 42:275, 1979.
33. Sun T: The clinical significance of plasma proteins. North Shore Univ Hosp Clin J 1:12, 1978.
34. Sun T: Laboratory diagnosis of multiple sclerosis. In "Special Topics Check Sample Critique, No. ST80-2." Chicago: American Society of Clinical Pathologists, 1980.
35. Sun T, Chan SK, Gross S: Evaluation of a high-resolution electrophoresis system. Am J Clin Pathol 67:247, 1977.
36. Sun T, Evans H, Degnan T: Acquired alpha-1 antitrypsin deficiency and dysgammaglobulinemia. Ann Clin Lab Sci 10:149, 1980.
37. Sun T, Kurtz S, Copeland BE: Alpha-1 antitrypsin deficiency and pulmonary disease. Am J Clin Pathol 62:725, 1974.
38. Sun T, Lien YY, Degnan T: Study of gammopathies with immunofixation electrophoresis. Am J Clin Pathol 72:5, 1979.
39. Sun T, Lien YY, Gross S: Clinical application of a high-resolution electrophoresis system. Ann Clin Lab Sci 8:219, 1978.
39a. Sun T, Lien YY: Reversed-polarity immunoelectrophoresis. Clin Chem 26:1763, 1980.
40. Sunderman FW: Studies of the serum proteins. VI. Recent advances in clinical interpretation of electrophoretic fractionations. Am J Clin Pathol 42:1, 1964.

41. Sunderman FW, Sunderman FW Jr: "Serum proteins and the Dysproteinemias." Philadelphia: Lippincott, 1964.
42. Tarnoky AL, Dowding B, Lakin AL: Eight types of bisalbuminemia. Nature 225:742, 1970.
43. Tourtellotte WW, Tavolato B, Parker J, Comiso P: Cerebrospinal fluid electroimmunodiffusion. Arch Neurol 25:345, 1971.
44. Werner M: Serum protein changes during the acute phase reaction. Clin Chim Acta 25:299, 1969.
45. Werner M, Brooks SH, Cohnen G: Diagnostic effectiveness of electrophoresis and specific protein assays, evaluated by discriminate analysis. Clin Chem 18:116, 1972.
46. Whicher JT: The value of complement assays in clinical chemistry. Clin Chem 24:7, 1978.
47. Zak B, Baginski ES, Epstein E: Associated problems of protein electrophoresis, staining and densitometry. Ann Clin Lab Sci 8:385, 1978.
48. Ritzmann SE, Fischer CL, Nakamura RM: Quantitative immunochemical procedures — Electroimmunodiffusion technique (EID). In Ritzmann SE, Daniels JC (eds): "Serum Protein Abnormalities, Diagnostic and Clinical Aspects," 2nd printing. New York: Alan R. Liss, Inc., 1982, pp 68–84.
49. Ritzmann SE: Bence Jones proteins. In Ritzmann SE, Tucker ES III (Directors): ASCP Workshop Manual "Identification and Significance of Protein Abnormalities," October 1980, pp 27–33.
50. Seligmann M (Chairman), Bentwich Z, Bianco N, et al: Use and abuse of laboratory tests in clinical immunology: critical considerations of eight widely used diagnostic procedures. Report of an IUIS/WHO Working Group. Clin Exp Immunol 46:662, 1981.

Physiology of Immunoglobulins: Diagnostic and
Clinical Aspects, pages 65–87
© 1982 Alan R. Liss, Inc., 150 Fifth Avenue, New York, NY 10011

3

High-Resolution Two-Dimensional Electrophoresis of Human Body Fluid Proteins

Gerald B. Dermer, PhD, John F. Chapman, Dr PH, Lawrence M.
Silverman, PhD

INTRODUCTION

Of the large number of different proteins in body fluids, electrophoresis, as performed in the clinical laboratory today, can resolve and estimate the concentration of only about 12 of these proteins under optimal conditions. Though this limited information has been helpful in the diagnosis and monitoring of many disorders, the ability to resolve a greater number of constituent proteins may enhance the diagnostic utility of this approach. High resolution two-dimensional electrophoresis in acrylamide gels, as described by O'Farrell [18], combines isoelectric focusing in one dimension and electrophoresis with sodium dodecyl sulfate (SDS) in the other dimension and can resolve complex mixtures of proteins. Anderson and Anderson have adapted O'Farrell's system for the analysis of human plasma [1] and urinary proteins [5] and have demonstrated that hundreds of proteins can be resolved and visualized with Coomassie blue. They have appreciated the wealth of analytical information provided and the implications for clinical diagnoses. The subsequent development of a silver stain [21] 100 times more sensitive than Coomassie blue indicates a still greater potential for protein detection and evaluation.

The pioneering efforts of the Andersons [1–6,10,11] and others [12,15,16,21] have prompted us to establish high-resolution two-dimensional electrophoresis and the silver stain in the clinical laboratories of North Carolina Memorial Hospital. Our efforts during the first year of this endeavor have been directed towards establishing two-dimensional protein maps of several types of normal body fluids. Variations in protein patterns are being determined and proteins which appear fluid type-specific are being catalogued. Procedures such as affinity chromatography, which are being used to prepare fluid fractions enriched in type-specific or other components, and electrophoretic blotting [23], which are being used to identify protein spots in two-dimensional patterns, are also being established. The aims of this work are 1) to establish a body of data concerning two-dimensional protein patterns of normal body fluids, 2) to develop a clinically useful system for detecting variations in two-dimensional patterns of body fluids which are associated with disease, 3) to identify those protein spots of diagnostic interest, and 4) to identify fluid type-specific proteins. Some of our experiences and results to date are discussed here. It is hoped that the chapter will provide an introduction to two-dimensional electrophoresis for the clinical scientist and convey our conviction that these analyses will become important in clinical chemistry and proteinology. Detailed procedures for two-dimensional electrophoresis are provided by references to the original literature.

SAMPLES

Our investigative efforts have concentrated on the analysis of human body fluids, including cerebrospinal fluid, amniotic fluid, synovial fluid, cervical mucous, pleural and peritoneal effusions, and fetal and adult serum. With the use of the extremely sensitive silver stain, samples containing only 50 μg total protein are electrophoresed. Under these conditions, more proteins are visible on second-dimension slabs than if 1–2 mg samples are electrophoresed and stained with Coomassie blue [1]. Thus, fluids low in protein, such as cerebrospinal fluid, do not have to be concentrated 50–100-fold as is customary for most electrophoretic techniques. We concentrate cerebrospinal fluid 4–8-fold resulting in 10–50 μl samples containing 50 μg protein. The use of small amounts of protein also eliminates artifacts due to overloading including horizontal and vertical streaking of proteins and poor migration of some sample proteins into first dimension isoelectric focusing gels. These proteins remain near the top of first dimension gels close to where samples are applied (the basic end) and form a stained streak down the basic side of slab gels after electrophoresis in the second dimension.

SAMPLE TREATMENT

Samples in volumes ranging from 10–50 μl are heated at 95°C for five minutes after the addition of 20 μl of sample buffer [1] containing 0.25% SDS (a strong anionic detergent), 10% glycerol, and 5% β-mercaptoethanol. This treatment converts disulphide bonds to free sulphydryls, destroys the three-dimensional structure of proteins and produces separate polypeptide chains with a constant weight ratio of bound SDS to protein.

First-Dimensional Isoelectric Focusing Separations

First-dimensional separations [3,18] are done in 3.0-mm diameter 120-mm-long acrylamide tube gels containing 9 mol/L urea, 2% Nonidet P-40 (a neutral detergent), and 2% ampholytes. We have found that a combination of pH 3–10 and pH 4–6 ampholytes in a ratio of 1:1 produces a pH gradient which resolves most of the proteins detected in body fluids. Electrophoresis of denatured samples is usually carried out overnight for a total of 6000 volt hours. Separation in the first dimension reflects the ratio of acidic and basic groups of unfolded peptide chains which in turn mirrors the amino acid composition of proteins. Amphoteric molecules such as proteins migrate in isoelectric focusing gels towards the pH where they have a zero net charge, and at their isoelectric points they become focused into narrow bands. These bands can be visualized by staining first-dimension gels. However, stained gels cannot be electrophoresed in the second dimension.

After isoelectric focusing, first-dimension gels are removed from their glass tubes and either loaded on second dimension slab gels or frozen at $-70°C$ for electrophoresis in the second dimension at a later time. Also, the pH gradient in tube gels is estimated by use of a microelectrode on one gel. This determination takes only a few minutes and does not damage the gel which can then be frozen or run in the second dimension. It is assumed that all gels electrophoresed at the same time and containing the same concentration of ampholytes exhibit identical pH gradients. We do not equilibrate first-dimension gels because protein is lost from gels by this treatment [18]. During isoelectric focusing, the bound SDS from the sample buffer is removed from proteins and focuses at the extreme acid end of the first-dimension gel producing a swollen plug which identifies that end of the gel. During second-dimension electrophoresis, this SDS migrates down the acid side of second-dimension slabs often distorting the appearance of very acidic proteins such as α_1-acid glycoprotein, which also focuses at the extreme acid end of our tube gels. This problem has been diminished by reducing the amount of SDS in the sample buffer from 2 to 0.25%. This change has not produced any detectable alterations in the two-dimensional patterns of body fluid proteins.

Second-Dimensional Molecular Mass Separations

Proteins or their subunits separated according to isoelectric point in the first dimension are then electrophoresed in a second direction in the presence of SDS. Separation in the second dimension occurs on the basis of molecular mass. Proteins covered by SDS have a constant charge to mass ratio and uniform shape and in free electrophoresis all of these particles have the same mobility regardless of size. However, in the microporous acrylamide slab gels, large particles move more slowly than small ones, so that separation takes place according to molecular weight. In practice, we use a 4.5% stacking gel and a running gel of 10% acrylamide. The dimensions of the stacking plus running gels are $1.5 \times 140 \times 160$ mm. The first-dimension tube gel, oriented by convention [1] with its acid end to the left, is laid out on the top of the stacking gel and cemented to it by a 1% agarose gel containing 10% glycerol and 2.3% SDS. We have eliminated β-mercaptoethanol from the agarose gel since it was responsible for the parallel horizontal lines visible after silver staining across the entire width of second-dimension gels. These lines, which have been noted by others [25], were at a molecular weight of about 50,000 to 60,000 daltons and increased in intensity with staining time. They were present on every gel and obscured the detection of proteins of similar molecular weight.

Estimation of molecular weights of proteins or their subunits is carried out by use of molecular weight standards (Bio-Rad) which are pipetted into the solidified agarose gel at a spot to the right of where the first-dimension gel is embedded. Also, since all body fluids contain serum proteins, many of which have a known molecular weight, identification of these proteins or their subunits can be used as internal molecular weight standards. Identification of these proteins is possible by comparing positions of spots on second dimension slabs to positions of known plasma proteins or their subunits as determined by Anderson and Anderson [1].

Fixing and Silver Staining

Second-dimension slab gels are fixed overnight in 50% methanol/acetic acid (90/10). They are rehydrated the next morning in distilled water for two hours with several changes. The staining method we use is based on a modification [17] of the original silver staining procedure [21] which is approximately 100 times more sensitive than Coomassie blue staining. It has been demonstrated that some proteins can be detected when as little as 0.5 ng are present in a sample [17]. We have also made some minor modifications to suit our 1.5-mm-thick slab gels and have developed a staining procedure which is very reproducible, with good contrast and little background.

As has been pointed out, successful staining is dependent on the freshness of the ammonium hydroxide solution [21]. We take an unopened pint-size bottle of ammonium hydroxide and distribute it in 20-ml scintillation vials. Parafilm is placed over the vial tops and the caps are screwed on tightly. Each vial is used only once and unused portions of ammonium hydroxide are discarded. Exposure to the ammonical-silver solution is for 30–40 minutes with the container being covered by aluminum foil. The clear ammonical-silver solution and the gel often take on a pale straw color after this time. We have found it convenient to use, as staining containers, disposable liners from Corning (catalogue No. 470162). Gels are transferred to new liners from the water wash (after the glutaraldehyde step in the Oakley procedure [17]) to the ammonical-silver, from the ammonical-silver to another water wash and from the water wash to the final reduction step in citric acid-formaldehyde. These changes of containers prevent silver deposition on the surface of gels. Also, the water wash after the ammonical-silver step has been lengthened from two minutes to one hour with three changes. Development of stain is halted by transferring gels to a 1% solution of acetic acid. We do not dry stained gels but store them wet in clear, 5 × 7 inch vinyl zipper bags from 20th Century Plastics (Los Angeles, CA 90016).

Apparatus

Most tube gel electrophoresis units are suitable for first-dimension separations. The unit we use is the GT3 model manufactured by Hoeffer Scientific Instruments (San Francisco, CA). It holds 18 glass tube gels of 3-mm inner diameter. A similar unit is also distributed by Bio-Rad Laboratories. The design of vertical slab gel electrophoresis units has recently been improved making the setup for second-dimension runs rather simple. Two uniform rectangular glass plates are used instead of beveled or grooved plates. Sealing the plates is also much easier than in older models. Two gels can be run in one chamber. Almost identical units are available from Hoeffer Scientific, Bio-Rad Laboratories, or LKB.

General Features of Two-Dimensional Patterns of Body Fluid Proteins

High-resolution two-dimensional protein patterns of cerebrospinal fluid, amniotic fluid, synovial fluid, cervical mucus, pleural and peritoneal effusions, and fetal and adult serum are complex but highly reproducible with usually two hundred or more spots visible in each. The vertical streaks associated with albumin in many samples are due to its overloading even though samples contain only 50 μg total protein. Most of the proteins in each fluid are assumed to be serum proteins since they occupy identical positions in gels to serum proteins. Patterns for each fluid appear type specific, however, since novel proteins are seen and certain characteristic serum proteins are not detected.

Not evident in the black and white prints is the fact that proteins are not all of the same color after silver staining. Each protein always exhibits the same color, however, which can be orange, red-orange, brown, dark brown, gray, black, and several even exhibit a greenish tint. Although to our knowledge no explanation for these color differences has been given, it seems likely that they, in some way, reflect the composition of proteins.

Many of the proteins, especially those larger than 30,000 daltons, are not made up of single spots but appear as families of spots due primarily to carbohydrate heterogeneity. Rows of spots that slope upward to the left indicate that the negative charge of the protein increases with molecular weight. This could be due to the addition of negatively charged sialic acid residues.

Diagnostic Potential of Two-Dimensional Electrophoresis

Several groups, but most notably that of N.G. and L.A. Anderson at the Argonne National Laboratory, have pioneered the search of reliable indicators of disease in two-dimensional protein patterns [4,5,11]. Their ambitious aim [1,4,6] is to map and catalogue most of the estimated 30,000–50,000 human protein gene products and to identify specific qualitative and quantitative changes in proteins which are related to disease. The use of high-resolution two-dimensional electrophoresis as a screen for genetic disease markers has been proposed [1,16], and investigations into Lesch-Nyhan Syndrome [14], cystic fibrosis [8], and muscular dystrophy [7] have begun. In cystic fibrosis [8], several low-molecular weight proteins have been reported in parotid saliva that are not detected in controls. We are also interested in genetic screening and are mapping and determining variations in the proteins of normal amniotic fluid. Samples are obtained from women being screened for abnormal levels of α-fetoprotein.

Anderson et al. [6] have suggested that high-resolution two-dimensional maps may have implications for cancer detection and evaluation of therapy. In support of this view, they have shown that the two-dimensional urinary protein pattern of a patient with bladder cancer [5] showed marked alterations in the pattern and the presence of multiple additional spots in comparison with the usual configuration. Perhaps one or more of these additional spots are tumor products that may become reliable diagnostic indicators. Recently, preliminary data have shown that in light chain myeloma [24], the isoelectric point of immunoglobulin light chains may have prognostic significance.

The search for protein tumor products in body fluids has also been of interest in our laboratory [9,22]. These early data showed that human adenocarcinomas synthesize and rapidly release glycoproteins into the extracellular environment. We have begun studying the malignant effusions by two-dimensional electrophoresis in an attempt to detect and characterize these tumor glycoproteins.

Two-dimensional electrophoresis may also aid in tumor classification. Proper classification is often a problem in poorly differentiated lesions and in those patients with proven metastatic disease where the site of the primary tumor is not known. Recent work suggests that two-dimensional patterns of cytosol proteins from several normal rat tissues are distinctive for each tissue [13]. Furthermore, the protein patterns of normal rat liver and some rat hepatomas are very similar [13]. Thus, it is possible that human tumors may retain patterns for cytosol proteins which reflect the cell type from which they are derived. Knowledge of the cell of origin is the basis for tumor classification.

High-resolution two-dimensional electrophoretic analysis of normal [10,11] and pathological [11] human skeletal muscle biopsies has also been undertaken by the Argonne group. Patterns for normal quadriceps show 100–200 proteins, and spots for several of the major contractile proteins and enzymes have been identified. Four of seven Duchenne muscular dystrophy samples exhibited decreased amounts of actin and myosin relative to normal muscle. Normal patterns were seen with myotonic dystrophy; but in nemaline rod myopathy, the pattern was deficient in two of the fast-type myosin light chains. Although the investigators conclude that the analysis by two-dimensional electrophoresis of human biopsy samples is feasible, they also realize that more studies are needed before the method becomes routine in the diagnosis of muscle disease.

High-Resolution Two-Dimensional Electrophoresis of Body Fluids

In this section, some results from exploratory studies using the methodology discussed will be presented. Typical patterns for several body fluids will be shown and some of their most salient features briefly discussed.

Serum

A typical silver stained pattern for a sample of 50 μg of serum proteins is shown in Figure 1. It is quite similar to the Coomassie blue stained pattern established by Anderson and Anderson [1]. The high sensitivity of the silver stain is illustrated by the fact that several proteins are observed in our gels which are not present in Coomassie blue stained gels even though the latter contain more than ten times the amount of protein. One of the proteins not in the published map of plasma proteins has a molecular weight of approximately 80,000 daltons and a very acidic isoelectric point. We have observed this protein in all sera, effusions, and cerebrospinal fluids. Creation of very acidic pH gradients in first-dimension gels, by employing pH 4–6 and 2–4 ampholytes in a ratio of 3:1, results in the resolution of this protein and α_1-acid glycoprotein into rows of spots that slope upward (Fig. 2). This is indicative of carbohydrate heterogeneity. The apparent identical isoelectric points of several members of these two families suggests that the high molecular weight protein may be a precursor of α_1-acid glycoprotein.

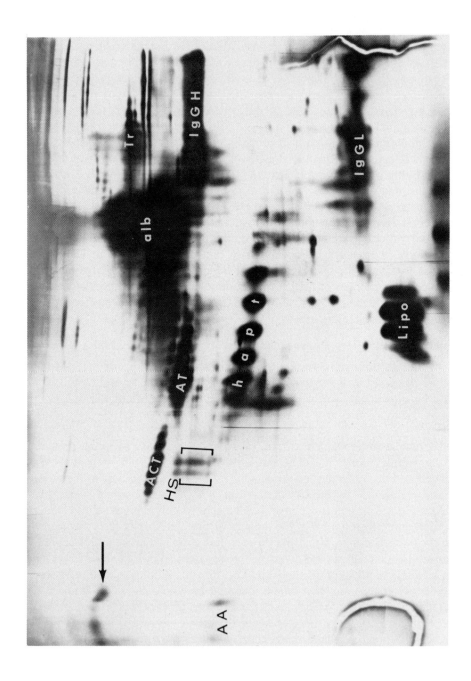

Our silver-stained gels also exhibit added complexity associated with α_2-HS glycoprotein (Fig. 1). Vertical streaks of stained material connect α_2-HS spots with a lower molecular weight family of spots. This lower molecular weight family is situated next to the most acidic member of haptoglobin β-chain spots and appears to increase the number of spots of the haptoglobin β-chain family. The streaks suggest a conversion of α_2-HS glycoprotein into a lower molecular weight form. Use of narrow acidic gradients in first-dimension gels also show these relationships (Fig. 2). Although our work also indicates the presence of additional new families not present in the published plasma protein map [1], these data will be presented elsewhere.

Fetal Blood

Blood was obtained from a living fetus and sent to us through the courtesy of Dr. M. J. Mahoney of Yale University Medical School. It provides an opportunity to examine the expression of serum protein genes at one developmental period. A high-resolution two-dimensional pattern is shown in Figure 3 which should be compared to the adult serum pattern (Fig. 1). Immediately evident is the simplicity of the fetal pattern due to the absence of several major serum proteins including IgG, haptoglobin, α_1-acid glycoprotein and α_1-antichymotrypsin. Second, several protein families are enriched in fetal blood and may represent fetal products since they have not been detected in adult serum. Third, fetal albumin appears to be composed of two forms which focus at different isoelectric points. Clearly, the ability to simultaneously analyze a large fraction of proteins at different developmental periods provides a way to discover how their expression is arranged during development.

Cerebrospinal Fluid

Patterns for cerebrospinal fluid (Fig. 4) are similar to those of serum. In addition, cerebrospinal fluid appears to contain several families of proteins which are not represented in serum [12]. One of these putative cerebrospinal

---

Fig. 1.   Two-dimensional pattern of serum proteins. Arrow indicates 80,000 dalton acidic protein not previously reported. Brackets indicate streaks which connect α_2-HS spots with a lower molecular weight family. Proteins have been identified by reference to the Anderson map of plasma [1]. AA, α_1-acid glycoprotein; alb, albumin; AT, α_1-antitrypsin; ACT, α_1-antichymotrypsin; HS, α_2-HS glycoprotein; hapt, haptoglobin; IgGH, IgG heavy chains; IgGL, IgG light chains; Lipo, A-I lipoprotein; Tr, transferrin. (For all the figures, more proteins are visible in gels than can be resolved in photographs. Proteins are visualized with a silver stain and unless otherwise stated, samples contain 50 μg total protein. The high molecular weight proteins are near the top of gels and acidic proteins to the left.)

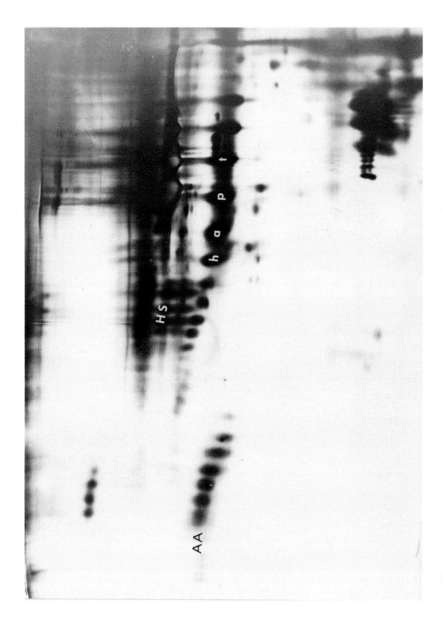

Fig. 2. Two-dimensional pattern of acidic serum proteins. Use of a very acidic pH gradient in first dimension gels resolves α_1-acid glycoprotein into a family of seven spots and the 80,000 dalton protein directly above it into a family of four spots. Vertical streaks connecting α_2-HS glycoprotein with a lower molecular weight family are clearly seen.

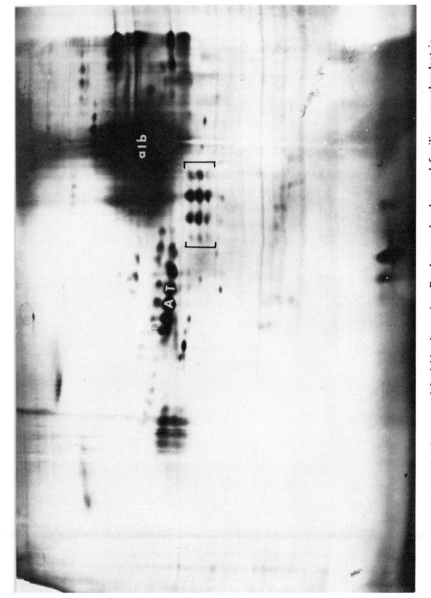

Fig. 3. Two-dimensional pattern of fetal blood proteins. Brackets enclosed several families more abundant in fetal than adult blood.

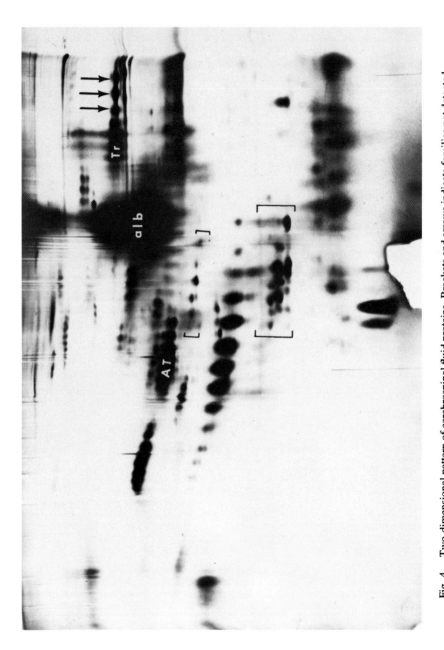

Fig. 4. Two-dimensional pattern of cerebrospinal fluid proteins. Brackets and arrows indicate families not detected in serum.

specific protein families has a molecular weight slightly less, and a pI slightly more basic, than transferrin. Another group appears to be composed of four families of proteins with molecular weights around 36,000. A third group is made up of six to eight spots and has a molecular weight of approximately 48,000. Removal of serum proteins before electrophoresis by affinity chromatography has given additional information about the nature and number of cerebrospinal fluid proteins and is discussed in a later section.

Cervical Mucus

Samples of cervical mucus have been examined and a representative two-dimensional pattern is shown in Figure 5. Several major serum proteins including α_1-acid glycoprotein, α_2-HS glycoprotein, haptoglobin, α_1-antichymotrypsin, and APO A-1 lipoprotein are either present in very low concentrations or not detectable. One major protein family of about 70,000 daltons with a pI slightly more acidic than albumin is enriched in cervical mucus, and it may be a unique component. It is composed of ten spots that slope upward to the left indicating the presence of carbohydrate. A finding of clinical interest is that the cervical mucus from two women with immunologic infertility had readily detectable amounts of IgG light and heavy chains. The other two-dimensional patterns, from normal women or those with infertility of another etiology, had barely detectable or undetectable amounts of IgG light and heavy chains. These observations suggest the presence of specific antibodies in the cervical mucus of women with immunologic infertility. Further work suggests that certain of these antibodies may be directed against the BB isoenzyme of creatine kinase, a normal component of prostatic fluid [19].

Synovial Fluid

Synovial fluid from patients with rheumatoid arthritis or degenerative joint disease has been examined at our institution. A two-dimensional pattern from a patient with active arthritis is shown in Figure 6. The pattern, not surprisingly, shows the presence of many serum proteins, including light and heavy chains of IgG. When compared to serum, there appears to be more complexity in an area associated with a molecular weight somewhat less than albumin. This complexity may be due to the presence of components more concentrated in synovial fluid. It will be interesting to compare these patterns to those of normal fluid to see if there are any differences associated with disease.

Effusions

Two-dimensional patterns of pleural and peritoneal effusions (Fig. 7) look very much like serum. To date, components not found in serum have not been identified.

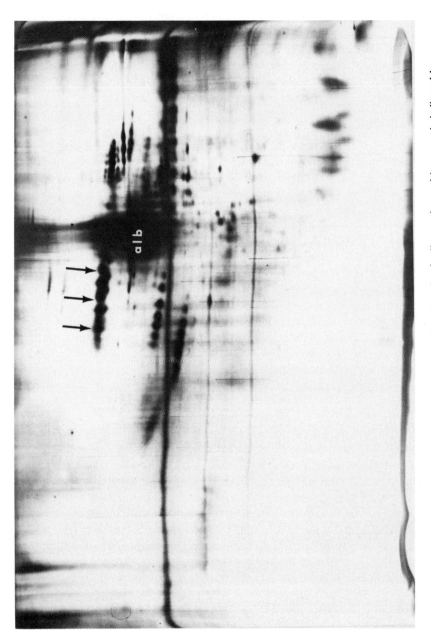

Fig. 5.   Two-dimensional gel of cervical mucus proteins. A major family not detected in serum is indicated by arrows.

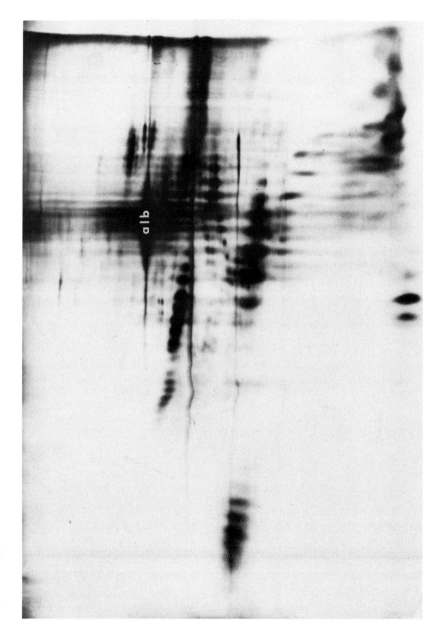

Fig. 6.   Two-dimensional gel of synovial fluid proteins.

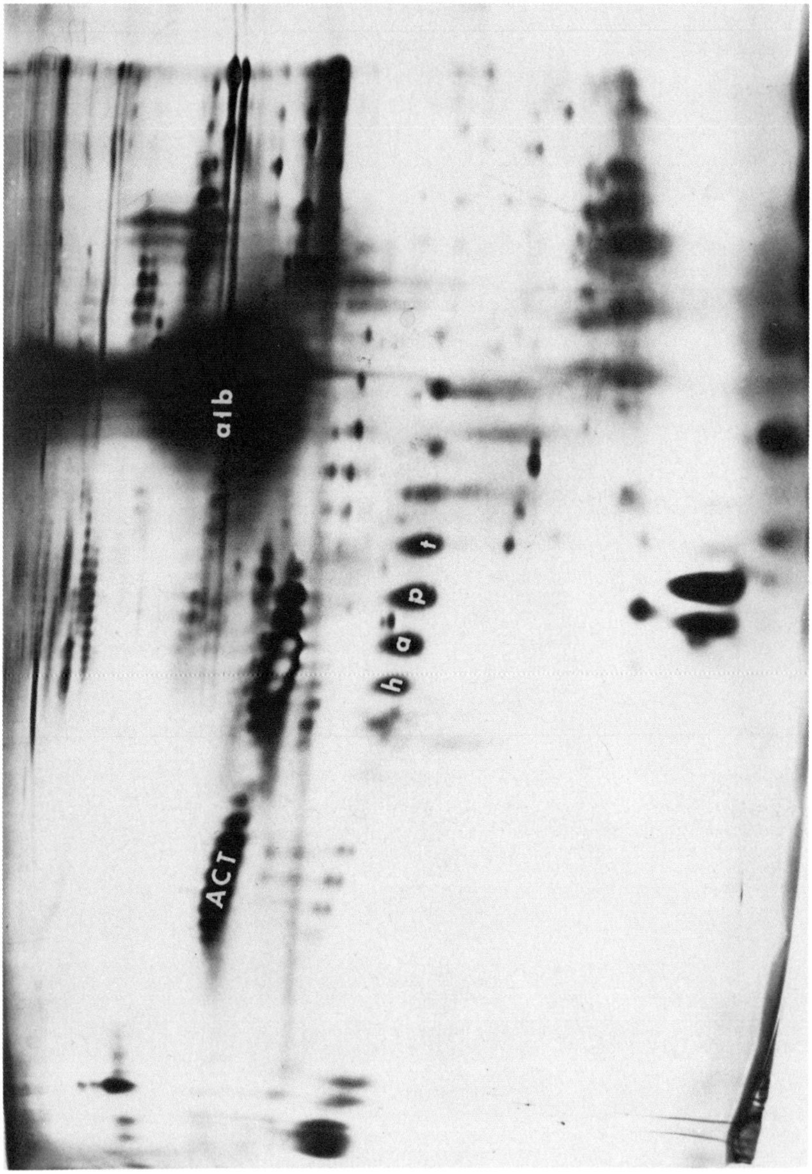

Fig. 7. Two-dimensional protein pattern of a pleural effusion.

Amniotic Fluid

Amniocentesis is commonly performed for detection of genetic disease at the 16–20 week gestational age period and these fluids have been examined by two-dimensional electrophoresis (Fig. 8). Since the major contribution to the proteins of amniotic fluid derives from the maternal circulation, most serum proteins are represented in two-dimensional patterns. Haptoglobin β-chains however are often present at barely detectable levels. Several protein families appear enriched in amniotic fluid when compared to serum, and further work will be required to show whether they are unique to amniotic fluid.

Future Directions

We are in the early stages of analyzing human body fluids by high-resolution two-dimensional electrophoresis, and at this stage are also exploring procedures that will increase the amount of information obtainable from the technique at the practical clinical laboratory level. Firstly, we want to maximize the number of proteins or their subunits visualized on gels in order to increase the probability of detecting proteins of diagnostic interest and those which might be unique to each fluid type. This can be done without applying more total protein which would overload gels and reduce resolution, by selectively removing albumin prior to electrophoresis. Such a procedure is currently being investigated in our laboratory, and it involves passing samples over columns of Cibacron Blue F3GA crosslinked to sepharose (Fig. 9). Albumin is strongly bound, but most proteins do not interact with the dye. Detection of proteins previously obscured by albumin is possible. Also, each 50 μg total protein sample contains higher concentrations of the remaining proteins which might permit the detection of new proteins.

We have found spots in each fluid type that are not seen in serum or any other kind of fluid, which, therefore, may represent type-specific proteins. To further probe the nature of these proteins, affinity columns of anti-human serum proteins coupled to CNBr-activated Sepharose 4B (Pharmacia) have been prepared. These immobilized antibody gels provide a method for the separation of fluid-specific proteins from serum constituents. Fluid fractions not bound to columns contain putative fluid-specific proteins which can be revealed by two-dimensional electrophoretic analysis. Specific proteins present in unfractionated fluids at concentrations below levels of detection may become detectable, since after the affinity step, samples for electrophoresis are enriched in these proteins.

Initial experiments using these affinity columns with cerebrospinal fluid have been encouraging. After reaction with immobilized antibodies, cerebrospinal fluids, as before, are concentrated and electrophoresed in two-dimensional gels. In Figure 10, a sample, which before depletion of serum

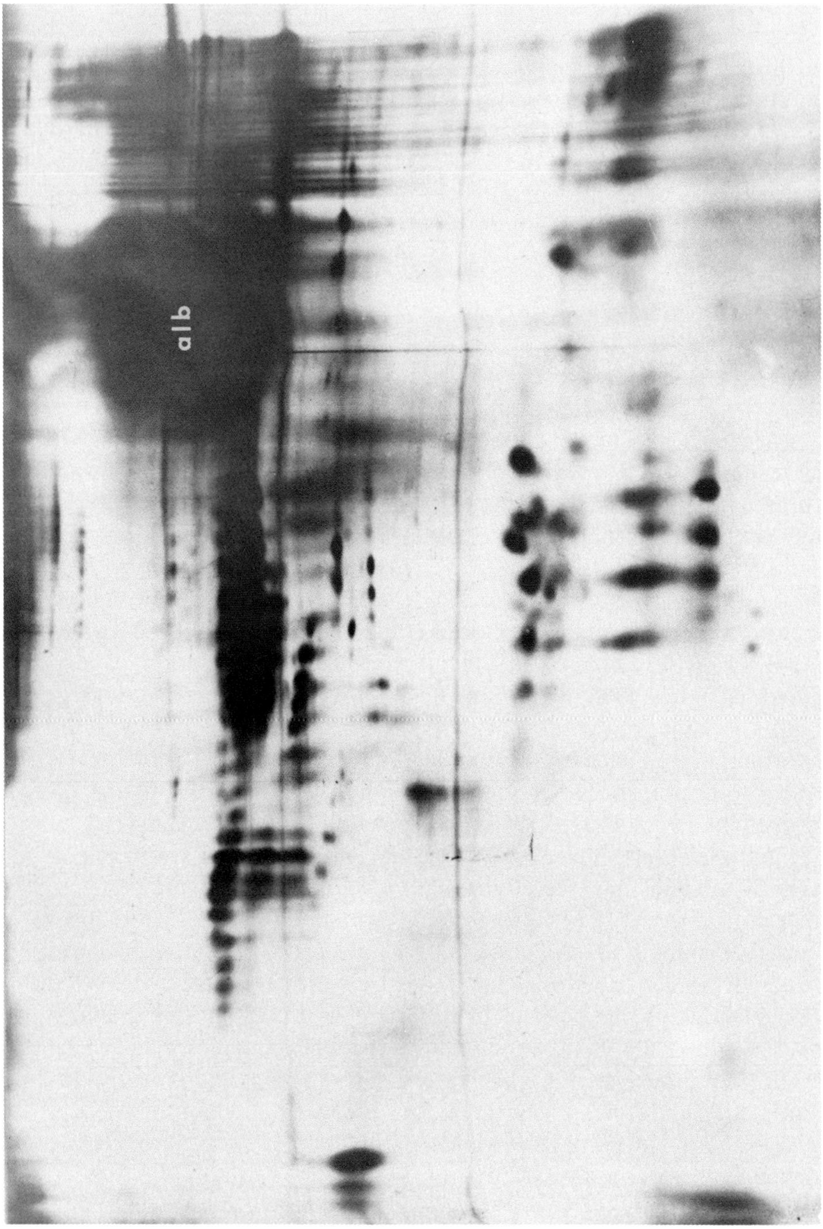

Fig. 8. Two-dimensional gel of amniotic fluid proteins.

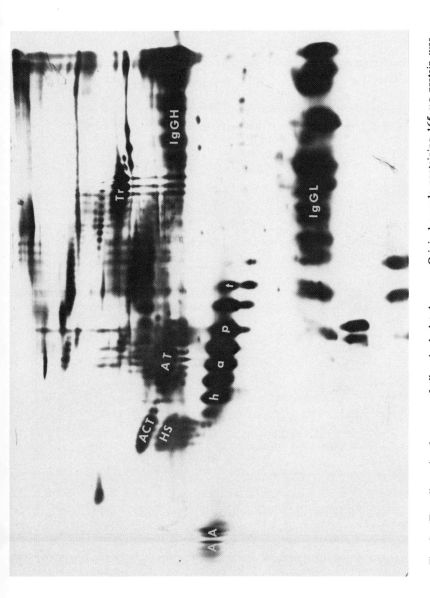

Fig. 9. Two-dimensional pattern of albumin-depleted serum. Original sample containing 165 μg protein was reacted with a Cibacron Blue-Sepharose column before electrophoresis. Protein families which are normally partially or totally obscured by albumin are now visible.

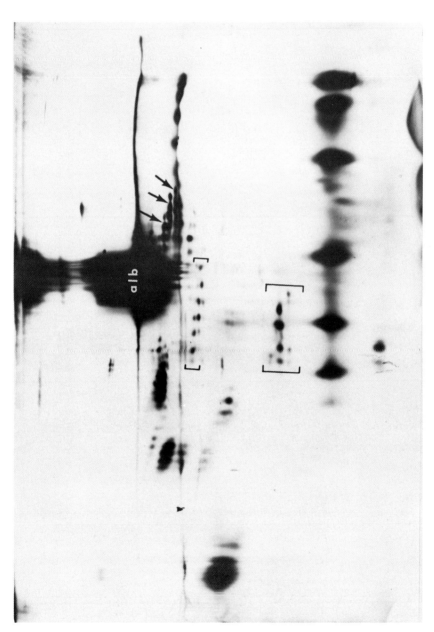

Fig. 10. Two-dimensional pattern of cerebrospinal fluid proteins partially depleted of serum proteins. Cerebrospinal fluid containing 210 μg protein was reacted with immobilized antihuman serum antibodies before electrophoresis. Brackets enclose protein families that are enriched in the sample after the affinity step. Families that have not been previously seen are indicated by arrows.

components contained 210 μg of protein, was used for two-dimensional analysis. This gel should be compared to the pattern produced by 50 μg of unfractionated cerebrospinal fluid (Fig. 4). Although the sample before the affinity step contained more than four times the amount of protein of unfractionated cerebrospinal fluid, its pattern is simpler. The absence of some components and a reduction in staining intensity of others is due to the removal of serum components by the antihuman serum antibodies. Much albumin remains because it made up about half of the total protein of the original sample and at that concentration could not be completely removed by the antisera. Passing samples over columns of Cibacron blue will reduce this problem. Transferrin and the family with a molecular weight slightly less and a pI slightly more basic than transferrin are not detectable. This family adjacent to transferrin is therefore not unique to cerebrospinal fluid, as was originally thought, but represents possibly a transferrin with lower sialic acid content. Such a component has been described in cerebrospinal fluid [20]. The other two families, which on study of unfractionated cerebrospinal fluid were thought to be unique to cerebrospinal fluid, may truly be central nervous system proteins since they are enriched in the pattern depleted of serum components.

After the affinity step, two-dimensional patterns of cerebrospinal fluid also exhibit protein families which are not detected in unfractionated cerebrospinal fluid. These new families may not have been seen before because they were obscured by serum components or present at concentrations too low to be detected in unfractionated cerebrospinal fluid. Particularly prominent are five or six families which have a molecular weight somewhat less and a PI slightly more basic than albumin. It is evident that combining affinity chromatography with two-dimensional analyses increases the amount of information obtainable and provides a means for partially purifying proteins of interest for further study.

Other data being sought are the identification of previously unclassified proteins in two-dimensional patterns. Spots for about 30 plasma proteins [1] and several muscle proteins [10] have been identified by co-electrophoresing known pure proteins with plasma or homogenized muscle to associate a particular protein with a given spot or by preparing immunoprecipitates with specific antibodies. The immunoprecipitates are analyzed by two-dimensional electrophoresis, and the location of the precipitated antigen spot or spots in the second-dimension gel can then be determined. Recently, a method called electrophoretic blotting [23] has been devised, which should greatly facilitate the identification of protein spots in two-dimensional patterns. The procedure, which is currently being developed in our laboratory, involves electrophoretically transferring proteins from second-dimension gels to sheets of nitrocellulose where they are immobilized. The nitrocellulose sheet is placed in contact with the gel surface after electrophoresis and the two are put into a blotting apparatus containing buffer. The proteins migrate from the gel into the nitrocellulose sheet when voltage is applied and an exact replica of the original gel is produced. The proteins on the nitrocellulose sheet can then be identified by immunological procedures.

Finally, Guevara [12a] has described a method by which spots can be removed from two-dimensional gels with hydroxyapatite. Proteins removed in this fashion can then be used for further identification or used as antigens in antibody production. Ideally, proteins purified in this fashion can then be used in hybridomas, yielding highly specific monoclonal antibodies.

REFERENCES

1. Anderson L, Anderson NG: High resolution two-dimensional electrophoresis of human plasma proteins. Proc Natl Acad Sci USA 74:5421–5425, 1977.
2. Anderson NL, Anderson NG: Analytical techniques for cell fractions. XXII. Two-dimensional analysis of serum and tissue proteins: Multiple gradient-slab gel electrophoresis. Anal Biochem 85:341–354, 1978.
3. Anderson NG, Anderson NL: Analytical techniques for cell fractions. XXI. Two-dimensional analysis of serum and tissue proteins: Multiple isoelectric focusing. Anal Biochem 85:331–340, 1978.
4. Anderson NG, Anderson NL: Molecular anatomy. Behring Inst Mitt 63:169–210, 1979.
5. Anderson NG, Anderson NL, Tollaksen L: Proteins of human urine. I. Concentration and analysis by two dimensional electrophoresis. Clin Chem 25:1199–1210, 1979.
6. Anderson NL, Edwards JJ, Giometti CS, Willard KE, Tollaksen SL, Nance SL, Hickman BJ, Taylor J, Coulter B, Scandora A, Anderson NG: High-resolution two-dimensional electrophoretic mapping of human proteins. In: Radola, BJ (ed.): "Electrophoresis '79, Advanced Methods, Biochemical and Clinical Applications." Berlin: Walter De Gruyter, 1980, pp 313–318.
7. Burghes AHM, Dunn MJ, Statham HE, Dubowitz V: Analysis of cultured skin fibroblasts from patients with Duchenne muscular dystrophy using electrophoretic technique. Electrophoresis '81, First Annual Meeting of the Electrophoresis Society, p 104, 1981.
8. Bustos SE, Fung L: Isoelectric focusing and two-dimensional maps of normal and cystic fibrosis saliva. Electrophoresis '81, First Annual Meeting of the Electrophoresis Society, p 105, 1981.
9. Dermer GB, Sherwin RP: Autoradiographic localization of glycoprotein in human breast cancer cells maintained in organ culture after incubation with fucose-^{3}H or glucosamine-^{3}H. Cancer Res 35:63–67, 1975.
10. Giometti CS, Anderson NG, Anderson NL: Muscle protein analysis. I. High-resolution two-dimensional electrophoresis of skeletal muscle proteins for analysis of small biopsy samples. Clin Chem 25:1877–1884, 1979.
11. Giometti CS, Barany M, Danon MJ, Anderson NG: Muscle protein analysis. II. Two-dimensional electrophoresis of normal and diseased human skeletal muscle. Clin Chem 26:1152–1155, 1980.
12. Goldman D, Merril CR, Ebert MH: Two-dimensional gel electrophoresis of cerebrospinal fluid proteins. Clin Chem 26:1317–1322, 1980.
12a. Guevara J, Chiocca EA, Clayton FC, von Eschenbach AC, Edwards JJ: A simple method for the elution of proteins from two-dimensional gels. Clin Chem 28:756–758, 1982.

13. Hirsch FW, Nall KN, Busch FN, Morris HP, Busch H: Comparison of abundant cytosol proteins in rat liver, Novikoff hepatoma, and Morris hepatoma by two-dimensional gel electrophoresis. Cancer Res 38:1514–1522, 1978.
14. Merril CR, Goldman D, Ebert M: Quantitative two-dimensional electrophoresis as a screen for genetic disease markers. Electrophoresis '81, First Annual Meeting of the Electrophoresis Society, p 24, 1981.
15. Merril CR, Goldman D, Sedman SA, Ebert MH: Ultrasensitive stain for proteins in polyacrylamide gels shows regional variation in cerebrospinal fluid proteins. Science 211:1437–1438, 1981.
16. Merril CR, Switzer RC, VanKeuren ML: Trace polypeptides in cellular extracts and human body fluids detected by two-dimensional electrophoresis and a highly sensitive silver stain. Proc Natl Acad Sci USA 76:4335–4339, 1979.
17. Oakley BR, Kirsch DR, Morris NR: A simplified ultrasensitive silver stain for detecting proteins in polyacrylamide gels. Anal Biochem 105:361–363, 1980.
18. O'Farrell PH: High resolution two-dimensional electrophoresis of proteins. J Biol Chem 250:4007–4021, 1975.
19. Silverman LM, Dermer GB, Zweig MH, Van Steirteghem AC, Tokes ZA: Creatine Kinase BB—A New Tumor Marker. Clin Chem 25:1432–1435, 1979.
20. Stibler H: The normal cerebrospinal fluid proteins identified by means of thin-layer isoelectric focusing and crossed immunoelectrofocusing. J Neurol Sci 36:273–288, 1978.
21. Switzer RC, Merril CR, Shifrin S: A highly sensitive silver stain for detecting proteins and peptides in polyacrylamide gels. Anal Biochem 98:231–237, 1979.
22. Tokes ZA, Dermer GB: Glycoprotein synthesis as a function of epithelial cell arrangement. Biosynthesis and release of glycoproteins by human breast and prostate cells in organ culture. J Supramol Struct 7:515–530, 1978.
23. Towbin H, Staehelin T, Gordon J: Electrophoretic transfer of proteins from polyacrylamide gels to nitrocellulose sheets: Procedure and some applications. Proc Natl Acad Sci USA 76:4350–4354, 1979.
24. Tracy RP, Currie R, Kyle R, Yound DS: 2-dimensional electrophoresis of specimens from patients with monoclonal gammopathies. Clin Chem 27:1065, 1981.
25. Merril CP: Personal communication.

Physiology of Immunoglobulins: Diagnostic and
Clinical Aspects, pages 89–96
© 1982 Alan R. Liss, Inc., 150 Fifth Avenue, New York, NY 10011

4

Two-Dimensional Immunoelectrophoretic Analysis of Body Fluid Proteins

L.M. Killingsworth, PhD, Mary M. Tyllia, BS, and Carol E.
Killingsworth, BS

INTRODUCTION

The technique of immunoelectrophoresis (IEP), in which protein antigens are allowed to react with antibody by passive diffusion after an electrophoretic separation step, has been used for over two decades to examine complex protein mixtures [6,15]. Several investigators recognized limitations in the technique shortly after its introduction, however, and modified the reaction steps [3,10,14]. They showed that resolution and sensitivity could be improved, and that the method could be rendered quantitative by forcing the antigens into an antibody-containing gel by a second electrophoresis step. This two-dimensional immunoelectrophoresis (2D-IEP) could be used to both measure and qualitatively evaluate proteins in various body fluids [4,5,13,18,20]. The highly technical nature of 2D-IEP has kept it from gaining widespread use in the clinical laboratory, but in recent years, attempts have been made to simplify the technique by changes in the support medium [1,7,12], or in the manner of peak area estimation [2,11]. A semiautomated approach has also been reported [19].

METHODOLOGY

Two-dimensional IEP is performed in two steps. In the first dimension, proteins are separated with respect to their net charge at pH 8.6. In the second step, these proteins are forced by electrophoresis to migrate at a right angle to their path of separation into an antibody-containing gel. The reactions which take place in the second gel result in areas of precipitate which reach a peak when all antigen has been complexed with antibody. When polyvalent anti-whole human serum is used as reagent, numerous specific proteins can be visualized and quantitated. Monospecific antiserum is used in the study of protein polymorphism, analysis of microheterogeneity, demonstration of complex formation, and activation of proteins by fragmentation [5,9,16].

Apparatus

Commercial agarose gel electrophoresis chambers, designed for water cooling and fitted with safety covers, are used for the separation and reaction steps. A constant electrical field is provided by a regulated high-voltage power supply and constant gel temperature is maintained at 7 °C by circulating water bath.

The agarose gels are cast on precoated plastic sheets with use of a 0.75-mm plastic frame, a plexiglass plate, and a glass backing plate. The casting assembly is held together with large binder clamps.

Reagents

Barbital buffer. The procedure is performed at pH 8.6 in barbital buffer. The buffer has a barbital concentration of 75 mmol/L, contains calcium lactate, and has an ionic strength of about 0.10.

Agarose. Purified agarose, with medium electroendosmosis ($-m_r$ = 0.16–0.19), is used for the electrophoretic gel, the antibody-containing reaction gel and the vertical wicks in the chamber.

Antibody. High titer polyvalent anti-whole human serum, produced in goats or rabbits, is used as reagent for the general evaluation of proteins in body fluids. Monospecific antisera are employed for the study of individual proteins.

Protein stain. After completion of the antigen-antibody reaction step and removal of nonprecipitated proteins, the complexes are stained with a 0.5 percent solution of Coomassie brilliant blue R.

Analysis with Polyvalent Antiserum

Procedure. The 2D-IEP gel is cast in two steps. First, a 1.0% solution of agarose is prepared by adding 0.5 g of agarose to 50 mL of buffer and boiling. This solution is then cooled to 56 °C and the appropriate amount of prewarmed antibody is immediately added and mixed well. In this procedure, a 10% solution of antibody was found to give the best resolution, peak area, and precipitate density. The antibody-containing gel is rapidly pipetted into the 10.6-cm square casting assembly and allowed to gel for one hour. In the second step, the casting assembly is opened and a 2.5-cm-wide strip of gel is removed from across the top. The casting assembly is then put back together and 1% agarose gel, containing no antibody, is pipetted into the top. After another one-hour cooling period, a 2-mm sample well is punched and the two-part gel is ready for use. This procedure of using a two-part gel is technically more straightforward than the conventional approach of performing electrophoresis in one gel, then cutting out a strip and placing it alongside the antibody-containing gel for the second electrophoresis.

The gel is placed in the electrophoresis chamber, making sure that good contact is made with the cooling surface. Horizontal wicks are then applied to assure good electrical connection between the gel and the vertical wicks which lead to the buffer chambers and power supply. A 2-μL sample of serum, cerebrospinal fluid (CSF), urine or other body fluid is applied to the well and the first electrophoresis is carried out at 25 V/cm for 45 minutes. These electrical conditions provide good protein separation and cause albumin to migrate about 6.5 cm from the point of application.

After the separation step, the gel is rotated 90°, the wicks are reattached, and the proteins are forced to migrate into the antibody-containing gel. The reaction step is best carried out at reduced voltage for a prolonged period (3 V/cm for 17 hours). Higher voltages and shorter times can be used, but the reaction precipitates are usually much fainter under these conditions.

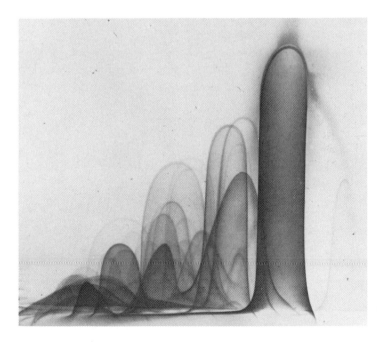

Fig. 1.   Two-dimensional immunoelectrophoresis of normal human serum.

Nonprecipitated protein, primarily from the antiserum, is removed by the usual press-drying procedure and the immunoprecipitates are visualized by staining with Coomassie brilliant blue R. After staining, polyvalent 2D-IEP patterns are either evaluated visually or peak areas are measured for quantitative analysis. Examples of typical patterns for normal serum, urine from a patient with glomerular proteinuria, and normal whole saliva are shown in Figures 1–3.

Applications. Visual evaluation of 2D-IEP patterns usually takes the form of contrasting various body fluids for differences in their protein composition. This can be a valuable teaching tool, since 2D-IEP provides a broad overview of both the electrophoretic location and relative concentration of most major proteins.

Polyvalent 2D-IEP provides the means for quantitation of many proteins in one sample from a single analytical run. With appropriate antiserum, distinct peaks for more than 50 proteins can be identified in human serum. Even though it would be impractical to quantitate them all, most of the higher concentration proteins can be measured.

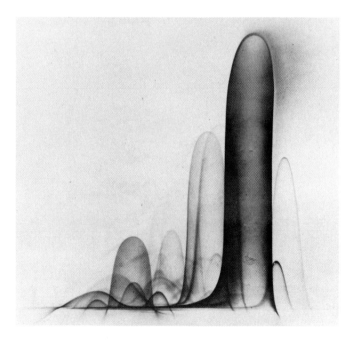

Fig. 2. Two-dimensional immunoelectrophoresis of urine from a patient with glomerular proteinuria.

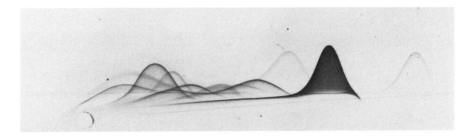

Fig. 3. Two-dimensional immunoelectrophoresis of normal whole human saliva. (From Killingsworth, LM: Review: Clinical applications of protein determinations in biological fluids other than blood. Clin Chem 28:1093, 1982. Reproduced by permission of the American Association for Clinical Chemistry.)

Analysis with Monospecific Antiserum

Procedure. This section illustrates how 2D-IEP can be used with monospecific antiserum to evaluate changes in a single protein. It also gives an example of how internal standardization can be accomplished through the addition of a known amount of nonhuman protein to the patient sample. The proteins to be assayed in this procedure are C3 and its major conversion products. The protein chosen for an internal standard is bovine serum albumin (BSA).

The procedure for monitoring C3 conversion is similar to that described above for analysis with polyvalent antiserum, but there are three substantial differences. First, the primary reagent is goat antihuman C3, which is monospecific for the C3 molecule, but also reacts against C3 conversion products. Second, addition of a constant, known amount of the reference protein BSA to the patient sample allows for expression of conversion product concentration in arbitrary units and normalizes for any changes in electrophoretic conditions. The reaction gel also contains a second antibody, rabbit antibovine albumin, which reacts with the internal standard, but not with any human proteins. Thirdly, the reaction buffer for these studies contains EDTA, which is necessary to complex any calcium present and prevent *in vitro* C3 breakdown. Reaction conditions for this procedure are outlined in Figure 4. Since migration distances in the second dimension are small, two samples can be assayed on each plate.

After the procedure is complete and the complexes have been stained, distinct peaks are visible for native C3, the BSA internal standard, and in cases with complement activation, the C3 conversion product C3c (Fig. 5). Peak areas are measured by planimetry and the conversion peak area is expressed as a percent of the internal standard area.

Application. Activation of the complement sequence *in vivo* can be monitored by measuring the conversion of the third component, C3. When the

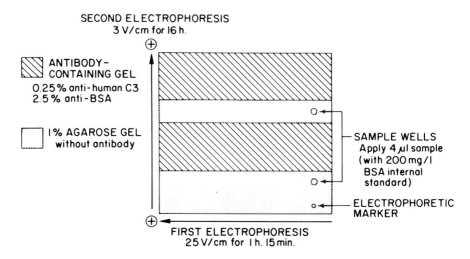

Fig. 4. Procedure for two-dimensional immunoelectrophoresis of C3 with BSA internal standard.

complement cascade is activated, either through the classic or alternative pathway, C3 is broken down into several conversion products which are thought to consist primarily of the fragments C3b, C3c, and C3d. The major fragment, C3c, has a faster electrophoretic mobility than the native C3 molecule, but is reactive to some anti-C3 antisera. Two-dimensional IEP with internal standardization is an excellent technique for the quantitative evaluation of *in vivo* C3 conversion, even in the presence of normal total C3 levels [9,16]. It can also be used to precisely follow serial changes in the degree of complement utilization in individual patients with various immunologic disorders.

SOURCES OF ERROR AND LIMITATIONS OF 2D-IEP

The technique of 2D-IEP is subject to many of the same errors as other immunochemical reactions in gel media. Most of these are technical in nature and include reagent reactivity and stability, temperature control in casting the gel and performing the two electrophoretic steps, proper mixing of antiserum with gel during casting, and control over electrical conditions. Anomalous migration of the proteins to be analyzed should also be taken into consideration as a factor that could lead to improper identification of a precipitate peak.

It should be noted that proteins which migrate toward the cathode under the specified reaction conditions, such as immunoglobulin G and C-reactive

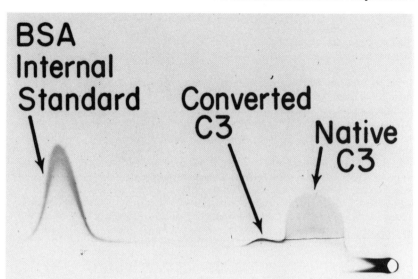

Fig. 5. Results of a C3 activation study on a patient with complement consumption. The peak designated as "converted C3" is the C3c (β-1-A) fragment (see [17]).

protein, are not present in the final patterns. Chemical modification of electrophoretic mobility by reaction with KCNO or addition of a cathodal antibody-containing gel are necessary for analysis of cathodal proteins [18].

Quantitation of proteins by 2D-IEP depends upon accurate and precise measurement of peak area. This can be done best by planimetry but photographic reproduction with weighing, estimation of peak area by measurement of peak height and width, and other approaches have been used. These methods are adequate when dealing with simple patterns, but they are not well suited for evaluating the multiple overlapping peaks in a polyvalent pattern. This imposes limitations on the use of 2D-IEP for simultaneous assay of numerous specific proteins, particularly when compared with the relative ease of analysis provided by automated nephelometric methods [8].

REFERENCES

1. Afonso E: Laurell's two-dimensional immunoelectrophoresis: Improved technique. Clin Chim Acta 54:123, 1974.
2. Bradwell AR, Burnett D: Improved methodology and precision using a straight baseline technique for the quantitation of proteins by two-dimensional immunoelectrophoresis. Clin Chim Acta 58:283, 1975.
3. Clarke HGM, Freeman TA: A quantitative immunoelectophoresis method (Laurell Electrophoresis). In Peeters H (ed): "Protides of the Biological Fluids." (Proceedings of the 14th Colloquium). Oxford: Pergamon Press, 1966, pp 503–509.

4. Cline LJ, Crowle AJ: Identification of α_1-lipoproteins in crossed immunoelectrophoresis. Clin Chem 25:1749, 1979.
5. Ganrot PO: Crossed immunoelectrophoresis. Scand J Clin Lab Invest 29 (suppl 124):39, 1972.
6. Grabar P, Williams CA: Methode permittant l'etude conjugee des proprietes electrophoretiques et immunochimique d'un melange de proteines. Application au serum sanguin. Biochem Biophys Acta 10:193, 1953.
7. Groc W, Harms A, Lahn W: Electrophoretic separation of serum proteins on cellulose acetate followed by electrophoresis in antibody-containing agarose gel. Clin Chim Acta 60:371, 1975.
8. Killingsworth LM: An automated approach to the preparation of plasma protein profiles. In Peeters H (ed): "Protides of the Biological Fluids." (Proceeding of the 23rd Colloquium). Oxford: Pergamon Press, 1976, pp 291–294.
9. Killingsworth LM, Britain CE: Internal standardization of gel immunoelectrophoretic procedures through the use of a dual antigen-antibody system. Clin Chem 22:1200, 1976.
10. Laurell C-B: Antigen-antibody crossed electrophoresis. Anal Biochem 10:358, 1965.
11. Markowski B: Zur Quantifizierung zur Zweidimensionalen Immuneletrophorese. Clin Chim Acta 44:319, 1973.
12. Pizzolato MA: Two-dimensional immunoelectrophoresis on cellulose acetate: Improved method for routine protein estimation. Clin Chim Acta 45:207, 1973.
13. Raisys V, Arvan D: Determination of proteins in biological fluids by electroimmunodiffusion and two-directional immunoelectrophoresis. Clin Chem 17:745, 1971.
14. Ressler N: Two-dimensional electrophoresis of protein antigens with an antibody containing buffer. Clin Chim Acta 5:795, 1960.
15. Scheidegger JJ Une micromethode de l'immunoelectrophorese. Int Arch Allergy Appl Immunol 7:103, 1955.
16. Teisberg P: In vivo activation of C3 revealed by crossed immunoelectrophoresis as a parameter of immunological activity in disease. Clin Chim Acta 62:35, 1975.
17. Tucker ES: Plasma complement analysis. In Nakamura RM, Dito WR, Tucker ES (eds): Immunoassays in the Clinical Laboratory. New York: Alan R. Liss, Inc., 1979, pp 273–279.
18. Verbruggen R: Quantitative immunoelectrophoretic methods: A literature survey. Clin Chem 21:5, 1975.
19. Versey JMB, Slater L and Hobbs JR: Semiautomated two dimensional immunoelectrophoresis. J Immunol Methods 3:63, 1973.
20. Weeke B: Crossed immunoelectrophoresis. In Axelsen NH, Kroll J, Weeke B (eds): "Quantitative Immunoelectrophoresis." Oslo: Universitets-forlaget, 1973, pp 47–56.

Physiology of Immunoglobulins: Diagnostic and
Clinical Aspects, pages 97–115
© 1982 Alan R. Liss, Inc., 150 Fifth Avenue, New York, NY 10011

5

Immunofixation Electrophoresis

Tsieh Sun, MD

INTRODUCTION

The most accurate way of identifying individual protein fractions, until
now, has been the simultaneous determination of their electrophoretic mobility and their antigenicity by immunochemical means. Immunoelectrophoresis (IEP) has been the most popular method based on this principle. The
popularity and practicality of the two-dimensional cross-immunoelectropho-
resis are impeded by its difficulty in both technique and interpretation.

Nevertheless, even the popular IEP has several faults. The major drawback
is its long diffusion process. As a result, when small amounts of protein are
to be identified, such as those found in oligoclonal or minimonoclonal gammopathy, they will be too diluted to be detected after an overnight diffusion
[5,25,33], resulting in a relatively low degree of sensitivity. In addition,
when two proteins share a partially identical antigenic component, such as
in IgM-κ and IgM-λ biclonal gammopathy, the two protein arcs may merge
into one precipitin arc, thus giving a false identity (Fig. 1A)[5,33]. Furthermore, in light chain typing, light chains from different immunoglobulins
form a single arc on IEP. If an abnormal light chain is present in small
quantity, for instance in the early stage of IgM-κ macroglobulinemia, the
small monoclonal κ-arc may be totally masked by the bulk of normal light
chains from other immunoglobulins (Fig 2). This is the so-called "umbrella
effect" [25,33].

In 1964, Afonso [1] and Wilson [4] described independently their modified
techniques of immunoelectrophoresis, which are considered the forerunners
of immunofixation electrophoresis (IFE). However, their utilization of polyvalent antiserum for immunofixation renders the results difficult to interpret.
Alper and Johnson [3] are given the credit for perfecting this technique by

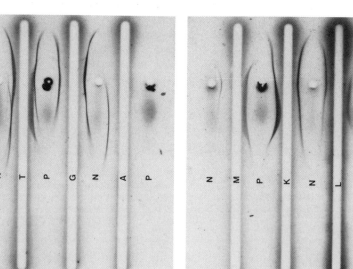

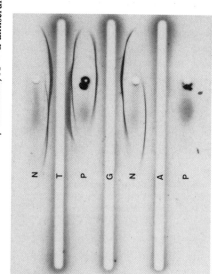

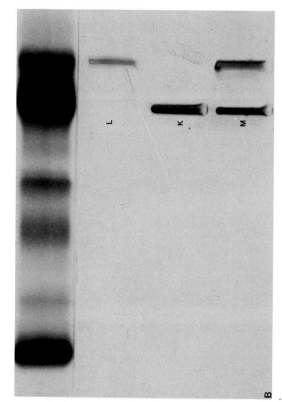

Fig. 1. (A) IgM-κ and IgM-λ biclonal gammopathy. Two IgM arcs merge into a single arc, giving a false identity as a monoclonal gammopathy (B) IgM-κ and IgM-λ biclonal gammopathy. Immunofixation pattern shows that one monoclonal band consists of IgM-κ, another IgM-λ. (Reproduced by permission from Sun, T. et al., Am. J. Clin. Pathol. 72:5, 1979).

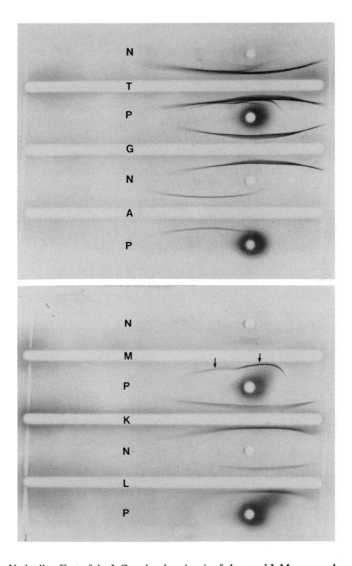

Fig. 2   Umbrella effect of the IgG molecules: A pair of abnormal IgM arcs are demonstrated (arrows). The one with faster electrophoretic mobility is composed of monomeric IgM molecules, the slower one consists of pentameric IgM. The κ-light chain arc assumes the IgG configuration, masking the abnormal κ-arcs from the abnormal IgM. The abnormal κ-arcs were identified by immunoelectrophoresis after the patient's serum was treated with 2,3-mercaptoethanol and also by immunofixation with the untreated serum.

using monospecific antisera, which render the technique with a high degree of sensitivity as well as high specificity [6].

IMMUNOFIXATION ELECTROPHORESIS PROCEDURES

Like IEP, IFE is essentially a two-step procedure. *The first step is electrophoresis* to accomplish the separation of different protein fractions. *The second step is application of the antiserum* that is monospecific for the particular protein of interest. If this particular protein is present, it will react with the antiserum, forming a precipitin band which may be visible with or without staining. Unlike IEP, the antiserum is applied directly onto the surface of the supporting medium, avoiding the lengthy diffusion process.

There are *several methods of antiserum application*. The original method is to flood the entire slide or the area of interest with antiserum [1,6,34]. This method requires a large amount of antiserum and is therefore costly. In addition, if the electrophoretic strips are not separated, the antiserum may flow onto the adjacent strip, giving misleading results [15]. The use of a camel's-hair brush can pinpoint the area of antiserum application, but it still requires a relatively large amount of antiserum [5]. For these reasons, the above methods are now rarely used. The most widely used method is that of Ritchie and Smith [25], which includes soaking a strip of cellulose acetate [25] or filter paper [5] with antiserum and placing it over the surface of the supporting medium. This method uses antiserum economically and is more versatile. For instance, one long cellulose acetate strip can be placed over several adjacent electrophoretic patterns or several small strips with different antisera can be laid on different protein bands of the same electrophoretic pattern.

In our laboratory, antiserum is applied through a slit in a plastic sheet onto the protein band of interest (Fig. 3). This method uses a minimal quantity of antiserum and yet produces a well-defined precipitin band. It is, therefore, used as an example to illustrate the detailed steps of IFE.

Agarose slides are recommended for IFE, especially in the study of gammopathies [29,33]. Agarose gel provides a higher resolution of individual protein fractions and more space between different bands than cellulose acetate slides. Polyacrylamide gel electrophoresis also provides high-resolution separation but has the inherent disadvantage of its lengthy procedure and its consumption of relatively large amounts of antiserum [14]. For the determination of one protein fraction, *at least two electrophoretic patterns should be obtained. An undiluted serum specimen is used for the first pattern,* which should be stained with Amido black. This pattern is for identifying and localizing the protein band of interest. *A diluted serum specimen from the same patient is used for the second pattern,* which is for the immuno-

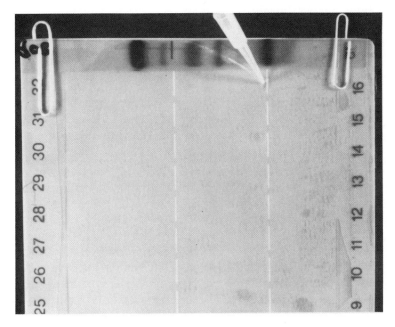

Fig. 3. Guided by a stained electrophoretic strip, monospecific antisera are applied through the slits of a plastic sheet onto unstained strips at the location corresponding to the monoclonal band.

fixation process and therefore should not be stained. The purpose of dilution is to eliminate antigen excess, and also to minimize the background protein, which is important, especially for the study of monoclonal bands in the γ-zone. Fivefold dilutions with saline are optimal in most cases, but titration may be necessary in some cases to determine the optimal antigen/antibody ratio. Dilutions as high as 1:64 may be required in some cases [31].

In the *study of monoclonal gammopathy,* at least *six patterns* should be obtained. The first strip is stained as a reference. Monospecific antisera for γ, α, μ, κ, and λ are to be applied to the other strips. δ-antisera should also be used if the possibility of IgD myeloma exists.

For other body fluid such as cerebrospinal fluid (CSF) and urine, when the protein concentration is lower than 1 g/dL, concentrated specimens should be used for the first pattern as a reference, and undiluted specimens should be applied for immunofixation. Coomassie brilliant blue is usually used for the staining of body fluids with low protein content.

After electrophoresis of the entire battery, the first pattern is cut out and stained with Amido black or Coomassie brilliant blue, while the other strips are kept in a moist chamber to avoid drying. The protein band of interest is then located from the stained strip and aligned with the unstained strips. Fifteen μL of antiserum are applied through the slit of a plastic sheet onto the unstained strip at the location corresponding to the abnormal band (Fig. 3). Excess antiserum is removed by blotting with filter paper 10–30 minutes after application. The agarose slide which contains several strips is pressed with one moist and four dry sheets of filter paper plus a weight of 1–2 kg for ten minutes. The slide is deproteinized with normal saline for 2–16 hours, rinsed with tap water for ten minutes, and finally dried with air and stained with Amido black or Coomassie brilliant blue. Immunoprecipitin bands are usually visible in unstained slides within an hour after antiserum application. However, weak immunoprecipitin can be demonstrated only in stained slides. The presence of a pale area in the center of the immunoprecipitin band usually indicates antigen excess (Fig. 4).

Although this IFE method has proved to be very useful, it is not applicable to the following situations: 1) when the protein fraction of interest is not visible in the electrophoretic pattern or is uncertain in location and 2) when the density of the background immunoglobulin approximates that of the paraprotein band, the background protein may also be stained even after dilution of the serum [33]. In these two situations, the method of Ritchie and Smith should be used. The antiserum-soaked cellulose acetate strip can cover a broader area, thus providing a better chance for the detection of the invisible band(s). A broader area coverage may also contrast the band of interest with the background by their difference in staining intensity.

CLINICAL APPLICATIONS

Quantitative and Qualitative Studies of Individual Protein Fractions

It was Afonso's initial intention to use IFE for quantitation of protein fractions separated by electrophoresis [1]. While the capability of IFE in quantitating protein bands by scanning is still one of its advantages over IEP, it should probably be reserved for the assay of minute amounts of proteins which are not measurable by other means. This statement is based on the fact that IFE is only a semiquantitative technique and that protein bands can be scanned after direct staining without immunofixation; the function of IFE in this respect is only to augment the invisible or weak protein bands. The most useful aspect of IFE, however, lies in its various qualitative functions. These include *identifying a protein band of unknown nature, demonstrating genetic variants, determining the status of enzymatic conversion, probing the possible causative agents of antibodies, and classifying as well as typing of immunoglobulins*. Although polyacrylamide gel is not recommended for

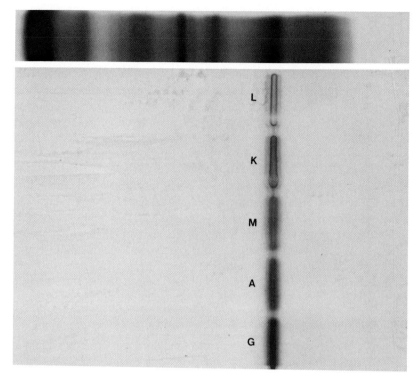

Fig. 4.   Immunofixation pattern of polyclonal gammopathy. A narrow band in the gamma region reacting to all antisera. Note that the pale centers of μ-, κ-, and λ-chains indicate antigen excess (Reproduced by permission from Sun T et al., Am. J. Clin Pathl. 72:5, 1979).

routine IFE, IFE may well be the right tool to solve the intriguing mystery of the numerous protein bands separated by polyacrylamide gel electrophoresis.

Study of Protein Polymorphism

In most of the early reports, IFE was utilized for the study of protein polymorphism [2,3,26]. The information thus obtained is useful for the phenotyping of certain proteins, and some genetic variants may be associated with certain diseases. For instance, a specific transferrin band (phenotype $B_{0-1}C$) is frequently observed in the CSF of patients with Maria-Sanger-Brown's ataxia [30]. Nevertheless, the most widely used application in this aspect is the *protease inhibitor typing (Pi typing)* for α_1-antitrypsin [4,11,26].

Pi typing is useful because of the close correlation between Pi types and clinical situations, for instance, the correlation of PiZ and early onset emphysema [21,32]. Phenotyping by IFE also has a great potential in cases of disputed paternity [9]. Other serum proteins that have been studied for their genetic variants include Gc-globulin, ceruloplasmin, complement, transferrin, α_2-macroglobulin, haptoglobin, α_1-acid glycoprotein, properdin factor B, and IgM [2,3,12,14,18,29]. Transferrin, α_2-macroglobulin, and haptoglobin in CSF [18,30] and Gc globulin in amniotic fluid [12] have also been investigated.

Determination of the Source of Specimen

Due to the presence of a genetic variant of transferrin in normal CSF [30], IFE can be used for the diagnosis of CSF leakage by identifying a pair of transferrin bands (β_1- and β_2-bands) in nasal fluid samples (rhinorrhea) or in those from the ear [10]. This variant of transferrin is deficient in neuraminic acid and is, therefore, located in the β_2-zone due to its resultant slow electrophoretic mobility [10]. The transferrin normally seen in serum is positioned in β_1-zone. Further exploration of genetic variants in different body fluids may provide helpful information for further distinctive characteristics.

Demonstration of Conversion Products of Proteins

So far, only the conversion products of the third component of complement have been studied [2,3]. The presence of these products indicate activation of the complement system. The capability of IFE in demonstrating a complex formed by two reacting elements is being used to determine the stoichiometry of the interaction of α_1-antitrypsin with elastase [4a]. Theoretically, conversion products of any protein can be studied by IFE. The study of conversion products of fibrinogen, for instance, may prove helpful in the diagnosis of disseminated intravascular coagulation (DIC).

Study of Gammopathies

It appears that the most useful application of IFE in clinical laboratories is for the classification and typing of immunoglobulins, especially in monoclonal gammopathies [5,20b,27,33]. IFE is a very sensitive technique for the screening of paraproteins. In a study of 100 sera from patients with chronic lymphocytic leukemia and suspected multiple myeloma, paraproteins were found in 39 sera by IFE, 33 sera by agarose gel electrophoresis, and 30 sera by immunoelectrophoresis [24]. In addition, more paraprotein bands, some of which were composed of light chains, were detected by IFE than the other two methods. The advantages of using IFE for the study of gammopathy are especially apparent in the following situations:

Oligoclonal and minimonoclonal gammopathies. These two terms are frequently used synonymously. In a strict sense, however, they are different. Oligoclonal gammopathy is traditionally defined as multiple, narrow, discrete, and faint bands in the γ-zone, usually seen in demyelinating disorders if detected in CSF, or as a nonspecific early immune response if seen in serum alone. Minimonoclonal gammopathy, on the other hand, may include oligoclonal gammopathy in a broad sense, but it usually indicates a single, discrete, inconspicuous protein band in the γ- or other electrophoretic zones, and frequently represents early changes associated with multiple myeloma or macroglobulinemia. IEP, more often than not, is unable to detect these bands in either case, because the antiserum used in IEP meets with only a portion of the low-level antigen after diffusion [5,33]; in contrast, IFE can readily identify the components of these bands. In this respect, most studies have been performed on oligoclonal bands encountered in patients with multiple sclerosis [5,13,19,20]. Early reports indicate that these bands are monoclonal IgG in nature [5]; a recent study, however, shows that IgA, IgM, and light chains and even polyclonal immunoglobulins can be detected in these bands [20].

Umbrella effect of IgG on light chain typing in monoclonal gammopathy. The light chain arcs detected by IEP are composed of the same type of light chains from different immunoglobulins. If the changes in light chains of IgM or IgA origin are not very prominent, these changes may be masked by the major light chain component from IgG (Fig. 2) [5,27,33]. This is a diagnostic problem encountered frequently in early cases of IgM macroglobulinemia and occasionally of IgA myeloma, leading to a wrong interpretation of polyclonal IgM or IgA gammopathy. The treatment of the patient's serum with 2,3-mercaptoethanol or boric acid precipitation can augment the light chain changes in cases of IgM macroglobulinemia or occasionally in polymerized IgA cases. However, IFE provides a more convenient and direct approach to solve this problem [33].

Equivocal biclonal gammopathy. When biclonal proteins assume close electrophoretic positions, a problem for the interpretation of the immunoelectrophoretogram exists [5,33]. When the two paraproteins share the same light chain (e.g., IgG-κ and IgM-κ), the phenomenon can be misinterpreted as an immune complex; on the other hand, when the heavy chain is the common antigenic component (e.g., IgM-κ and IgM-λ), one of the light chains may be mistaken for Bence Jones protein (Fig. 1A). However, IFE allows the identification of the biclonal immunoglobulins unequivocally as two separate proteins (Fig. 1B).

Immune complexes. As the clinical significance of immune complexes are being gradually recognized, their determination is being requested more

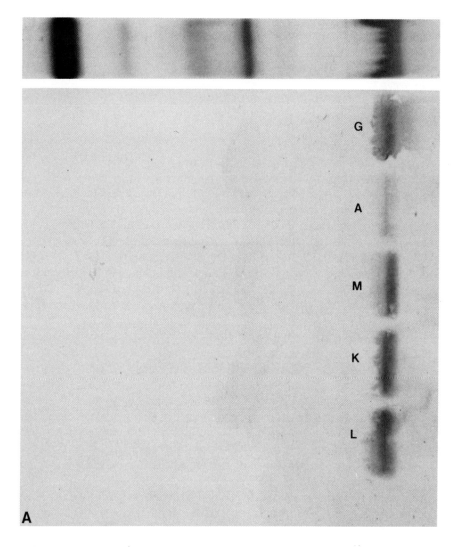

Fig. 5. (A) Immune-complex disease. Immunofixation shows γ-, μ-, κ-, and λ-chains, indicating a polyclonal immune complex. (B) Immune complex disease. Immunoelectrophoretic pattern shows prominent arcs of μ, κ and λ at the same position, indicating polyclonal IgM gammopathy. Note that the κ- and λ-light chain antisera react with the immune complexes (arrows), and these additional precipitin arcs are distinguished from the normal κ- and λ-arcs. Alternatively, a monoclonal rheumatoid factor may act as an antibody against components in κ and λ-antisera. (Reproduced by permission from Sun T et al., Am. J. Clin. Pathol. 72:5, 1979).

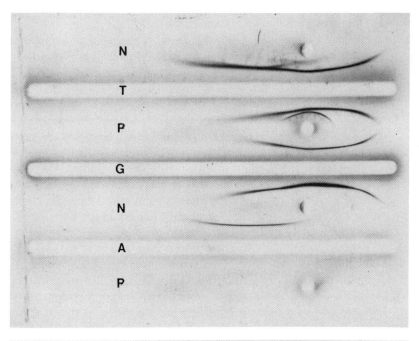

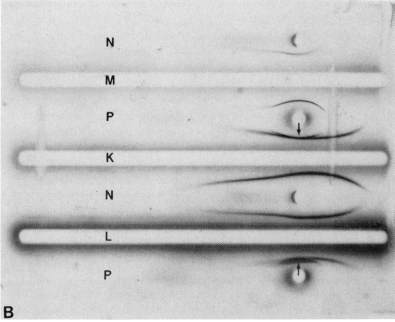

frequently than ever before by clinicians. Although there are several tests available for this purpose, none of them can detect all the immune complexes. For instance, the Clq methods detect mainly large complexes containing IgM or other polymeric immunoglobulins (>19S); whereas rheumatoid factor assays mainly demonstrate the small IgG-containing complexes [17]. IFE is a reliable technique for the detection of immune complexes, which are visible in electrophoretograms as discrete bands [17,27,33] (Fig. 5A). They usually represent monoclonal IgM rheumatoid factors forming immune complexes with the patient's autologous IgG which is polyclonal. Cryoglobulin is often present and hepatitis-associated antigen is not infrequently demonstrated. For immune complexes, IEP is capable of showing the monoclonal component (Fig. 5B), and theoretically it may also reveal a distorted IgG arc which would return to normal configuration after being released from the complex by reducing IgM with 2,3-mercaptoethanol [23]; in our experience, however, this phenomenon rarely occurs. The IFE, on the other hand, may detect all the components, but it fails to show which component is monoclonal or polyclonal (Fig. 5A). For instance, if the immune complex contains mon-oclonal IgM-κ and polyclonal IgG, the IFE will show that the complex is composed of μ, γ, κ, and λ chains. Therefore, the combination of using both IFE and IEP to provide a complete picture of the analyzed immune complex is recommended. IFE is also useful in delineating other protein complexes, such as lactate dehydrogenase/IgG, alkaline phosphatase/IgG, and IgG/lipoprotein complexes [5].

Controversial Bence Jones protein. A small amount of light chains can be present in the urine of patients with renal diseases as well as under normal conditions. These light chains are usually polyclonal in nature and thus are nonspecific, unless a considerable amount is detected, such as in systemic lupus erythematosus [28]. The light chains are subject to digestion by ly-sozymes and bacterial enzymes in urine and the relatively smaller amount of λ-light chains will disappear first, leaving the relatively larger amount of κ-light chains as the only light chains detectable in the immunoelectrophor-etogram (Fig. 6). As a result, the presence of κ-chain may be misinterpreted as "monoclonal free light chains" or Bence Jones protein. With IFE, the small amount of λ-light chains as well as heavy chains can also be discovered

Fig. 6. Equivocal case of Bence Jones proteinuria. The immunoelectrophoretic pattern shows only a κ-light chain without a corresponding heavy chain or λ-light chain. Note a fragment of heavy chain (h) is present with a fast electrophoretic mobility indicating enzymatic cleavage has taken place. Electrophoretic pattern shows minimonoclonal banding, which was identified by immunofixation as polyclonal in nature (Reproduced by permission from Sun T et al., Am. J. Clin. Pathol. 72:5, 1979).

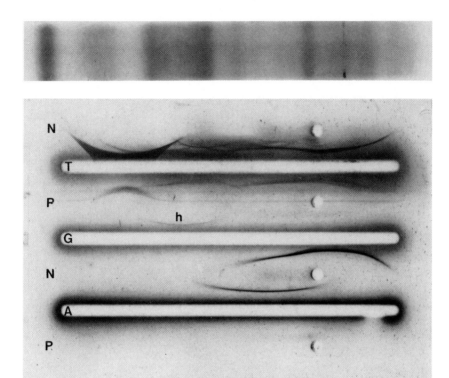

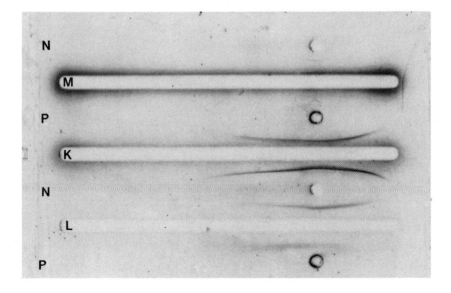

from urine, thus showing the polyclonal feature and excluding the diagnosis of Bence Jones protein [33]. In our experience, if a monoclonal band is not demonstrated in the electrophoretogram, the "free" κ-chain shown in IEP is usually due to the above mentioned phenomenon and IFE verification may not be necessary.

Occult paraprotein bands. Occult paraprotein bands or M-proteins are most frequently encountered in light chain disease, and to a lesser extent, in IgD myeloma and heavy chain disease [5,27,28,33]. The inability of electrophoresis to demonstrate the paraprotein is either due to the limitation of its resolution power for a protein with a low concentration, or the paraprotein is hidden under a normal band. On most occasions, however, IEP is able to detect those occult paraproteins, but it may miss small quantities of light chains that are present in the serum of myeloma cases or Bence Jones proteinemia. The merit of IFE is not only in the detection of these otherwise missed Bence Jones proteins but also in pinpointing the locations of the hidden or occult paraproteins in the electrophoretogram [33] (Fig. 7). While the searching for the location of paraprotein may be partly an exercise in academic curiosity, it is, nevertheless, helpful for quantitation purposes. All the quantitative methods that are available cannot distinguish normal immunoglobulins from myeloma protein of the same class. When the quantity of paraprotein is small, a relatively accurate way for quantitation is to multiply the percentage of the paraprotein band, obtained by scanning, by the quantity of total protein [8].

Exploration of the Causative Agents of the Disease

IFE can be performed not only by using a monospecific antiserum but also by using an antigen for the detection of antibody [7,16,22]. In the latter case, it is called *reverse IFE*. The most attractive finding in this field so far has been the discovery of antimeasles antibodies in the oligoclonal bands present in the CSF from patients with subacute sclerosing panencephalitis [22]. It is obvious that this approach opens a broad field for meaningful exploration.

THE ROLE OF IFE IN CLINICAL LABORATORIES

While some IFE advocators assert the pending demise of IEP, many experienced immunochemists still value IEP. There is no doubt that these

Fig. 7. IgG-λ myeloma. A monoclonal protein band is present at an atypical region overlapping with β_2, which is identified by immunofixation as IgG-λ (only γ-antiserum is illustrated) (Reproduced by permission from Sun T et al., Am. J. Clin. Pathol. 72:5, 1979).

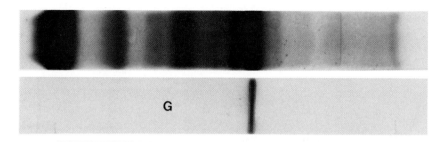

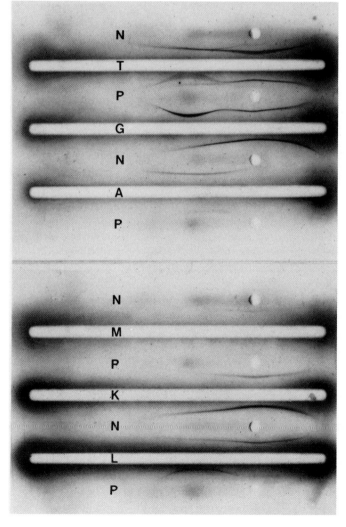

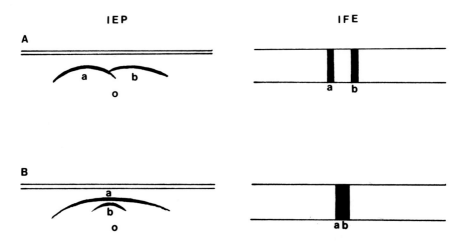

Fig. 8.   (A) Two different antigens (a and b) react with the same antiserum. The two precipitin arcs formed in IEP show a reaction of partial identity as evidenced by the presence of a spur. Two precipitin bands are also formed in IFE, but one cannot tell whether there is complete or partial identity. (B) Two antigens (a and b) react with the same antiserum forming two precipitin arcs in IEP, but only one precipitin band in IFE, as the two antigens have the same electrophoretic mobility (same isoelectric point).

two procedures are complementary, and each one has its own merits. The problem remains, however, whether the IEP or the IFE should be the routine test [35,35a].

While the interpretation of IFE is more straightforward, it is technically more difficult than IEP. *For experienced immunochemists, IEP is undoubtedly more informative* [5,20b]. IEP clearly distinguishes a normal immunoprecipitin arc from an abnormal arc and a pure protein from a contaminated protein (Fig. 8). In Figure 5B, the arcs of a rheumatoid factor are clearly distinguished from those of the remaining IgM-κ by their location and configuration in the immunoelectrophoretogram, whereas IFE can hardly distinguish the rheumatoid factor from the normal IgM-κ, as they are overlapping in position and share the same antigenicity (Fig. 5A). An experienced interpreter can tell the difference between a monomeric IgM from a pentameric one by IEP (Fig. 2) and may even sometimes be able to predict the malignant nature of a monoclonal gammopathy by observing the subtle changes in an immunoelectrophoretogram. On the other hand, there are no changes in configuration of the precipitin bands to express the extent of deviation from normal in IFE. IFE also poses some difficulty in delineating a monoclonal band against a heavy γ-globulin background.

Technically, IFE is less reproducible than IEP. The major reason seems to be due to the existence of a narrow range of optimal antigen-antibody ratios for the formation of immunoprecipitates in IFE [31,33]. In IEP, antigen and antibody are simultaneously diluted as they migrate in the support medium during the incubation period, which acts as a mechanism of titration. This mechanism does not exist in IFE. Therefore, IFE is more demanding than IEP for the required quality of antiserum in terms of high titer and avidity. Unfortunately, many commercial products are not of the highest standard [3]. Therefore, the recommended dilutions for patients' sera reported from the literature are frequently not applicable and readjustments have to be made on an individual basis after a titration trial in each laboratory.

In the clinical application of IFE it appears mandatory to provide side-by-side comparison between the patient's serum and a normal control. As mentioned before, most of the commercially available antisera do not have a sufficiently high antibody titer, therefore, a positive control, such as a case of monoclonal gammopathy, is probably needed to exclude false-negative results.

When the antigen-antibody ratio is routinely titrated on an individual basis, and when positive and negative controls are set up, routinely, IFE will appear too time-consuming to serve as a practical screening test in the clinical laboratory.

THE POTENTIALS OF IFE

Although we do not recommend IFE as a routine test in its present stage, it may find its way to clinical laboratories in due time, as IFE is a test of great potential. This potential depends on the combination of IFE with other tests. To enhance the sensitivity of IFE, the antibodies or second antibodies can be labeled with enzymes, radioisotopes, or fluorescein dyes [5,12]. Conversely, the antigens labeled with the above mentioned enhancing reagents can be used to detect the function of the antibodies [7,16,22]. The combination of immunofixation with isoelectric focusing provides an even higher resolution of protein components than can be obtained with electrophoresis and is especially suitable for the study of protein polymorphism [4,12,18,29,30]. Furthermore, the immunofixation print techniques developed by Arnaud et al. produces a sharper pattern than that of the isoelectric focusing-immunofixation technique and is probably more promising in the field of protein polymorphism [4].

In summary, IFE is an excellent tool for the study of protein polymorphism, gammopathies, and conversion products of proteins. It has also been applied successfully, on a limited basis, for the determination of the source of body fluids, and the function of antibodies. Although, in our opinion, at present, IEP is still the method of choice for the routine study of gammopathies, IFE will undoubtedly receive wider acceptance in clinical laboratories in the near future, and it should certainly be used as a supplementary test to solve ambiguous problems in the various cases as discussed in the section on Clinical Applications.

REFERENCES

1. Afonso E: Quantitative immunoelectrophoresis of serum proteins. Clin Chim Acta 10:114–122, 1964.
2. Alper CA: Genetic polymorphism of complement components as a probe of structure and function. In Amos B (ed): "Progress in Immunology, First International Congress of Immunology." New York: Academic Press, 1971, pp 609–624.
3. Alper CA, Johnson AM: Immunofixation electrophoresis: A technique for the study of protein polymorphism. Vox Sang 17:445, 1969.
4. Arnaud P, Wilson GB, Koistinen J, Fudenberg HH: Immunofixation after electrofocusing: Improved method for specific detection of serum proteins with determination of isoelectric points. I. Immunofixation print technique for detection of alpha-1 protease inhibitor. J Immunol Methods 16:221, 1977.
4a. Baumstark JS: Quantitative immunofixation of protein following zone electrophoresis in agarose gel: Application to the determination of the stoichiometry of the α1-antitrypsin with elastase interaction. J Immunol Methods 23:78, 1978.
5. Cawley LP, Minard BJ, Tourtellote WW, Ma BI, Chelle C: Immunofixation electrophoretic techniques applied to identification of proteins in serum and cerebrospinal fluid. Clin Chem 22:1262, 1976.
6. Change CH, Inglis NR: Convenient immunofixation electrophoresis on cellulose acetate membrane. Clin Chim Acta 65:91, 1975.
7. Cotton RGH, Milstein C: Immunoreactive precipitation of protein components after isoelectric focusing. J Chromatogr 86:219, 1973.
8. Daniels JC, Vyvial TM, Levin WC, Ritzmann SE: Methodologic differences in values for M-proteins in serum, as measured by three techniques. Clin Chem 21:243, 1975.
9. Hoste B: Group-specific component (Gc) and transferrin (Tf) subtypes ascertained by isoelectric focusing: A simple nonimmunological staining procedure for Gc. Hum Genet 50:75, 1979.
10. Irjala K, Suonpaa J, Laurent B: Identification of CSF leakage by immunofixation. Arch Otolaryngol 105:447, 1979.
11. Johnson AM: Genetic typing of alpha-1 antitrypsin in immunofixation electrophoresis. Identification of subtypes of PiM. J Lab Clin Med 87:152, 1976.
12. Johnson AM: Immunofixation following electrophoresis or isoelectric focusing for identification and phenotyping of proteins. Ann Clin Lab Sci 8:195, 1978.
13. Johnson KP, Arrigo SC, Nelson BJ: Agarose electrophoresis of cerebrospinal fluid in multiple sclerosis. Neurology 27:273, 1977.
14. Kahn SN, Thompson EJ: Rapid quantitative surface immunofixation of proteins in polyacrylamide gels. Clin Chim Acta 89:253, 1978.
15. Karinkanta HH, Nieminen EJ: An improved technique for immunofixation of electrophoretograms. Clin Chem 24:1639, 1978.
16. Keck K, Grossberg AL, Pressman P: Specific characterization of isoelectric-focused immunoglobulins in polyacrylamide gel by reactions with ^{125}I-labeled protein antigens or antibodies. Eur J Immunol 3:99, 1973.

17. Kelly RH, Scholl MA, Harvey VS, Devenyi AG: Quantitative testing for circulating immune complexes by use of zone electrophoresis on agarose. Clin Chem 26:396, 1980.
18. Lawrenzi MA, Link H: Characterization of the mobility on isoelectric focusing of individual proteins in CSF and serum by immunofixation. J Neurol Neurosurg Psychiatry 42:368, 1979.
19. Leterre EC, Callawaert A, Heremans JF, Sfaello Z: Electrophoretic morphology of gamma globulins in cerebrospinal fluid of multiple sclerosis and other diseases of the nervous system. Neurology 20:982, 1970.
20. Link H, Laurenzi MA: Immunoglobulin class and light chain type of oligoclonal bands in CSF in multiple sclerosis determined by agarose gel electrophoresis and immunofixation. Ann Neurol 6:107, 1978.
20a. Marshall MO: Comparison of immunofixation and immunoelectrophoresis methods in the identification of monoclonal immunoglobulins in serum. Clin Chim Acta 104:1, 1980.
20b. Merlini G, Piro P, Pavesi F et al: Detection and identification of monoclonal components: IEP on agarose gel and immunofixation on cellulose acetate compared. Clin Chem 27:1862, 1981.
21. Morse, JO: Alpha-1 antitrypsin deficiency. N Engl J Med 299:1045, 1099, 1978.
22. Nordal HJ, Vandvik B, Norrby E: Demonstration of electrophoretically restricted virus-specific antibodies in serum and cerebrospinal fluid by imprint electroimmunofixation. Scand J Immunol 7:381, 1978.
23. Penn GM, Davis T: "Identification of myeloma protein." Chicago: American Society of Clinical Pathologists, 1976, pp 26–27.
24. Pedersen NS, Axelsen NH: Detection of M-components by an easy immunofixation procedure: Comparison with agarose gel electrophoresis and classical immunoelectrophoresis. J Immunol Methods 30:257, 1979.
25. Ritchie RF, Smith R: Immunofixation I. General principles and application to agarose gel electrophoresis. Clin Chem 22:497, 1976.
26. Ritchie RF, Smith R: Immunofixation II. Application to typing of alpha-1 antitrypsin at acid pH. Clin Chem 22:1735, 1976.
27. Ritchie RF, Smith R: Immunofixation III. Application to the study of monoclonal proteins. Clin Chem 22:1982, 1976.
28. Ritzmann SE: Immunoglobulin abnormalities. In Ritzmann SE, Daniels JC (eds): "Serum Protein Abnormalities, Diagnostic and Clinical Aspects," 2nd printing. New York: Alan R. Liss, Inc., 1982, pp 351–485.
29. Rosen A, Ek K, Aman P: Agarose isoelectric focusing of native human immunoglobulin M and alpha-2 macroglobulin. J Immunol Methods 28:1, 1979.
30. Stiber H: Direct immunofixation after isoelectric focusing: An improved method for identification of cerebrospinal fluid and serum proteins. J Neurol Sci 42:275, 1979.
31. Sufuge K: Immunofixation electrophoresis. J Med Tech 23:881, 1979 (in Japanese).
32. Sun T, Kurtz S, Copeland BE: Alpha-1-antitrypsin deficiency and pulmonary disease. Am J Clin Pathol 62:725, 1974.
33. Sun T, Lien YY, Degnan T: Study of gammopathies with immunofixation electrophoresis. Am J Clin Pathol 72:5, 1979.
34. Wilson AT: Direct immunoelectrophoresis. J Immunol 92:431, 1964.
35. Seligmann M (chairman), Bentwich Z, Bianco N et al: The use and abuse of immunological tests. A report of an IUIS/WHO working group on critical considerations of eight widely used diagnostic procedures. Clin Exp Immunol 46:662–674, 1981.
35a. Clinical immunology laboratory tests—a growth industry. (Ed.) Lancet II:1269, 1981.

DIAGNOSTIC METHODOLOGY AND INTERPRETATION

Immunochemical Quantitation of Serum Proteins

Physiology of Immunoglobulins: Diagnostic and
Clinical Aspects, pages 119-137
© 1982 Alan R. Liss, Inc., 150 Fifth Avenue, New York, NY 10011

6

Quantitation of Serum Proteins by Centrifugal Fast Analyzer

William R. Dito, MD

INTRODUCTION

Quantitative measurements of specific serum or plasma proteins by immunochemical means are currently widely utilized in research and clinical practice [1,5,8–13]. Both manual and variably automated methods are available as commercial kits and are based upon differing means to detect and quantify the immunoprecipitin reaction. This chapter deals with one method of automating the assay of comparatively large numbers of different plasma or serum proteins employing a centrifugal fast analyzer (CFA). Manual and other methods of automation are described elsewhere in this text. All are adaptable to both research and clinical environments; method and technique selection are often made on the basis of throughput requirements, available financial support, personal preference, and convenience.

THE CENTRIFUGAL FAST ANALYZER

The CFA has been utilized in clinical laboratories for more than a decade, and excellent detailed descriptions are available for review [2,4]. Although significant differences may exist between the various commercial instruments available, the principles of operation are shared and these will be briefly reviewed.

The CFA is a modular instrument composed of five basic parts. These include a rotor assembly, optical detection system, temperature control assembly, computational module, and a pipetting station. All must operate in an integrated and sequentially controlled system.

The rotor assembly is the basic unit that provides for transfer and mixing of samples and reagents to a cuvette compartment by means of centrifugation.

A transfer disc, which may be made of a disposable plastic, nondisposable Teflon, or an integral part of the rotor assembly, is loaded with sample(s) and reagent(s) either manually or at a pipetting station. Specimen separation is accomplished by the use of radially arranged wells, pockets of which contain the individual assay sample(s) and reagent(s). With centrifugation, partial mixing occurs during passage to the cuvette, full mixing being later accomplished by agitation with siphoned air bubbles. This process is significantly influenced by the diameter of the transfer disc and a series of accelerations and decelerations of rotor speed. Each manufacturer provides detailed information regarding these specifications for their individual instrument, including time and procedural sequences to accomplish the initial mixing and agitation of a sample and reagent.

Most of the current CFAs utilize spectrophotometers with either an interference filter or a diffraction grating to accomplish wavelength isolation. Newer versions have incorporated fluorescence detection (Instrumentation Laboratories) with compatible instrument geometry. Laser light sources have also been employed (American Instrument Co.) and require the use of a special postcuvette filter (Darkfield type) [3].

Temperature control monitoring, accomplished by means of a variety of methods and thermisters, is an important segment of instrument design and cannot be overemphasized for application to kinetic or rate analysis.

The computational module provides the means for process control, data acquisition and reduction, and the incorporation of various reporting forms. Its importance to instrument performance, control, and flexibility is well documented. Briefly, timing and numbers of data points, detection of signal errors and electronic drifts, maintenance of sample and blank identity, and selection of a variety of calculation modes and data storage (e.g., controls, patients) are but a few of the areas where the computational module (frequently a minicomputer or microprocessor with variable disk or tape storage device) provides invaluable assistance. Without it, the CFA would be severely crippled and, frankly, of little functional use.

Again, critical to the successful operation of a CFA, the pipetting station provides the user with the opportunity to autoload a transfer disc with appropriate standards, patient samples, controls, and reagents. Accurate volume delivery is essential, as is the identity of the appropriate radially arranged wells. Although manual reagent and sample delivery is feasible, it is often tedious and more subject to sample identity error.

MINIMUM INSTRUMENTATION REQUIREMENTS

As there are a number of CFAs available commercially, certain characteristics of instrument performance make their adaptation to specific protein analysis more feasible. These include the following:

1) an accurate automatic pipetting device for sample and reagent delivery to transfer discs;
2) accurate temperature control of the cuvette chambers;
3) the capability to make a variable number of individual cuvette readings at variable time intervals;
4) either the capability to program the interfaced processor device to perform the desired mathematical manipulations and report formats by laboratory personnel or availability of such a program for purchase from the commercial supplier. In its absence, it will be necessary to manually calculate (or graph) resultant standard curves as well as sample data. In addition, manual (visual) detection of sample turbidity interference (sample blank requirements) and the detection of antigen excess will be required.

A limiting factor to adapting the initial specific protein assay to a CFA is the provision for technical simplicity and continued quality assurance of assay performance by the microprocessor module. It must be programmed to properly process control the assay and provide the mathematical manipulations inherent in the kinetics of the immunoprecipitin reaction. The basis for this effort can be derived from the following descriptive requirements.

ASSAY ADAPTATION REQUIREMENTS

The adaptation of an immunoprecipitin reaction to the CFA for quantification of a specific macromolecular antigen presents several problems. The problems are identical for each assay application but must be individualized to the characteristics of the specific reaction and its reagents.

Problem areas include the following:

1) antibody specificity;
2) antibody concentration;
3) quality of reference standards;
4) clarity of reagents;
5) lot-to-lot antibody variation;
6) final selection of antibody reagent dilution must provide a useful assay range, not only for clinical utility but for practical time requirements for instrumental analysis;
7) assay conditions (e.g., pH, ionic strength of buffer, need for polymer enhancement) may be individualized for optimum test performance;
8) an appropriate mathematical model must be selected, preferably programmed into the computer device used within the CFA;
9) antigen excess error detection methods must be incorporated;
10) an assessment of need for serum blank corrections must be made and implemented, preferably by use of the computer modality.

Following initial solution of these problems, antibody and reference standard constituents will require constant surveillance in order to achieve comparability of assay results over time. Antibody reagents may be highly variable between lots and require comparatively frequent reassessment of dilutional requirements.

Similarly, with the passage of time, the characteristics of the antiserum may change, most perceptibly with improper handling and storage.

With these concepts in mind, the following detailed descriptions of one method of adaptation [7] will be described. This system was employed with both the Rotochem II and IIA models of American Instrument Co. (Silver Spring, MD).

ASSAY PRINCIPLE

The assay of specific plasma (serum) proteins by CFA is based upon the formation of an insoluble immune complex resulting from a specific immunoprecipitin reaction [7]. Increasing changes in absorbance at 340 nm over assay-specific time intervals, corrected for both antibody and serum blank values, are related to antigen concentration by use of a logit-log transformation. A minimum of three standards, preferably four, covering an assay-related range of values are used, and following regression analysis unknown concentrations are calculated from the expression $Y = e^{(a + bx)}$ where $x =$ logit of unknown change in absorbance.

Reagents providing the capability of quantitation of various specific plasma proteins by centrifugal fast analyzer are not currently widely available in kit form. In many instances, the user must evaluate any commercially available antisera and standards in order to assure adequate and comparable reactivity for clinical application. In addition, *once* a commercial *reagent source* is *identified, continued surveillance* is necessary for maintenance of assay comparability from lot to lot. Generally, the employment of appropriate assay controls during the use of a specific antibody lot will serve to detect decay of the antibody reagent with specific attention to its reactivity. This method can be made sensitive to protein concentrations in the range of 2–3 mg/dL in serum. Thus protein concentrations less than those of C_4 may not be clinically reliable by this technique.

GENERALITIES REGARDING METHOD
Selection of Antibody Reagents

There are certain minimal criteria which must be met by the antibody reagent. These include the following:

1) a minimum change of 0.001 Å/mg of protein between the low and high standard concentration employed (following mathematical linearization);
2) a reflection of at least 0.05 Å by the low standard prior to the high standard reaching its peak absorbance following corrections for both sample and antibody blanks.

In addition, once assay conditions are determined with a specific lot of antibody, the peak times of absorbance using the high and middle standards of the assay are recorded for future reference in relating new antibody lots. This will help to maintain comparable assay conditions for specific protein quantitations of both controls and samples. Later comparisons with these data will allow detection of antibody quality shifts over time when assay results seem spurious.

These relationships are studied in the following way:

Commercial antisera to the specific protein to be assayed is diluted in pH 8.0 barbital buffer containing 4% polyethylene glycol-6000 (infravide). Following dilution, the antibody reagent is allowed to stand and is subsequently subjected to microfiltration.

Multiple antigen dilutions are made covering a wide range of concentration, viz., from very low to very high in approximately 20% of normal range increments. They are individually studied over a time interval of approximately ten minutes. Transfer discs are set up such that sample and barbital buffer are placed in the middle well and the antibody reagent is placed in the inner well.

The computational module is programmed to obtain the maximum number of absorbance readings over a time frame with intervals that will allow detection of peak absorbance times for each individual antigen concentration. Ideally, a program should be available which will allow the taking of approximately 30 data points beginning at a lag time of 10 seconds at intervals of 30 seconds or less.

The resultant absorbance data is plotted on linear-log graph paper (Fig. 1) as absorbance (Y-axis) vs. time in seconds (X-axis). In this way the individual curvilinear response of each antigen concentration is plotted and its peak absorbance time identified.

Once the peak absorbance time of each antigen concentration is determined, a second graph (linear/linear) is made (Fig. 2) plotting antigen concentration (Y-axis) versus peak absorbance time (X-axis). This results in a parabolic curve, the vertex of which represents the point of antigen-antibody equivalency. A concentration of approximately 20–25% less than the antigen concentration represented at the vertex is employed as a high standard and its peak time (in seconds) recorded for future reference. The low standard

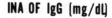

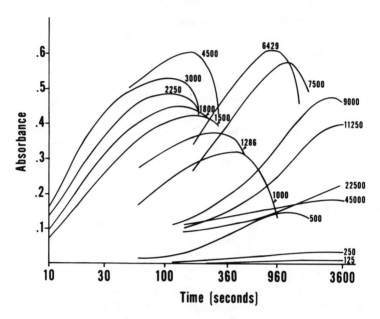

Fig. 1. The immunoprecipitin reaction occurring between antihuman IgG (goat) concentration and variable human IgG reference material at the indicated concentrations is shown above. Spectrophotometric detection at 340 nm was employed in a CFA to study induced turbidity reflected in absorbance changes over time. Note that the time of absorbance plateau (antigen-antibody equivalency) varies according to antigen concentration. Ionic strength of buffer, pH, degree of polymer enhancement, and assay volume are constant. (Used with permission [6].)

is selected at any point where a minimal deflection of 0.05 absorbance units is seen prior to the peak time obtained with the high standard chosen (when appropriately corrected).

Middle standards are chosen at an appropriate interval between the low and high standard, roughly representing either halfway between or in increments of one third if one is using three or four standards, respectively. It is preferable to use as many as six standards. Unfortunately, a greater number of standards will allow less sample throughput. The selected low and high standards should cover a range of not less than 2 standard deviations (SD) above and below the anticipated or recorded normal range for the specific protein in question.

If all the abovementioned criteria are not met, including the minimum absorbance change/mgm of protein 0.001 Å, appropriate dilution of the

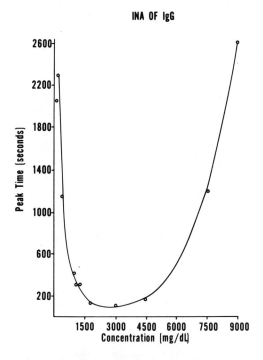

INA OF IgG

Fig. 2. The parabolic relationship of peak time (seconds) vs. antigen concentration is demonstrated above. Peak values are derived from the time of absorbance plateaus identified in Figure 1. (Used with permission [6].)

antibody to allow for shortening or delaying peak absorbance intervals must be made and the entire procedure repeated.

Once assay range at the antibody reagent dilution selected is determined and the sensitivity of the assay is deemed acceptable, aliquots of diluted standards selected may be frozen at −70°C indefinitely for use. Similarly, all stock antibody *must* be stored at −70°C to prevent early decay of antibody reactivity—preferably in aliquots appropriate for anticipated daily use.

Assay Performance

In the organizational approach to the assay of specific proteins by CFA, we have chosen to prepare polymer (polyethylene glycol-6000)-enhanced reagent within the preceding 24 hours of use. All assays are performed in a batch made using buffer and antibody blanks followed by a series of standards (three or four) and two dilutions of each sample to be assayed. Two runs

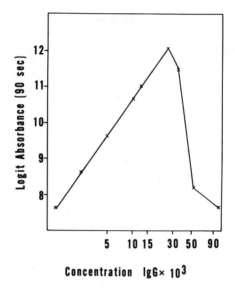

Fig. 3. A representative plot of data derived by assay of known concentrations of IgG through antigen excess. Logit-log mathematics are employed for linearization and serve to accentuate an abrupt change following the equivalency point (Used with permission [6].)

are required, one as a sample blank, using buffer in place of the antibody reagent. Following printout of absorbance data, calculations of unknown concentrations are either done manually employing a graph (logit-log) or by use of a previously programmed calculator device or by the computer module of the CFA if it is appropriately programmed.

Antigen excess is recognized by corrected absorbance values being less or greater than low or high standards, respectively. With lower absorbance readings, it may also indicate absent or low protein concentrations. By use of two dilutions and mathematical assurance that resultant assay values are appropriately proportional, one can confirm that antigen excess is not a problem with the serum being assayed (Fig. 3). We have also inspected a protein electrophoresis strip for evidence of M spikes or obvious abnormal protein content particularly when performing large panel groupings. We have used a 580 μL total volume, 80 μL of which represents a diluted sample (standard) with its attendant wash solution (nonpolymer enhanced buffer). Assay condition of pH (8.0), temperature (37°C), degree of polymer enhancement (4% PEG-6000), and ionic strength of buffer (barbital-HCl) have been essentially similar for each protein we had studied. The variables involved included the degree of sample dilution (1/10, 1/20, etc.) with non-polymer-enhanced buffer, the volume of its aliquot, the volume of wash solution (to make a total sample and wash volume of 80 μL) and the selected dilution of the antibody reagent with polymer-enhanced buffer.

SPECIFIC EXAMPLE OF METHOD DEVELOPMENT

Detailed Description of Antibody Selection

The immunoprecipitin reaction for IgG has been chosen as a model for description. Principles derived from this model can be directly applied to all other immunoprecipitin reactions differing obviously in the antigen/antibody system and the appropriate selection of antigen concentration based upon normal levels in anticipated clinical ranges.

In this example, we have obtained an anti-IgG antibody from a commercial source (Atlantic Antibodies, Inc.), said to be of nephelometric grade and derived by immunization of goats with human IgG. Standard materials from a human source was similarly obtained.

Reagents and Their Preparation

Polyethylene glycol-6000 (PEG) can be obtained from Union Carbide, New York, New York. *Non-PEG barbital buffer, pH 8.0* (2 L) can be prepared by mixing 1412 mL of 0.1 mol/L sodium barbital (20.62 g/L) with 588 mL of 0.1 mol/L hydrochloric acid. To prepare *4% PEG in pH 8.0 barbital buffer (wt/vol)* dissolve 40 g of PEG by dilution to 1 L with non-PEG pH 8.0 barbital buffer with mixing. Filter through a 0.22-μmol/L filter to remove particulate matter that may interfere with the assay. To obtain *antisera reagent* for IgG, make a 1/20 (vol/vol) dilution with 4% PEG-barbital buffer (for all other antisera, begin with a 1/10 dilution).

Allow to stand two to four hours at room temperature. Filter through a 0.22-μmol/L filter to remove precipitated immune complexes. This nonspecific turbidity will interfere with the assay. A wide range of *standard concentrations* covering clinical assay values and some degree of antigen excess are required to evaluate an antiserum for potential use.

In the case of IgG, *assuming our standard material is said to represent 2500 mg/dL,* prepare the following series of standards:

Concentration (mg/dL)	2500 mg/d standard (μL)	Barbital buffer (μL)
250	100	900
500	200	800
750	300	700
1000	400	600
1250	500	500
1500	600	400
1750	700	300
2000	800	200
2250	900	100
2500	1000	0

Note: All standards can be preserved at -70 °C indefinitely.

Aliquots of each of the above standards are diluted 1/20 (vol/vol) with non-PEG barbital buffer for study.

Higher representative concentrations to cover anticipated areas of antigen excess should also be prepared by appropriate variations in the dilution procedure.

Pipetting Station Setup

Arrange sample cups in dilutor ring in a manner which will provide for evaluation of the following:

Example

Well	Content
0	buffer blank
1	antibody blank
2–14	various standards
15	buffer blank
16	antibody blank
17–end	various standards

Set up dilutor to deliver 40 μl of sample and a 40 μl wash of non-PEG barbital buffer to the middle well of the transfer disc. Antibody reagent should be delivered to the inner well using either the pipetting station or manually in the volume of 500 μl. Note that the number of standards studied will vary in each run depending upon the maximum number of samples a transfer disc can accommodate.

Notes Regarding Transfer Discs

1) Preincubate empty transfer discs in a 37°C oven for at least ten minutes.
2) Following delivery of reagents and samples to transfer disc, again incubate the *covered* disc in a 37°C oven for ten minutes.

Process Control Settings for Computational Module

Software that provides for the printout of multiple absorbance readings per cuvette, preferably in the range of 15–30 readings, should be used. The KR-I software of American Instrument's Rotochem II or IIA provides access to a maximum of nine readings/cuvette. In order to more accurately identify the peak time of absorbance, one may be forced to use one run to localize it to a 1.5-minute time interval, followed by a second assay taking nine readings within that specific time period.

Assuming the use of the KR-I program, settings should be as follows: lag time: 4 seconds; reading interval: 20 seconds; temperature: 37°C.

This provides a study time of only 180 seconds following mixing in the centrifuge assembly. If, under these conditions, peak times are not in evidence, a subsequent run using a more delayed lag time to cover an additional 3–4 minutes of study would be appropriate for some antigen-antibody systems. Following localization of a peak time occurring within a 1.5-minute time frame, repeat the study using an appropriate lag time and nine readings, ten seconds apart to more accurately pick the peak absorbance time. This value should be assessed to ± ten seconds.

The study should obtain a printout of all absorbance readings taken from individual cuvettes for subsequent plotting.

Preparation of Graphic Plots

Correct all observations by subtracting antibody blank readings. Note that with Aminco software the buffer blank can be automatically subtracted from all cuvette readings.

On linear-log graph paper, plot corrected absorbance readings on the Y-axis (linear) and read time on the X-axis (log) in seconds. Plot data from each cuvette on the identical graph (Fig. 1), labeling concentrations represented appropriately. Draw best-fit curves correcting points such that peak absorbance times are best estimated.

On linear/linear graph paper, plot resultant peak times on the Y-axis and representative concentrations on the X-axis. This should result in a parabola (Fig. 2), the vertex of which represents the point antigen-antibody equivalency under the assay conditions of pH, ionic strength of buffer, PEG content, temperature, and sample dilutions.

Evaluation

Read the antigen concentration represented by the vertex of the parabola obtained from the second graph. Find the antigen concentration represented by subtracting 20–25% from this value.

Choose a read time that occurs *prior* to this concentration reaching its peak (Fig. 1). Find the lowest concentration that shows a reflection of at least 0.05 Å prior to this indicated peak time. These values represent the range of the assay under these conditions. Ideally they should cover 2 SD both in excess and below the anticipated normal range for the protein being assayed.

The change is absorbance represented by the chosen low and high concentration should not be less than 0.001 Å/mg of protein following mathematical linearization for all proteins *except* IgG and C_4. With IgG, values of 0.0004 Å/mg of protein (3 mg/0.001 Å) have proven adequate for clinical reliability of the assay.

With proteins other than IgG and C_4, a change of 0.01 Å represents 10 mg protein/dL. If this is not acceptable clinically for an individual protein, with low serum concentrations (e.g., C_4), minimal absorbance change must be increased to fulfill the clinical sensibility requirement (e.g., 0.003 Å, where 0.01 Å will represent 3.3 mg protein).

Procedural Alterations Following Evaluation

If the minimum criteria outlined above are not met, the following procedural alterations can be made:

1) Antibody dilution may be changed so that its concentration is increased. This provides a greater range of absorbance change per unit of time and the entire assay study repeated. It also shortens the time required to reach peak absorbance. A more dilute antibody solution will provide for the converse observations.
2) Sample size may be decreased, with appropriate increase of wash volume, and the entire study repeated. This will increase the range of assay but tend to make detection of lower concentrations less sensitive. It will also increase the time interval required to reach peak absorbance. The converse is true with increased sample size.
3) Any combination of the above. Assay pH, ionic strength of the buffer, PEG content and reaction to temperature are already optimized. Further increases in PEG content have little or no effect on changing absorbance readings.

Final Choice of Individual Assay Read Time

Allowing that the antibody reagent and standards selected meet the criteria listed above, choice of assay read time is based on an evaluation of individual data points over a period of 60 seconds prior to the peak absorbance time reached by the high standard. In most instances there is at least a 20–30-second window over which linearity of the curve and resultant assay values are acceptable.

Assay Procedures and Mathematical Evaluation

Set up the assay with a buffer blank (well 0), antibody blank (well 1), three selected standards (wells 2–4), and a series of known-valued antigen concentrations covering the range of the assay in the remainder of the well positions.

Perform a blank run using the previously determined sample size and dilution, wash volume (e.g., 40 μL of a 1/20 serum sample and 40 μL wash) in the sample well (middle) and 500 μL of non-PEG barbital buffer in the reagent well. Use a 10-second lag time and a 10-second interval to cover a 100-second time frame, if appropriate, based on the known peak absorbance time of your high standard. If it occurs later than 100 seconds, vary the lag and interval time of the immediately preceding 60-second time frame to the time of peak absorbance of the high standard.

Using a programmable calculator (or manually by use of logit-log paper) determine the concentration of your unknowns by individual data points. It is simpler to use a calculator programmed to perform a regression analysis, calculating several appropriate statistical parameters for curve analysis with subsequent calculation of the unknown. The calculator should be programmed to do the following:

1) Enter and store antibody blank absorbance.
2) Enter and store standard and sample blank absorbances.
3) Compute individual cuvette corrected-absorbance by subtracting values of both antibody and sample blanks from observed sample absorbance.
4) Compute modified logit value of each corrected absorbance by

$$L = 10 + \frac{A* 1000}{1000 - (A* 1000)}$$

where L = modified logit value and A = corrected absorbance.
5) Do a regression analysis on a curve points:
   a) Accumulate sum of $\log_e$ standard concentrations (EY) and their squares individually (EY^2).
   b) Accumulate sum of modified logit values (EX) and their squares (EX^2).
   c) Accumulate sum of product of modified logit and $\log_e$ standard concentration (EXY).
   d) Calculate intercept (I) and slope (S) by

$$I = \frac{(EY)(EX^2) - (EX)(EY)}{N(EX^2) - (EX)^2}$$

$$S = \frac{N(EXY) - (EX)(EY)}{N(EX^2) - (EX)^2}$$

   where N = number of standards employed.
   e) Calculate correlation coefficient (r) of curve by

$$r = \frac{N(EXY) - (EX)(EY)}{\{N(EX^2) - (EX^2)\}* \{N(EY^2) - (EY^2)\}}$$

For apparently acceptable linearity, r must be greater than or equal to 0.98.
   f) Calculate and store individual standard concentration (C) by appropriate value substitution in the following exponential expression:

$$C = e^{(I + SL)}$$

where L = modified logit of individual standard data point and C = calculated concentration

g) Compute standard error of the estimate of Y on X (S_{yx}) by the following equation:

$$S_{yx} = \frac{E(Y - Yest)^2}{N}$$

where Y = known standard concentration and Yest = calculated standard concentration from regression analysis.

The S_{yx} is a measure of the error potential of the regression analysis using this logit-log fit. This is similar to standard deviation in that 68% of the time values between one such band width will be on each side of the regression line; 95% within two bands when N is large. With the N values we are using, a value no greater than 10% of the actual determinate standard (high) has been accepted.

h) Calculate unknown values from equation 5f for the selected data point.

i) Do (S_{sx}) again for the known assay values, using equation S_g where Y = known concentrations and Yest = calculated concentrations. This S_{yx} value must not exceed 10% of the mean value of the known concentrations.

j) Using equation 5e calculate the coefficient of correlation where X = known values and Y = calculated values. The r value should be greater than 0.99.

k) Repeat calculations and analyses on individual read time data points until these minimal criteria are met.

Examples of our results employing one commercial grade antiserum for each of eleven serum proteins are indicated in Tables I–III.

Actual Assay Procedures

Having now selected suitable antibody and sample dilutions as well as the appropriate read times, you should be ready to assay the antigen studied and compare the results with a previous methodology.

The general setup previously outlined is followed except that the unknowns are substituted for known-valued materials in dual dilutions to provide recognition of antigen excess.

1) Prepare diluted antibody reagent (as previously determined) using 4% PEG-barbital buffer (pH 8.0). Let stand two to four hours at room temperature. Remove precipitated immune complexes by filtration through a 0.22-μmol/L Millipore™ filter.

TABLE I. Absorbance Peak Times Employed for Assay of Eleven Serum Proteins

	Middle standard		High standard	
Protein	Concentration (mg/dL)	Peak time postmix (seconds)	Concentration (mg/dL)	Peak time postmix (seconds)
C_3	138	175	206	140
C_4	25	230	49	160
IgG	1125	130	2045	180
IgA	287	235	390	140
IgM	150	290	240	180
α_1-Antitrypsin	287	145	430	120
α_2-Macroglobulin	254	200	436	120
Transferrin	308	200	463	90
Haptoglobin	120	130	200	95
Orosomucoid	106	450	159	340
Low-density Lipoprotein	116	370	193	280

TABLE II. Sample Procedural Requirements for Assay of Eleven Serum Proteins

Protein	Sample dilution in buffer	AB dilution in buffer	Sample size (μL)	Wash size (μL)	Read time (s)	Standard concentrations (mg/dL)	Absorbance change/mg of protein
C_3	1:5	1:10	40	40	30	206/138/69	0.001
C_4	1:2	1:10	40	40	30	49/25/10	0.001
IgG	1:20	1:20	20	60	90	2045/1125/281	0.003
IgA	1:10	1:10	40	40	100	390/287/72	0.001
IgM	1:5	1:10	50	30	60	240/150/50	0.001
α_1-Antitrypsin	1:10	1:10	40	40	130	430/287/143	0.001
α_2-Macroglobulin	1:5	1:10	40	40	50	436/254/109	0.001
Transferrin	1:5	1:10	40	40	50	436/308/154	0.002
Haptoglobin	1:10	1:10	40	40	30	200/120/30	0.003
Orosomucoid	1:10	1:10	40	40	130	159/106/32	0.002
Low-density Lipoprotein	1:10	1:10	50	30	80	193/116/41	0.002

These requirements pertain to an Aminco Rotochem II centrifugal fast analyzer. All antibody reagents are prepared by dilution with pH 8.0 barbital buffer containing 4% PEG. All samples are diluted in pH 8.0 barbital buffer without PEG. Standard concentrations and absorbance change per mg of protein/dL are expressed in light of current log numbers of antibody. Volume of diluted antibody solution used for all studied = 500 μL.

TABLE III. Comparative Data for Eleven Specific Plasma Proteins Assayed by the Described Immunoturbidimetric Technique

Protein	Normal[a] range (mg/dL)	Comparison method[b]	Intercept (a)	Slope (b)	Correlation coefficient (r)	Coefficient of variations[c] (%)
C_3	80–168	A	15.2	0.93	0.90	6.6
C_4	14–38	A	3.0	1.01	0.91	7.2
IgG	708–1648	R	−85.2	1.04	0.98	4.6
IgA	138–350	R	−26.5	1.06	0.97	6.9
IgM	42–210	R	−2.2	0.98	0.96	7.4
α_1-Antitrypsin	160–325	R	13.1	0.93	0.97	6.8
α_2-Macroglobulin	109–324	R	16.1	0.99	0.96	8.1
Transferrin	205–361	R	−41.6	1.09	0.95	5.5
Haptoglobin	30–174	R	0.7	1.06	0.95	7.1
Orosomucoid	21–101	R	−3.0	1.04	0.92	8.0
Low-density lipoprotein	82–210	R	2.0	0.90	0.89	6.8

[a]Normal ranges were calculated (mean ± 2 SD) following assay of 30 fasting sera (15 each, male and female, adult) with completely normal SMA-12 screening tests.

[b]A = automated immunoprecipitin test; R = radial immunodiffusion.

[c]Coefficient of variations was obtained by assay of 30 replicate samples over a ten-day working period.

2) Prepare and filter through 0.22-μmol/L Millipore™ filter the appropriate standards.
3) Preincubate two transfer discs at 37 °C for ten minutes.
4) Set up pipetting station to deliver the selected sample size and wash to middle well of transfer disc (total volume, 80 μL). Set up reagent pump to deliver 500 μL to inner well.
5) Prime both pumps using non-PEG pH 8.0 barbital buffer.
6) Set up transfer ring with sample cups containing:

Example

Well	Contents
0	antibody blank
1	low standard
2	middle standard
3	high standard
4	human control valued material
5	sample 1, regular dilution
6	sample 1, one-half of regular dilution
7	sample 2, regular dilution
8	sample 2, one-half regular dilution
9–end	repeat in indicated pairs

7) Load transfer discs for blank run using non-PEG barbital buffer in reagent pump. Note that this buffer is used to fill *all* inner wells.
8) Incubate loaded, covered transfer disc in 37°C oven for ten minutes.
9) Using five-second lag time and five-second interval, print out absorbance and store for later use.
10) Load second transfer disc with 500 μL of antibody reagent in all inner wells.
11) Incubate covered, loaded transfer disc in 37°C oven for ten minutes.
12) Run assay using appropriate lag and interval times as previously determined. Print out absorbances. It is advisable to select for printout three or four data points both before and after the selected read time such that, if desired, the actual reaction can be later studied.
13) Using the logit transformation, regression, and correlation formulas indicated earlier, calculate I, S, and r. The r value must be 0.98 or greater. These values are obtained by using the appropriate data point observation corrected both for antibody and its sample blocks.
14) Compute the value of the unknowns according to equation 5f. Note: If the second sample, multiplied by two (example uses a one half dilution), results in comparable quantitation value indicated by first sample, there is no evidence of antigen excess and the result of the first sample is used for reporting purposes. With discrepancy, additional dilutions must be run until this criterion is met and the final result is appropriately corrected for dilution and repeated.

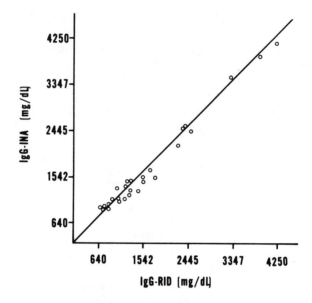

Fig. 4.   Representative scattergram of comparison data for IgG (CFA vs. RID). (Used with permission [6].)

Replicate analysis of control materials have shown coefficients of variation less than 10% in our hands for proteins studied. A sample scattergram of our results versus a commercial radioimmunodiffusion (RID) procedure is indicated in Figure 4.

Notes on Antigen Excess Detection

By proper selection of the high standard concentration, n_3, 20–25% below the value obtained at the vertex of the peak time versus absorbance graph (Fig. 2), most pathophysiologic states of antigen excess can be detected. Absorbance values above that obtained with the higher standard are indicative of this phenomenon. This is graphically shown in Figure 4. Note that assuming a 2500 mg/dL high standard is employed, IgG concentrations as high as approximately 4000 mg/dL will be excluded. Figure 4 also indicates the problem with higher levels of concentration, thus necessitating the use of at least two sample dilutions to provide reasonable assurance that a condition of antigen excess is not present.

SUMMARY

Details of the evolution of an immunoturbidimetric method for specific protein quantitation on a CFA have been presented. Most clinical laboratories will find this approach a difficult one that requires constant surveillance in all its parameters. Commercial manufacturers of antisera and reference materials may supply application sheets for various protein analytes in which these reagent evaluation efforts have already been accomplished for specific CFAs. The reader should maintain a constant awareness of the evolution of other semi- or fully automated instruments which have been specifically developed for immunonephelometric analysis to include commercially available kits for a more basic laboratory application.

REFERENCES

1. Alper CA: Automated nephelometric determination of haptoglobin, C3, and α_1-antitrypsin. In Barton CE et al. (eds): "Advances in Automated Analysis, Technicon International Congress 1970." Miami: Thurman Associates, 1971.
2. Anderson NG: Analytical techniques for cell fractions. XII. A multiple-cuvet rotor for a new microanalytical system. Anal Biochem 28:545, 1969.
3. Buffone GJ, Savory J, Cross RE: Use of a laser modified centrifugal analyzer for kinetic measurement of serum IgG. Clin Chem 20:1320, 1974.
4. Cross RE: "Centrifugal Fast Analyzers. Technical Improvement Service, No. 25." Chicago: American Society of Clinical Pathologists, 1976.
5. Deaton CD, Maxwell KW, Mith RS, Creveling RC: Use of laser nephelometry in the measurement of serum proteins. Clin Chem 22:1465, 1976.
6. Dito WR: Rapid immunonephelometric quantitation of eleven serum proteins by centrifugal fast analyzer. Am J Clin Pathol 71:301, 1979.
7. Goldberg RJ, Campbell DH: The light scattering properties of an antigen-antibody reaction. J Immunol 66:79, 1951.
8. Killingsworth LM, Buffone GJ, Sonaware MB, Lundsford GC: Optimizing nephelometric measurement of specific serum proteins: Evaluation of three diluents. Clin Chem 20:1548, 1974.
9. Killingsworth LM, Savory J: Nephelometric studies of the precipitin reaction: A model system for specific protein measurements. Clin Chem 19:403, 1973.
10. Killingsworth LM, Savory J: Automated immunochemical procedures for measurement of immunoglobulins IgG, IgA and IgM in human serum. Clin Chem 17:936, 1971.
11. Mancini G, Vaerman JP, Carbonara AO, Heremans J: A single radial diffusion method for immunological qantitation of proteins. Protides Biol Fluids 11:370, 1963.
12. Ritchie RF, Alper CA, Graves J, Pearson N, Larson C: Automated quantitation of serum proteins in serum and other biological fluids. Am J Clin Pathol 59:151, 1973.
13. Sternberg JC: A rate nephelometer for measuring specific proteins by immunoprecipitin reactions. Clin Chem 23:1456, 1977.

Physiology of Immunoglobulins: Diagnostic and
Clinical Aspects, pages 139-156
© 1982 Alan R. Liss, Inc., 150 Fifth Avenue, New York, NY 10011

7

Quantitation of Normal and Abnormal Serum Immunoglobulins G, A, and M by Radial Immunodiffusion, Nephelometry, and Turbidimetry

Stephan E. Ritzmann, MD, James J. Aguanno, PhD, Melodie A. Finney,
MEd, and R. Condon Hughes III, MD

INTRODUCTION

The introduction of radial immunodiffusion (RID) in 1965 [1,2] has rendered the quantitation of serum proteins practical and economical in the routine clinical laboratory. Its application to the assays of normal and abnormal immunoglobulins G, A, and M has aided in the laboratory diagnosis and monitoring of numerous disorders [3–5]. Previously, we have documented [6] differences in values for M-proteins as measured by RID, electroimmunodiffusion (EID) [7,8], and cellulose acetate serum protein electrophoresis (SPE) [9]. There exist unpredictable and marked intermethod and interlaboratory discrepancies of results obtained by these various methods. These differences were not attributable to specimen preparation, immunoglobulin (Ig) classes or types, or electrophoretic mobility [3,6]. It was postulated that subclass differences, polymerization states, and antibody properties could, in large measure, account for these discrepancies [3,6]. It was concluded that SPE provides an objective technique and is the preferred technique for the quantitation of M-proteins. The use of RID, however, was considered to yield relative values of M-proteins that, if used consistently in a given patient, could still provide reliable, clinically relevant information.

Recently, newer automated immunoassay techniques have been introduced which may potentially replace previously used methods [13–15,17–19]. Their application in the clinical laboratory requires baseline information regarding possible interassay deviations, methodological correlation of results, and clinical reliance.

EVALUATION OF NORMAL AND ABNORMAL SERUM IgG, IgA, AND IgM BY RADIAL IMMUNODIFFUSION, NEPHELOMETRY, AND TURBIDIMETRY

Normal control serum samples (n = 213) from local volunteer blood donors were selected after they were shown by SPE (Helena), immunoelectrophoresis (IEP), and Ouchterlony technique (OT) to contain no M-proteins. They included 149 male and 64 female donors, aged 18–65 years. The majority (91%) were Caucasian, with 3% Hispanic and 6% Black comprising the remainder. These normal specimens were assayed for IgG, IgA, and IgM by endpoint RID (Kallestad), rate nephelometry (Beckman ICS II) [10] and endpoint turbidimetry (duPont ACA) [11]. Each technique was performed according to the manufacturer's instructions.

Additionally, serum samples were identified by SPE, IEP, and OT from patients with hypo-γ-globulinemia (< 0.8 g/dL γ-globulin concentration), normal γ-globulins, polyclonal hyper-γ-globulinemia (> 1.6 g/dL γ-globulin), and monoclonal IgG, IgA, or IgM M-proteins. Each of these specimens was analyzed for all three immunoglobulins G, A, *and* M, by RID, ICS and ACA; whereas the monoclonal sera were quantitated only for their M-proteins (i.e., IgG, IgA, *or* IgM) by SPE, RID, ICS and ACA.

Normal Values in Adults

The normal values in adults for serum IgG, IgA, and IgM, as obtained by the ACA, ICS, and RID are presented in Table I, and the distribution ranges are shown in Figure 1. The results show method-dependent normal ranges for IgG, IgA, and IgM. Similar observations have been made by Dito et al. [18].

TABLE I. Normal Adult Values for Serum IgG, IgA, and IgM, as Obtained by Radial Immunodiffusion (RID), Kinetic Nephelometry (ICS), and Endpoint Turbidimetry (ACA)

	IgG (mg/dL)		IgA (mg/dL)		IgM (mg/dL)	
	Median	Range	Median	Range	Median	Range
ACA	911	568–1483	202	57–414	111	20–274
ICS	997	606–1570	196	65–405	126	53–276
RID	1145	750–1880	192	65–407	122	30–252

The results, based on 213 serum samples and expressed in mg/dL, are shown as median and 95th percentile ranges.

Hypo-γ-Globulinemia and Polyclonal Gammopathy

The three assay methods (RID, ICS, and ACA) provide comparable results for IgG, IgA, and IgM in the normal, hypo-γ-globulinemic, and increased ranges of polyclonal gammopathies [3,9] (Fig. 2a,b—IgG; 3a,b—IgA; 4a,b—IgM).

Normal Values in Children

Normal IgG, IgA, and IgM (and C3 and C4) values have recently been established by Jolliff et al. [12] for pediatric (and adult) age ranges (Table II) using the ICS assay method. Dito et al. [18] have reported adult male reference values for IgG, IgA, and IgM by RID, centrifugal fast analyzer,[1] and a kinetic laser nephelometer. There exist slight variations of these results with those presented in Table I and Figures 1a–c; however, such deviations are expected in the various laboratories, necessitating the establishment of normal values in each laboratory [18].

Monoclonal Gammopathies

Quantitative results of IgG, IgA, and IgM M-proteins by RID, ICS, and ACA are shown in Table III and the inserts of Figures 2a,b; 3a,b; and 4a,b. These *statistical summary data* show an excellent correlation with the possible exception of SPE versus RID for IgM patients. The accuracy varies considerably for the various parameters with the ACA showing the best overall accuracy for IgG, IgA, and IgM, followed by RID and ICS (Figs. 5a,b,c; 6a,b,c; 7a,b,c). Such summary data, however, may be misleading since marked variations of correlative data may occur in *individual patients*. Consequently, the results from individual patients with IgG, IgA, and IgM M-proteins, obtained with the various assay techniques, were correlated (Figs. 8a,b,c). These data demonstrate in individual patients either a straight-line relationship between M-protein values obtained by SPE, RID, ICS, and ACA, or, more frequently, a moderate to marked variation towards increased or decreased levels.

IgG M-proteins. In the case of *IgG monoclonal gammopathies* (Fig. 8a), RID often yields slightly higher values than does SPE, while nephelometry produces distinctly higher levels especially in the higher concentration ranges. This differences may relate to different diffusion characteristics among IgG subclasses in the agar gel of RID and to differences in the concentrations of IgG subclasses. RID plates for the quantitation of IgG should contain antibodies to all four subclasses, reflecting their approximate normal relative

---

[1]*Ed. note:* See also Chapter 6.

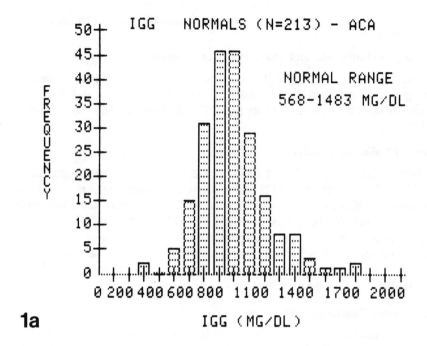

1a

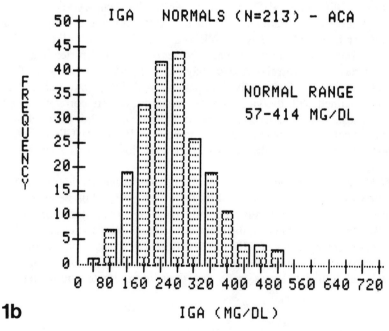

1b

Fig. 1.   Histograms for normal levels of IgG (a), IgA (b), and IgM (c) obtained by endpoint turbidimetry (ACA).

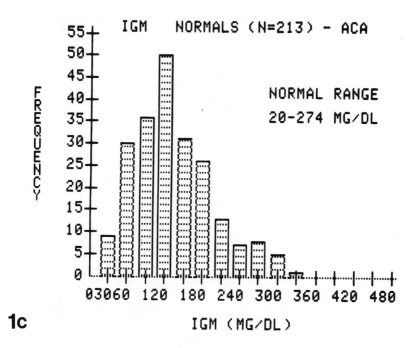

1c

concentrations of $IgG_{1,2,3,4}$ (i.e., 70%, 20%, 6%, and 4%, respectively). In a patient with an IgG_4 M-protein, for example, RID quantitation may lead to selective overutilization of the antibody moiety to its subclass (i.e., anti-IgG_4), resulting in greater immunodiffusion distances, increased precipitin rings and, consequently, spuriously high values. Unfortunately, commercially available antisera are not required to be tested for IgG_{1-4} subclass activity although they may be recommended by manufacturers for the quantitation of M-proteins that may be of any IgG subclass. The disporportionate correlation of SPE and nephelometry data may be explained by a similar overutilization of specific antibody moieties by high concentrations of respective M-proteins, when analyzed by nephelometry. Distorting effects of antibody affinity to these immunoglobulins must also be considered in this context. Results have been obtained with a turbidimetric technique adapted to the duPont ACA that are comparable to SPE-derived data in the lower and middle concentration ranges, but also are somewhat higher at elevated IgG M-protein levels.

IgA M-proteins. In *IgA monoclonal gammopathies* (Fig. 8b), the RID results may vary somewhat from those obtained by SPE. Spuriously low results are probably due to the presence of high molecular-weight IgA polymers,[2] while higher values may be due to antiserum overutilization and/or absolute relative subclass deficiency of antisera for IgA_1 and IgA_2 moieties.

---

[2]*Ed. note:* See also Ritzmann and Nakamura in Ritzmann and Daniels (eds.): "Serum Protein Abnormalities, Diagnostic and Clinical Aspects" [20].

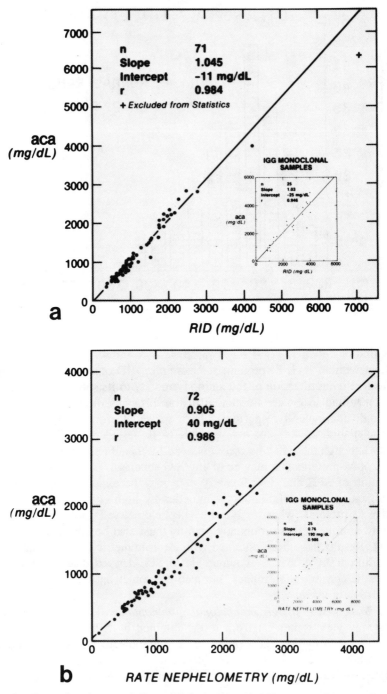

Fig. 2. Comparison between IgG results obtained by (a) RID versus ACA (n = 71), and (b) ICS versus ACA (n = 72) for the hypo-γ-globulinemic, normal, and polyclonal gammopathy ranges. The insert represents the correlation for IgG M-proteins (n = 25 for RID and ICS comparisons).

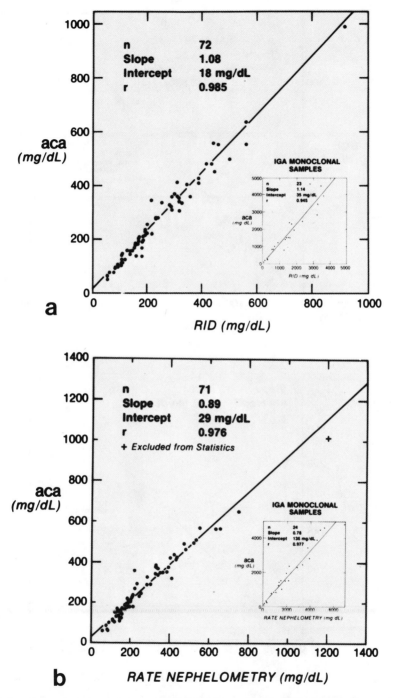

Fig. 3. Comparison between IgA results obtained by (a) RID versus ACA (n = 72), and (b) ICS versus ACA (n = 71) for the hypo-γ-globulinemic, normal, and polyclonal gammopathy ranges. The insert represents the correlation for IgA M-proteins (n = 23 for RID, n = 24 for ICS comparisons).

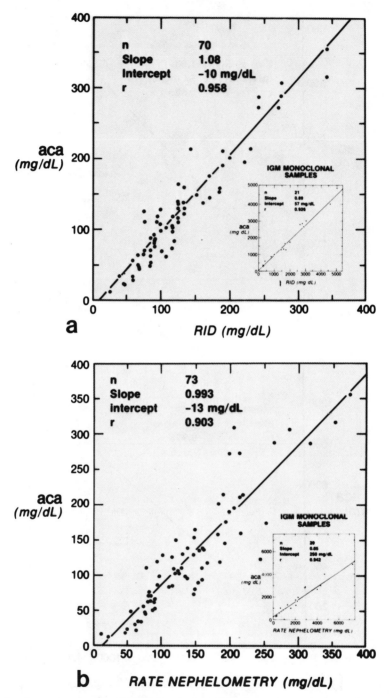

Fig. 4. Comparison between IgM results obtained by (a) RID versus ACA (n = 70) and (b) ICS versus ACA (n = 73) for the hypo-γ-globulinemic, normal, and polyclonal gammopathy ranges. The insert represents the correlation for IgM M-proteins (n = 21 for RID, n = 20 for ICS comparisons).

TABLE II. Mean and 95th Percentile Ranges for IgG, IgA, and IgM (Together With C3 and C4) in Relation to Age by the ICS Assay

	n	IgG Mean g/L	IgG 95% range g/L	IgA Mean g/L	IgA 95% range g/L	IgM Mean g/L	IgM 95% range g/L	C3 Mean g/L	C3 95% range g/L	C4 Mean g/L	C4 95% range g/L
Cord blood	50	11.21	6.36–16.06	0.023	0.014–0.036	0.13	0.063–0.25	0.83	0.57–1.16	0.13	0.066–0.23
1 month	50	5.03	2.51–9.06	0.13	0.013–0.53	0.45	0.20–0.87	0.83	0.53–1.24	0.14	0.070–0.25
2 months	50	3.65	2.06–6.01	0.15	0.028–0.47	0.46	0.17–1.05	0.96	0.59–1.49	0.15	0.074–0.28
3 months	50	3.34	1.76–5.81	0.17	0.046–0.46	0.49	0.24–0.89	0.94	0.64–1.31	0.16	0.087–0.27
4 months	50	3.43	1.96–5.58	0.23	0.044–0.73	0.55	0.27–1.01	1.07	0.62–1.75	0.19	0.083–0.38
5 months	50	4.03	1.72–8.14	0.31	0.081–0.84	0.62	0.33–1.08	1.07	0.64–1.67	0.18	0.071–0.36
6 months	50	4.07	2.15–7.04	0.25	0.081–0.68	0.62	0.35–1.02	1.15	0.74–1.71	0.21	0.086–0.42
7–9 months	50	4.75	2.17–9.04	0.36	0.11–0.90	0.80	0.34–1.26[a]	1.13	0.75–1.66	0.20	0.095–0.37
10–12 months	50	5.94	2.94–10.69	0.40	0.16–0.84	0.82	0.41–1.49	1.26	0.73–1.80[a]	0.22	0.12–0.39
1 year	50	6.79	3.45–12.13	0.44	0.14–1.06	0.93	0.43–1.73	1.29	0.84–1.74[a]	0.23	0.12–0.40
2 years	50	6.85	4.24–10.51	0.47	0.14–1.23	0.95	0.48–1.68	1.20	0.81–1.70	0.19	0.092–0.34
3 years	50	7.28	4.41–11.35	0.66	0.22–1.59	1.04	0.47–2.00	1.17	0.77–1.71	0.20	0.097–0.36
4–5 years	50	7.80	4.63–12.36	0.68	0.25–1.54	0.99	0.43–1.96	1.21	0.86–1.66	0.21	0.13–0.32
6–8 years	50	9.15	6.33–12.80	0.90	0.33–2.02	1.07	0.48–2.07	1.18	0.88–1.55	0.20	0.12–0.32
9–10 years	50	10.07	6.08–15.72	1.13	0.45–2.36	1.21	0.52–2.42	1.34	0.89–1.95	0.22	0.10–0.40
Adult	120	9.94	6.39–13.49	1.71	0.70–3.12	1.56	0.56–3.52	1.25	0.83–1.77	0.28	0.15–0.45

The data, expressed in g/L, were obtained from 870 normal individuals (by permission [12])

[a]All ranges based on a log transformation of the data to eliminate skewness except ranges indicated, which were distributed in a gaussian fashion.

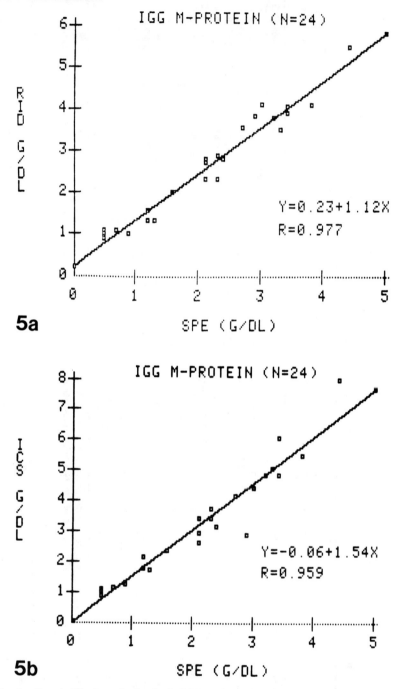

Fig. 5. Correlation of results for the IgG M-products (n = 24) between SPE and (a) RID, (b) ICS, and (c) ACA.

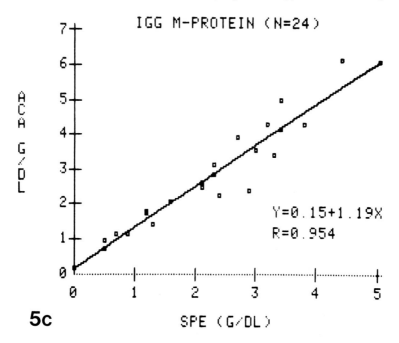

5c

IgM M-proteins. Conversely, in certain sera of *IgM monoclonal gammopathies* (Fig. 8c), the higher RID, ACA, and particularly, the nephelometric values may be due to the presence of low molecular-weight IgM-monomers or other poorly defined parameters. The distorting effects of high molecular-weight IgM polymers, including certain rheumatoid factors and other circulating immune complexes, also require consideration.

These foregoing observations and considerations reinforce the fact that antisera used for quantitation of immunoglobulins in general, and M-proteins in particular, must contain appropriate antibody specificity, potency, affinity, avidity,[3] and activity to the subclasses of IgG and IgA, and possibly IgM. In this context it should be noted that the use of monoclonal antibodies for the quantitation of IgG in normal serum and IgG-subclass M-proteins, can seriously underestimate their true concentration [21].

---

[3]*Ed. note: Avidity* in this context is defined [16] both in terms of *intrinsic affinity* instead of avidity (i.e., average association constant on molecular interaction between a single antibody combining site and a single antigenic determinant at equilibrium), and *functional affinity* in lieu of avidity (i.e., average association constant of molecular interaction between a divalent antibody molecule and an antigen possessing a number of combining sites, including all nonspecific interactions).

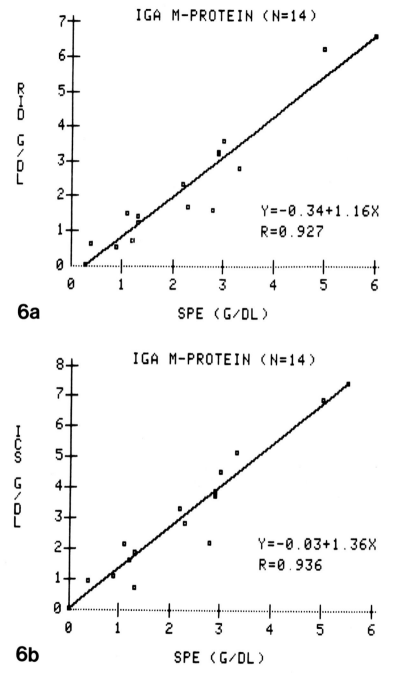

Fig. 6.   Correlation of results for IgA M-proteins (n = 14) between SPE and (a) RID, (b) ICS, and (c) ACA.

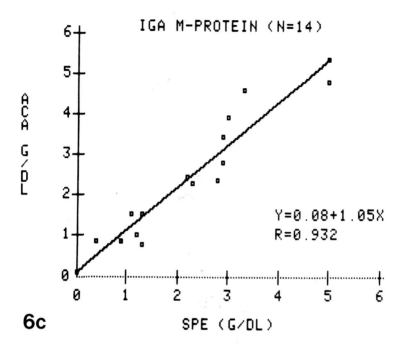

6c

TABLE III. Comparison of M-Protein Concentrations by Radial Immunodiffusion (RID), Kinetic Nonlaser Nephelometry (ICS), and Endpoint Turbidimetry (ACA), With Cellulose Acetate Electrophoresis (SPE) as the Reference Method

	RID			ICS			ACA		
	IgG	IgA	IgM	IgG	IgA	IgM	IgG	IgA	IgM
Slope	1.12	1.16	1.20	1.54	1.36	2.61	1.19	1.05	1.41
Intercept (g/dL)	0.23	−0.34	0.40	−0.06	−0.03	−1.27	0.15	0.08	−0.16
r	0.977	0.927	0.793	0.959	0.936	0.951	0.954	0.932	0.922

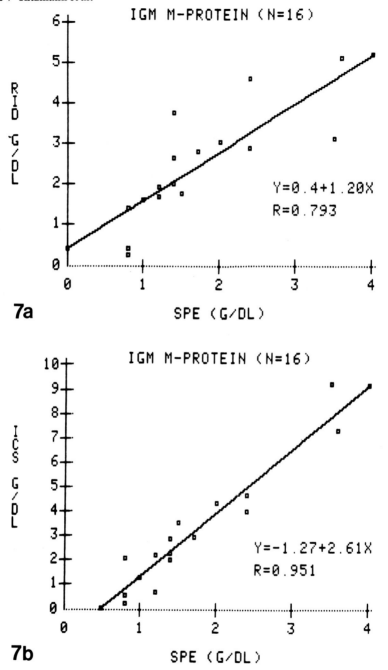

Fig. 7.   Correlation of results for IgM M-proteins (n = 16) between SPE and (a) RID, (b) ICS, and (c) ACA.

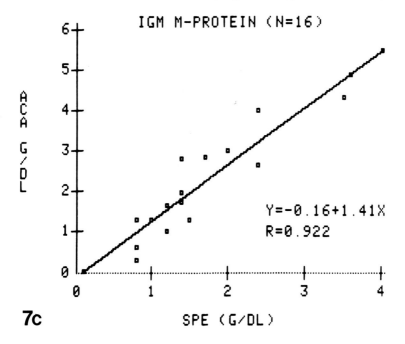

IGM M-PROTEIN (N=16)

$Y=-0.16+1.41X$

$R=0.922$

7c SPE (G/DL)

Reproducibility

Within-run and run-to-run variations are presented in Table IV. The coefficients of variations (CV%) for the within-run determinations on both normal and abnormal (monoclonal) specimens were all within the clinically useful range (with the possible exception of abnormal IgM by RID). The ACA showed the best overall within-run precision for both normal and abnormal samples. The run-to-run precision data yielded similar results with RID showing the poorest overall results with the ACA having the lowest CV values.

CONCLUSION

Normal values of IgG, A and M in adults vary somewhat according to the immunoassay techniques applied. The various RID, nephelometric, and turbidimetric methods are applicable to normal, decreased, and polyclonally increased IgG, IgA, and IgM values, although the results obtained differ somewhat between these techniques. For the quantitation of M-proteins of the IgG, IgA, and IgM classes, which are notoriously difficult to quantitate, these immunochemical methods frequently yield data that are divergent from those obtained by SPE. Because of the clinical significance of M-protein levels and the frequent need for their serial assays, a single method should be selected for quantitative monitoring in a given patient. *It appears that*

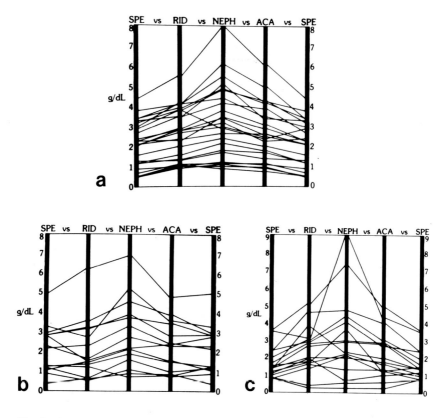

Fig. 8. Methodological correlation of M-protein concentration of (a) IgG, (b) IgA, and (c) IgM by SPE, RID, rate nephelometry, and endpoint turbidimetry. Monoclonal serum samples were analyzed by radial immunodiffusion (RID), rate nonlaser nephelometry (NEPH), and endpoint turbidimetry (ACA), with integration of the cellulose acetate protein electrophoretic "spike" (SPE) as the reference technique. Results for each sample are indicated by the connecting lines (Reproduced with permission: Ritzmann SE, Aguanno JJ: "Immunoglobulins in Health and Disease," duPont de Nemours, 1981.)

SPE offers a reliable means of absolute M-protein quantitation in patients with definite M-proteins. However, techniques such as nephelometry and turbidimetry (especially when automated) are viable alternatives to SPE. They possess the additional advantage of being less technically demanding and more rapid than SPE or RID. These assays, if used consistently for a given patient, will reflect the actual, albeit "relative" changes of M-protein levels resulting from either disease progression or therapeutic response.

TABLE IV. Within-Run and Run-to-Run Precision Data Obtained for Normal and Abnormal Sera With SPE, RID, Nephelometry, and Turbidimetry

	Normal (CV%)			Abnormal (CV%)		
	IgG	IgA	IgM	IgG	IgA	IgM
WITHIN-RUN PRECISION						
Radial immunodiffusion (RID) [17]	4.0	3.7	5.1	9.0	8.1	10.3
Nephelometry						
Endpoint						
Calbiochem–Behring [17]	4.0	3.0	4.1	4.5	3.8	4.0
Hyland [17]	2.5	2.5	5.0	4.7	3.5	4.2
Kinetic						
Beckman ICS [17]	2.8	3.0	3.6	3.3	3.7	3.0
Centrifugal fast analyzer[a]						
duPont ACA [11]	2.5	2.4	2.0	1.6	1.1	0.5
RUN-TO-RUN PRECISION						
Radial immunodiffusion (RID) [17]	9.0	7.1	12.0			
Nephelometry						
Endpoint						
Calbiochem–Behring [17]	7.1	8.4	7.1			
Hyland [17]	6.5	7.1	7.5			
Kinetic						
Beckman ICS [17]	2.9	3.1	3.7			
Centrifugal fast analyzer[a]	4.6	6.9	7.4			
duPont ACA [11]	3.0	1.4	2.6			

[a]From Chapter 6.

REFERENCES

1. Fahey JL, McKelvey E: Quantitative determination of serum immunoglobulins in antibody–agar plates. J Immunol 94:84, 1965.
2. Mancini B, Carbonara AO, Heremans JF: Immunochemical quantitation of antigens by single radial immunodiffusion. Immunochemistry 2:235, 1965.
3. Ritzmann SE: Radial immunodiffusion–revisited. ASCP Lab Med Vol. 9, Part 1, 7:23–33; Part 2, 8:27–40, 1978.
4. Fudenberg HH, Stites DP, Caldwell JL, Wells JV (eds): "Basic and Clinical Immunology," 3rd ed. Los Altos, CA: Lange Medical Publications, 1980, 782 pp.
5. Roitt IM: "Essential Immunology," 3rd ed. London: Blackwell, 1977, 324 pp.
6. Daniels JC, Vyvial TM, Levin WC, Ritzmann SE: Methodological differences in values for M-proteins in serum as measured by three techniques. Clin Chem 21:243–248, 1975.
7. Laurell CB: Quantitative estimation of proteins by electrophoresis in agarose gel containing antibodies. Anal Biochem 15:45, 1966.

8. Merrill DA, Hartley TF, Claman HN: Electroimmunodiffusion (EID). A simple rapid method for quantitation of immunoglobulins. J Lab Clin Med 69:151, 1967.
9. Ritzmann SE, Daniels JC (eds): "Serum Protein Abnormalities, Diagnostic and Clinical Aspects," 2nd printing. New York: Alan R. Liss, Inc., 1982, 550 pp.
10. Sternberg J: A rate nephelometer for measuring specific proteins by immunoprecipitin reactions. Clin Chem 23:1456–1464, 1977.
11. Ritzmann SE, Aguanno JJ, Ash KO, Wenk RE: An evaluation of the immunoglobulin G, A, and M Methods and calibrators for the duPont ACA. Wilmington: duPont de Nemours, 1981.
12. Jolliff CR, Cost KM, Stivrins PC, et al: Reference intervals for serum IgG, IgA, IgM, C3 and C4 as determined by rate nephelometry. Clin Chem 28:126–128, 1982.
13. Ritchie RF: "Automated Immunoanalysis." New York: Marcel Dekker, 1978, Part 1, pp 1–333; Part 2, pp 335–620.
14. Nakamura RM, Dito WR, Tucker ES III (eds): "Immunoassays in the Clinical Laboratory." New York: Alan R. Liss, Inc., 1979, 366 pp.
15. Nakamura RM, Dito WR, Tucker ES III (eds): "Immunoassays. Clinical Laboratory Techniques for the 1980's." New York: Alan R. Liss, 1980, 464 pp.
16. Hornick CL, Karush F: Antibody affinity. III. The role of multivalence. Immunochemistry 9:325, 1972.
17. Cloppet H, Francina A, Coquelin H, et al: Laser nephelometry and radial immunodiffusion compared for immunoglobulin quantification in pathological sera. Clin Chem 28:180–182, 1982.
18. Dito WR, Tucker ES III, Nakamura RM: Comparative evaluation of an automated kinetic laser nephelometer with other immunoprecipitin technics for the assay of serum immunoglobulins. Amer J Clin Pathol 76:753–759, 1981.
19. Virella G, Fudenberg HH: Comparison of immunoglobulin determination in pathological sera by radial immunodiffusion and laser nephelometry. Clin Chem 23:1925–1928, 1977.
20. Ritzmann SE, Nakamura RM: Analytical Centrifugation. In Ritzmann SE, Daniels JC (eds): "Serum Protein Abnormalities, Diagnostic and Clinical Aspects," 2nd printing. New York: Alan R. Liss, Inc., 1982, pp 107–120.
21. Devarill I, Jefferis R, Ling NR, Reeves WG: Monoclonal antibodies to human IgG: Reaction characteristics in the centrifugal analyzer. Clin Chem 27:2044–2047, 1981.

DIAGNOSTIC METHODOLOGY AND INTERPRETATION

Interpretation of Serum Protein Values

Physiology of Immunoglobulins: Diagnostic and
Clinical Aspects, pages 159–190
© 1982 Alan R. Liss, Inc., 150 Fifth Avenue, New York, NY 10011

8

Interpretation of Serum Protein Values

Robert F. Ritchie, MD, with the assistance of Dwight E. Smith, Wilfred
P. Turgeon, and Glenn Palomaki

INTRODUCTION

Numerical values remain only data with little useful dimension until they
are given relevance through interpretation. Data then becomes information.
Unfortunately, labortory science, for the most part, produces data and not
information. The reason is easily understood, but it is deplorable nevertheless.
The programs required to place a single laboratory result into proper clinical
perspective requires that at a minimum, the knowledge of values to be expected for a series of age- and sex-matched "normal" individuals must be
firmly established. Once a value has been found to be abnormal, a search
for clinical and laboratory conditions that may produce the affect can be
made. Both steps are arduous, expensive, and, to many investigators and
laboratory personnel, boring as well.

Laboratories too often slavishly embrace the limited information supplied
by manufacturers in the package insert, a generally incomplete and vague
document whose primary purpose is to satisfy the federal bureaucracy. The
laboratory looks to the manufacturer for the key—the Rosetta Stone—in-
forming them of what the value means for their patients. What most laboratories fail to recognize is that each laboratory serves a unique population
and must establish its own patient experience before releasing a test to their
communities. Manufacturers data, while not completely without value, represent a minimal effort to validate the kit for regulatory reasons. The task is
not a simple one to be sure. The laboratory feels the manufacturer is responsible and so does the government. Professional societies feel that the

laboratory shares in the responsibility. Federal, professional, and health-oriented granting agencies have little interest in supporting such mundane and expensive studies even though the very foundation of laboratory science depends upon them. The result of this fingerpointing is obvious. Information about the clinical relevance of the millions of even commonplace laboratory tests performed each day is scanty, and what there is exists scattered through hundreds of publications. This chapter, while focusing upon serum proteins, attempts to explain a mechanism by which any form of laboratory data can be converted to clinically useful information in a precise and repeatable manner by a process involving only modestly intricate computer programs; that is to say algorithms. In addition, some data will be included, presented in a variety of formats, that allow the observers to judge where, in a given population, significant new information lies hidden from conventional statistical analysis.

METHODS AND MATERIALS

Serum protein values that form the data base used in this chapter were analyzed in a modified Technicon AIP system [6,7]. Raw analogue data were transferred directly to a dedicated PDP-8 computer for data reduction [9], temporary storage, statistics, and final electronic transfer to a central system, a PDP-11/40 (Digital Equipment Corp. (DEC), Maynard, MA). Testing was performed employing nephelometric grade monospecific antisera from Atlantic Antibodies, Scarborough, ME.

Serum samples were received from a variety of sources in the Eastern United States with a majority originating in the state of Maine. They were analyzed on the day following receipt, with interim storage at 4°C. Demographic information obtained from the sample was entered directly into a DEC PDP-11/40. Immediate retrival for all specimen data since 1975 was possible with the total number of records exceeding 135,000 (as of July 1981). Data from individuals with serum levels of monoclonal immunoglobulins exceeding 2 g/L were excluded from this study.

Data on patients were extracted from the master file and transferred to a DEC PDP-11/34 for statistical analysis under the BMDP statistical package obtained from UCLA [1]. All programs for graphic display and analysis were developed by the FBR computer staff and produced on a Calcomp 565 plotter (California Computer Products, Inc., Anaheim, CA or a Hewlett–Packard (HP) 2648A/HP2631G video terminal (Hewett–Packard Co., Cupertino, CA) hard copy combination.

A lengthy program, written in BASIC PLUS (DEC) was assembled over a 4-year period relying on data collected up to the point of completion in 1977. During this period, and the subsequent years, the text produced by the algorithm has been subjected to clinical validation on a daily basis by a group of up to four clinicians. Errors were corrected and modification made at the time the problem report was generated. A complete revision of the program is underway, encompassing new data, some of which are referenced in this chapter.

Two batches of a reference calibrator were used throughout the study. Lengthy cross-correlation studies were carried out before and during the transition from the first to the second batch. To ensure unrecognized drift in values with time, the data reduction program calculated mean patient values for each working day, a value that was monitored over the 6 years. While day-to-day variations were occasionally wide, due to the changing characteristic of the tested population, regression analysis over long periods of time would have clearly shown drift or changes due to instrument maintenance or changes in calibrator and antiserum.

DEFINITION OF "NORMAL"

The word "normal" refers to "a standard, not deviating from a norm, regular, naturally occurring, average." Unfortunately, the natural state of human affairs is to be abnormal, to harbor some unrecognized or even recognized condition or to be in some way at variance by virtue of genetic makeup. In fact, to use the word "normal" is of very little help if not actually misleading. The great majority of studies describing the "normal range" for an analyte have selected a small number of available serum donors, usually young, alleged not to be under a physician's care, but not documentably well either. Their ethnic and racial background is carefully not considered, and their use of ubiquitous substances are ignored. In some cases, sex and age have been requested, but in general, they are considered equal in the eyes of the tester.

How valid is this type of approach? Has it merit of being a satisfactory first step in setting the stage for using a test in the community? Experience has shown that it is a reasonable effort by manufacturers and regulators but it cannot be construed in any way as being anything more than the first step with subsequent refinements being a function of the individual laboratory and the medical community as a whole.

METHODS OF DATA REVIEW AND DISPLAY
Restrictions

The great majority of data are analyzed by highly defined and relatively inflexible statistical routines available to virtually all through even the simplest of desktop calculators. For investigators with at least minicomputer capabilities, sophisticated packages can be obtained to enhance their capabilities. Nevertheless, these programs do not allow capitalization on man's ability to extract information through pattern recognition. Two- and three-dimensional displays of complex data often uncover new information of importance.

For example, to study the obvious relationship between total serum protein and serum albumin in samples not containing monoclonal immunoglobulins at levels greater than 2 g/L, a simple analysis yields information:

$$\text{Sample size} = 31,339$$
$$\text{Mean total protein} = 68.2 \text{ g/L}$$
$$\text{Mean albumin} = 41.7 \text{ g/L}$$
$$\text{Correlation coefficient} = 0.798$$

A better representation that explains the nature of the correlation is a two-dimensional plot as shown in Figure 1. It is clear that the distribution is skewed to the upper left as the result of other serum proteins contributing a substantial portion of the total in certain instances. We can also see that this skewing is greatest in absolute terms in the 25–35 g albumin/L range but in relative terms appears to be the same throughout the lower ranges.

The visual image would be further enhanced by representing the same data in three dimensions: total protein versus albumin versus the number of samples in each cell of the matrix (Fig. 2). The skewing is now clearly visible (Fig. 2A,C) as the data mass is rotated for better visualization, however, in the other dimension, there seems to be an even distribution (Fig. 2B,D). By employing a dot matrix or coarse grey-scale (Fig. 3) the distribution becomes visually more efficient but continues to lack specific definition. By connecting points of equal value by lines (Fig. 4) a better representation of the smooth relationship between these two tests appears clearly: in this large sample, no subpopulation of clinical interest appears.

Moving from two parameters with a clear correlation to another pair where a possible association might be seen, the same types of display might be valuable. Figures 5 and 6 show, in two dimensions, the association of serum transferrin and immunoglobulin A in males only. In three dimensions (Fig. 7), additional information appears suggesting more than one group along the IgA axis between a transferrin concentration of 2.0 and 3.4 g/L. An obvious next step in this form of data analysis where masses of data in a large matrix can be processed is computer enhancement so elegantly employed in the photo rendition of data released by NASA.

Intercorrelations

As stated earlier, the interpretation of a single serum protein analysis rarely yields useful information. Perspective can only be obtained by ex-

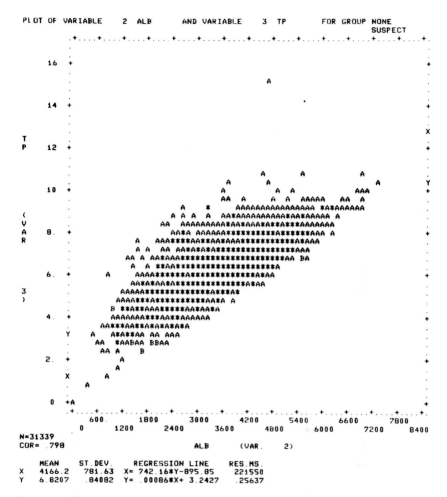

Fig. 1. Two-dimensional plot of total serum protein vs. serum albumin. A = 1–10 cases in a given cell; * = greater than 10 entries.

amining other proteins in the same sample or, in certain cases, many sequential analyses of a single protein over a sufficient length of time. The use of multivariant analysis as a further extension is beyond the scope of this chapter, however, it has been employed to advantage with multiple serum protein analyses as a marker of cancer of the breast [11].

As a first rough step in searching for proteins with a high degree of correlation Table I demonstrates that even without restriction for age or disease category, this analysis yields confirmation of several known associations (e.g., C3 vs. C4, albumin vs. transferrin, haptoglobin vs. oroso-

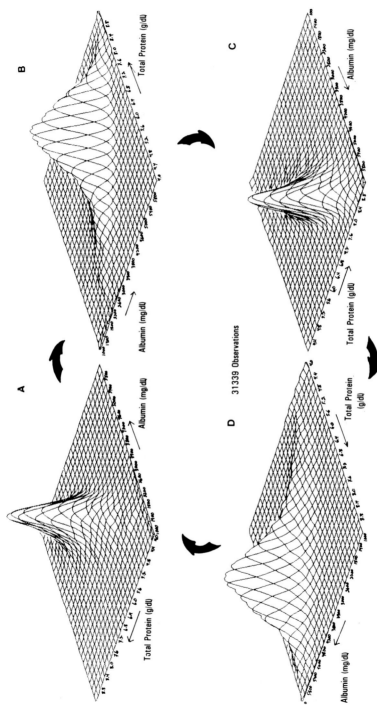

Fig. 2. Three-dimensional plot of data shown in Figure 1. Each frame is a view rotated 90° clockwise from A to D. The height of each grid intersection represents the number of entries into that cell.

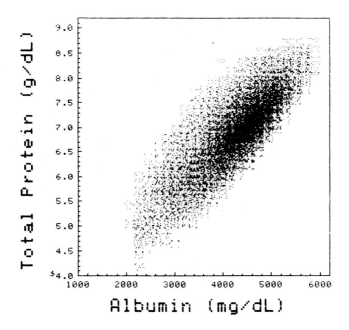

Fig. 3. Two-dimensional plot of serum total protein versus albumin using the dot matrix.

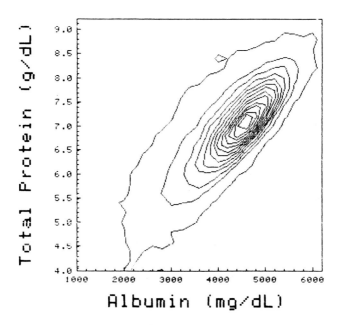

Fig. 4. Two-dimensional plot of data presented in Figure 3. Lines connect points of equal value and enclose area equal to or greater than a given value.

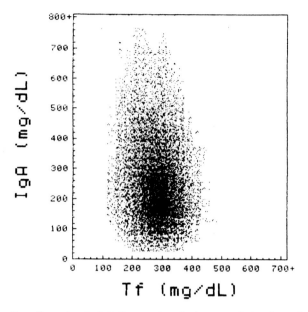

Fig. 5.   Two-dimensional plot of serum transferrin versus IgA using a dot matrix.

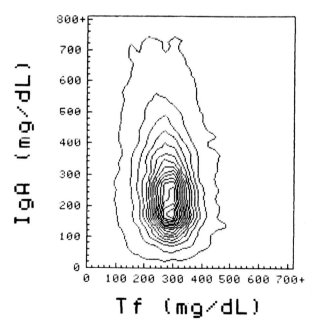

Fig. 6.   Two-dimensional plot of data in Figure 5 using lines connecting points of equal value.

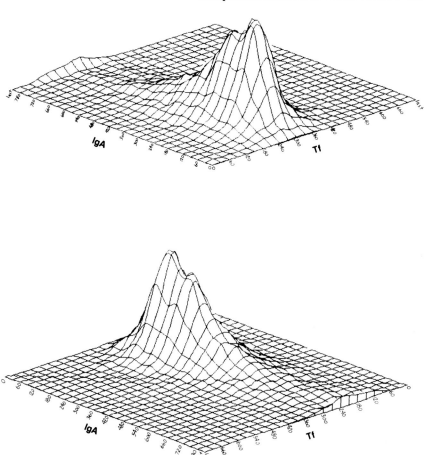

Fig. 7.   Three-dimensional display of the data shown in Figures 5 and 6.

mucoid (α_1-acid glycoprotein)). Some associations at a lower level of confidence were not expected and suggest that a more careful study of certain parameters restricted by age or sex may be fruitful (e.g., LDL vs. C3). A more efficient means of displaying these data is shown in Figure 8 by employing a coarse grey-scale.

The Overall Computer System

The multiple computer system in use at present is large by comparison to what would be needed if no developmental or statistical work were required. For example, the next generation of data processing systems envisioned for

TABLE I. Correlation Between All Proteins—Adult Males (Correlation Matrix)

	AGE 3	IGA 5	IGM 6	C3 7	HPT 8	TF 9	A2M 10	IGG 11	A1AT 12	ALB 13
AGE 3	1.0000									
IGA 5	-0.2315	1.0000								
IGM 6	-0.1234	0.0924	1.0000							
C3 7	-0.0035	0.1069	0.0373	1.0000						
HPT 8	0.1962	0.1408	-0.0146	0.4090	1.0000					
TF 9	-0.2204	-0.0859	0.0877	0.1487	-0.1598	1.0000				
A2M 10	0.0894	0.1168	0.2012	-0.0558	-0.0475	0.0152	1.0000			
IGG 11	0.0652	0.4011	0.2012	0.1168	0.0376	-0.0068	0.0928	1.0000		
A1AT 12	0.2771	0.1859	-0.0253	0.1978	0.5243	-0.2492	0.1174	0.0680	1.0000	
ALB 13	-0.4606	-0.2397	0.0724	-0.0120	-0.3914	0.4592	-0.0088	0.0337	-0.4730	1.0000
C4 14	-0.0036	0.0358	0.0048	0.4720	0.2293	0.0850	-0.0178	-0.0234	-0.0984	-0.0128
LDL 15	0.0077	-0.0440	0.1079	0.3177	-0.0132	0.2704	0.0031	-0.0416	-0.1456	-0.1658
ORO 16	0.1897	0.1596	0.1596	0.3678	0.6329	-0.2346	-0.0808	0.0759	0.5989	-0.4269
BL 17	-0.0537	-0.0715	0.1434	0.2353	-0.0791	0.2009	-0.0742	-0.0222	-0.1900	0.1873
IA1 18	-0.0046	-0.0019	0.0061	0.0069	-0.0018	0.0088	0.0125	0.0082	-0.0100	-0.0093
IA2 19	-0.0053	0.0027	0.0107	-0.0164	-0.0174	-0.0094	-0.0063	0.0028	-0.0149	-0.0061
TOT PROT 20	-0.3233	0.1402	0.2321	0.1913	-0.1431	0.4567	0.1312	0.4931	-0.2162	0.8327

	C4 14	LDL 15	ORO 16	BL 17	IA1 18	IA2 19	TOT PROT 20
C4 14	1.0000						
LDL 15	0.3434	1.0000					
ORO 16	0.2643	-0.0206	1.0000				
BL 17	0.1980	0.5635	-0.0088	1.0000			
IA1 18	0.0255	0.0028	-0.0059	0.0060	1.0000		
IA2 19	-0.0144	-0.0104	-0.0182	0.0009	0.0013	1.0000	
TOT PROT 20	0.0795	0.2061	-0.1808	0.1828	-0.0045	0.0013	1.0000

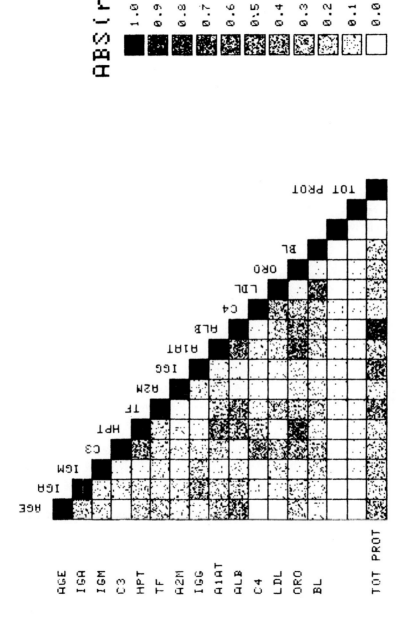

Fig. 8.   A visual representation of the data shown in Table I, employing a grey scale. The darker the cell, the greater the correlation either positive or negative.

the Beckman Immunochemistry System will be capable of creating a similar interpretive report for blocks of six proteins. Figure 9 is a block diagram of the complete system.

Normalization

Based upon large population studies, one develops a defined expectation. In the past, some analytic data were presented as percent of normal or, in effect, the patient value expressed as a percent of a "normal value" or "mean value" for a defined normal population:

$$\text{Reported value} = \frac{\text{Patient value}}{\text{Normal value}} \times 100 = \% \text{ Normal}$$

While this approach fell into disfavor as analyses shifted towards more precise methods and widely accepted reference materials, it is being revived as computers are used increasingly to solve the intricate problem of expressing test values as a function of demographic information such as age and sex. In other words, the report of a serum albumin value of 3700 mg/dL is of limited use to the clinician if that value is affected by individualization. The fact that the value is 100% of normal for a 73-year-old woman and 77% of normal for a 24-year-old man is more important and more comprehensible than is the absolute numerical value. Furthermore, reducing an analytic value in mass units to an arbitrary unit expressed in terms of an equivalent population becomes far more manageable for computerization where many parameters will be taken into consideration. This is the process of normalization. These values become increasingly important when the laboratory wishes to produce a visually efficient report such as shown in Figures 10 and 11.

Constructing the computer ability to normalize a value requires that either of two approaches be taken. The first is that a grid or two-dimensional matrix be created which represents the conversion of each value from its original form, for cxample 3700 mg/dL albumin to 100% for the grid at 73 years of age. This requires a matrix for each age group and for males and females. A more efficient approach is to convert the curves to a mathematical formula into which age can be inserted, recovering the desired value. Such an equation is illustrated in Figure 12 for IgG. Additional equations, adjusting for any parameter for which data exist, can be constructed and incorporated into even small computational devices. An example and block diagram of such a flow chart is shown in Figure 13 for serum IgG.

The importance of a particular normalized value in terms of standard deviation may be useful; ultimately, however, significance in clinical terms is needed. Evaluating results in this manner is termed "weighting" and can be given numerical values useful in generating clinical tests. From the clinical point of view a value is absent, very low, low, equivocal, below normal,

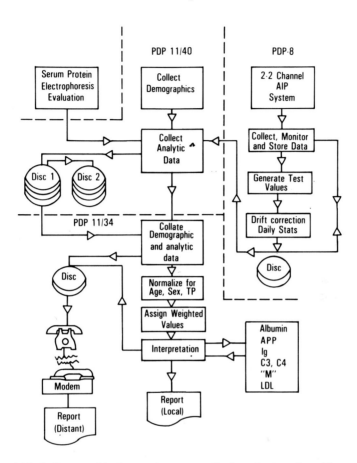

Fig. 9.   A block diagram of the interpretive program for the reduction of specific protein data to clinically relevant text.

normal, high normal, equivocal, high, or very high. Each category can be assigned delimiters, describing "normal" as falling between two analytic values, therefore assigning a numerical value to clinical judgement. In this manner, a series of protein values considered to be normal can be summarized easily at the end of the clinical weighting program by dividing the sum of all weighted values by the total number of assays. For example, if "normal" is assigned a value of 9.00 and 14 proteins are to be analyzed, the sum of the weighted value should equal 126. If the sum is 124, one or two analytes gave nonnormal values, and the examination of a single number separates normal from nonnormal.

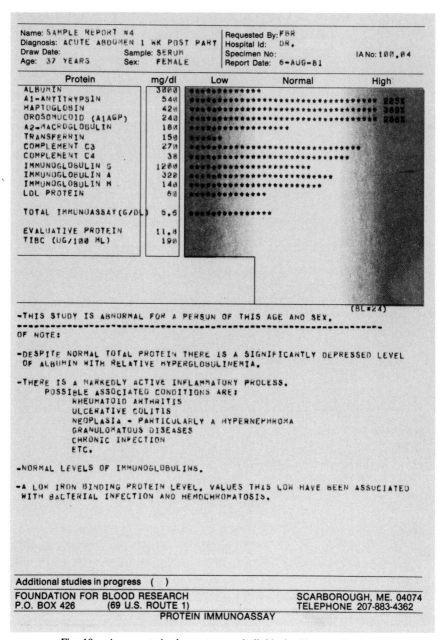

Name: SAMPLE REPORT #4
Diagnosis: ACUTE ABDOMEN 1 WK POST PART
Draw Date: Sample: SERUM
Age: 37 YEARS   Sex: FEMALE

Requested By: FBR
Hospital Id: DR.
Specimen No: IA No: 100.04
Report Date: 6-AUG-81

Protein	mg/dl	Low	Normal	High
ALBUMIN	3000			
A1-ANTITRYPSIN	540			225%
HAPTOGLOBIN	420			360%
OROSOMUCOID (A1AGP)	240			280%
A2-MACROGLOBULIN	180			
TRANSFERRIN	150			
COMPLEMENT C3	270			
COMPLEMENT C4	38			
IMMUNOGLOBULIN G	1200			
IMMUNOGLOBULIN A	320			
IMMUNOGLOBULIN M	140			
LDL PROTEIN	60			
TOTAL IMMUNOASSAY(G/DL)	5.6			
EVALUATIVE PROTEIN	11.8			
TIBC (UG/100 ML)	190			

(BL#24)

-THIS STUDY IS ABNORMAL FOR A PERSON OF THIS AGE AND SEX.

OF NOTE:

-DESPITE NORMAL TOTAL PROTEIN THERE IS A SIGNIFICANTLY DEPRESSED LEVEL
OF ALBUMIN WITH RELATIVE HYPERGLOBULINEMIA.

-THERE IS A MARKEDLY ACTIVE INFLAMMATORY PROCESS.
        POSSIBLE ASSOCIATED CONDITIONS ARE:
             RHEUMATOID ARTHRITIS
             ULCERATIVE COLITIS
             NEOPLASIA - PARTICULARLY A HYPERNEPHROMA
             GRANULOMATOUS DISEASES
             CHRONIC INFECTION
             ETC.

-NORMAL LEVELS OF IMMUNOGLOBULINS.

-A LOW IRON BINDING PROTEIN LEVEL. VALUES THIS LOW HAVE BEEN ASSOCIATED
WITH BACTERIAL INFECTION AND HEMOCHROMATOSIS.

Additional studies in progress ( )

FOUNDATION FOR BLOOD RESEARCH
P.O. BOX 426   (69 U.S. ROUTE 1)

SCARBOROUGH, ME. 04074
TELEPHONE 207-883-4362

PROTEIN IMMUNOASSAY

Fig. 10.   A computerized report on an individual with normal values.

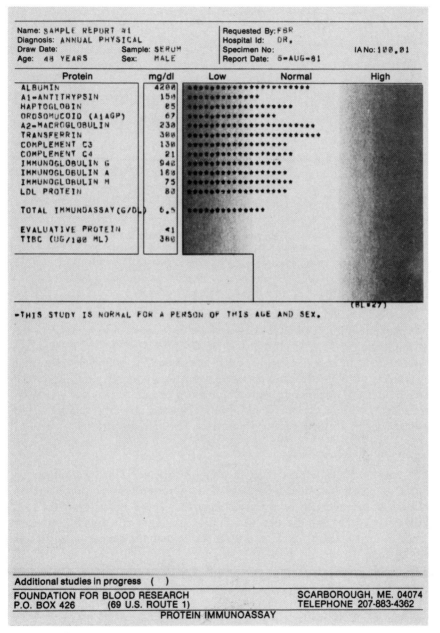

Fig. 11.   A computerized report on a patient with a severe inflammatory process. The diagnosis was a perforated uterus and peritonitis following a septic abortion.

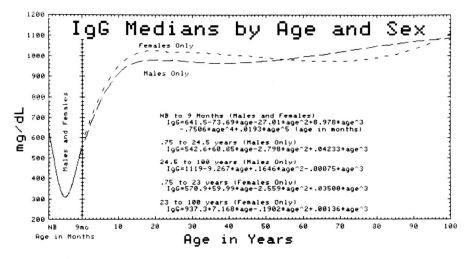

Fig. 12. The curve representing the IgG values from age 1 to 100 years.

The selection of delimiters for each clinical category can easily be changed if the delimiters are stored in a special file of variables. A change in the variable therefore requires only that a single entry into a file be altered, not at every point in an extensive program where that variable appears as part of an algorithm. Of future importance, is that weighting factors become the entry point into a common pathway for the interpretive program. New information resulting in refinements of normalization programs can be added without causing major revisions in the interpretive segments.

Developing the Flowchart

As mentioned earlier, starting to unravel such an ill-defined subject as clinical interpretation of a laboratory finding presents serious problems to both the uninitiated and experienced logician. There are many paths to a particular segment and the first functional algorithm will bear little resemblance to the first draft or to what will be the penultimate version. (In this subject there will be no "final versions.")

Figure 14 is a brief representation of a segment that could be used to evaluate serum haptoglobin. The flow diagram could represent the entry into a much broader evaluation program to test for the presence of inflammation. Any one of the decision points in the logic tree is expandable to add more detail. Each of the referenced subroutines at the margins may consist of dozens or, in some cases, hundreds of logic steps. For simplicity in this diagram, absolute values are shown which, in a more sophisticated form, will

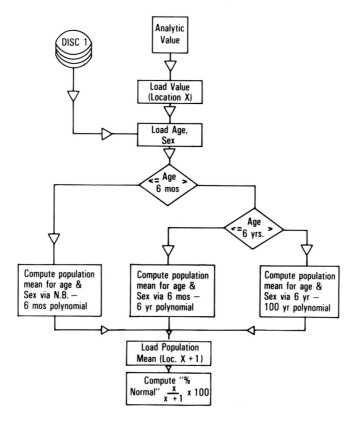

Fig. 13. A block diagram of the normalization of serum IgG values.

usually appear as weighted or, at the very least, normalized values. At two points, information from serum protein electrophoresis is incorporated for illustration. The presence of a monoclonal immunoglobulin may have a massive effect on the entire interpretive process and must be incorporated into the evaluation. *To attempt specific protein interpretation without serum protein electrophoresis information is futile even for nonimmunoglobulins.* In our system, serum protein electrophoresis information is available before specific protein analyses are completed and is visually assessed and manually entered into the data base in numerical form. The information is called upon at several points during the program. Perhaps the most dramatic effect can be seen in the instance when a modestly sized M-component is present and all serum protein analytic values fall into the "normal range." Without this objective information that an M component exists, the report would read that

AN EXAMPLE OF AN ABBREVIATED LOGIC "TREE" FOR A SERUM PROTEIN EVALUATION

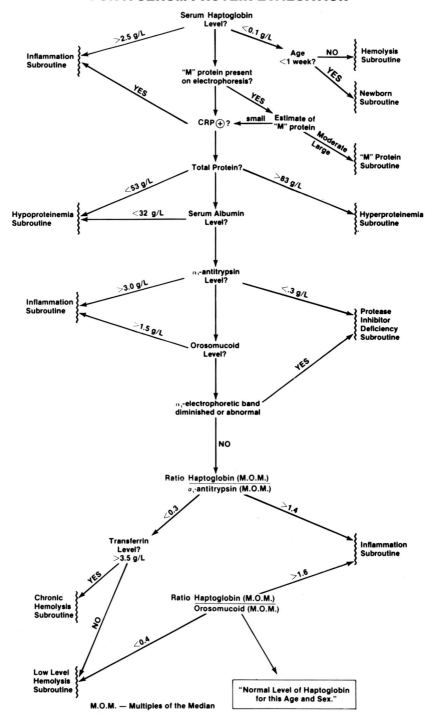

M.O.M. — Multiples of the Median

the study is normal. However, the entry that an M-component is present produces several paragraphs of text after the introductory statement indicating that the study is, in fact, abnormal.

Producing Text

The most flexible format for laboratory data is written text but it is the most difficult to generate. It contains the greatest amount of information for the clinician whereas the usual numerical report, no matter how precise, contains the least.

Text can be produced in two ways. The most commonly employed method is "canned text" or parallel format. Complete paragraphs are called from a mass storage device when certain specific conditions have been met. The approach is only possible when the number of permutations for a paragraph is relatively small or unlimited storage capacity is available. In the case of our program, the evaluation of eleven serum proteins produces 3.6×10^9 possible text sequences, some being two typewritten pages long.

A much more efficient format but also more difficult to create is an algorithm that produces text linearly or word by word, depending upon discrete pieces of data. For example, the statement:

This study is normal for a person of this age and sex.

contains a variable word. The word location filled by "normal" could change to:

. . . probably normal . . .

. . . possibly abnormal . . .

. . . probably abnormal . . .

. . . abnormal . . .

Five complete sentences plus the logic to decide which is correct must occupy memory or storage space. For segments where paragraphs are long and the number of permutations reaches into the hundreds, as for the immunoglobulins, storage space required for "canned" paragraphs become unreasonable even for large devices.

In the linear format, the phrase

This study is . . .

becomes part of the entry point into the program and the words

. . . for a patient of this age and sex.

is part of the exit from the segment. Both are common to all variations. Only the judgmental word changes and is incorporated into the actual algorithm without any recourse to calling text from memory, an action that may slow

---

Fig. 14. A simplified flow diagram for the clinical interpertation of serum haptoglobin.

processing time significantly, particularly on a busy time-sharing system. A more complex example of such a linear text printing format is shown in Figure 15.

Again, from the standpoint that these clinical statements are often in a constant state of change, altering a portion of the linear text producing program is far more practical than altering a word in many stored paragraphs. For example, the word "person" has disturbed some readers. "Person" should be used for the "normal reports" and "patient" for those that contain the word "abnormal." Others feel that the statement should be more personalized, e.g., "a newborn," "an infant," "a child," "an adolescent," "a young woman," "a young man," "a woman," "a man," "an elderly woman," "an elderly man," etc. The possibilities could be endless. The five lines, effectively 304 characters of stored text, now require 50 lines, or over 13,500 stored characters to accomodate the new words in the parallel format, whereas the linear format applying the same question sequence and less than 50 characters of live text, still requires no stored text.

THE REPORT

As the speed and sophistication of computer controlled printers increases the costs are decreasing. Furthermore, the price of inflexible printed forms has dramatically increased, leading data processing users to increasingly use reports generated on inexpensive blank paper. Some features of the printed form remain beyond the reach of reasonably priced hard-copy devices (shading and color). The former has already been successfully addressed as shown in Figures 3, 5, and 8, but the process is slow. Color printers are available but relatively crude and very expensive; however, the drive to make available visually efficient colored reports will overcome these objectives quickly and economically. Figures 10 and 11 illustrate how specific protein data can be presented on printed forms with today's equipment.

OTHER CONSIDERATIONS
Analytical Precision

Methodology for specific protein testing is moving rapidly away from inaccurate and imprecise manual technology to increasingly automated instruments. This presents an anacronism. Analytic precision has reached well below the 5% level in some instruments [10] while clinical precision remains rough. The situation, I believe, is a classical "Catch-22." Laboratory methods have been imprecise. Clinicians have expected no more, since precision at the bedside is an art form, ergo there is no incentive to improve laboratory performance. An interesting phenomenon has occurred, however. As the

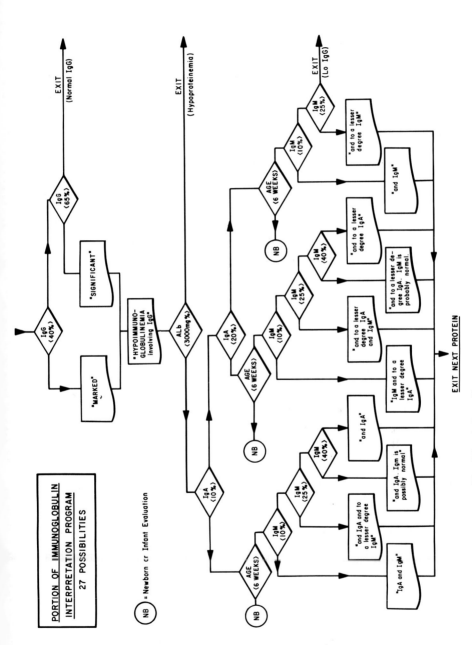

Fig. 15. A flow diagram for generating text relevant to serum IgA.

result of inexpensive microprocessors that can take over much of the drudgery at the laboratory bench, devices are becoming increasingly more automated to the delight of all laboratorians. Performance of the instrument is clearly superior with high precision, low error rates, and as yet, not fully appreciated by laboratory technologists, the need for highly trained personnel is decreasing. Reexamination of areas where imprecise specific protein analyses has not been fruitful, discloses that, in fact, important information can be obtained; it was obscured by poor performance of available commercial kits. Inevitably, a new cycle of reevaluation of serum protein analytes will gather momentum and uncover the extent of the clinical value. As a sequel to new information will come increasing usage and greater pressure to interpret the results properly.

Analytical Accuracy

Of major concern in specific protein analysis is the lack of readily available universal reference materials. Manufacturers of specific protein kits include calibrators in their products; however, in spite of the limited availability of international reference materials from the World Health Organization [8] and the Center for Disease Control [4], little agreement is evident. As shown by Reimer et al. [5], relative agreement for IgA exists but in many other cases, C3 and α_1-antitrypsin for example, agreement is virtually nonexistent with the highest value being over twice that of the lowest. Even IgG showed a spread of 1.5 times between the highest and lowest manufacturer assigned values. All other values were spread between. Of even further concern is the fact that in many instances, even under the careful conditions of the effort, it is clear that our ability in the laboratory to perform even simple dilutions and analyses at different levels is often embarrassingly poor.

In September of 1981, the College of American Pathologists released for general consumption the first reference preparation for serum proteins [3]. The values both in mass units and International Units were the results of efforts by 24 collaborators, manufacturers and experts, who assayed special serum preparations under strict conditions. The resulting concentration values are given on the package insert of the CAP Reference Preparation for Serum Protein vials. It is hoped that this material, which is also linked to the WHO and CDC reference materials, will become the basis for improving accuracy of many specific protein assays and reduce the evident wide spread seen in each CAP quarterly survey report [2].

INTERPRETATIVE LOGIC FOR SERUM PROTEINS

Because of the magnitude of our computer program, only very limited information will be included here as an illustration of a method of interpretation for serum proteins. It should be stressed that many logic sequences can be envisioned. Our approach has been to follow a data-processing sequence for each protein. Although the underlying sequence is identical in each instance, each segment is unique and based upon the knowledge of the analyte and its presentation in a population with and without pathology. The program has been in operation for several years, but is in transition to more efficient algorithms incorporating new laboratory and clinical data.

The First Steps

In spite of the depressingly complex problem of interpreting clinical laboratory data, the reader should be reminded that no problem is so complex that it cannot be reduced to a series of questions with *only yes* and *no* as alternatives. The discovery that certain information required for an appropriate response is lacking is extremely important and can generate a search for that answer. In the final analysis, there are no *maybes,* equivocals, or other such vagaries. The answer is either *yes* or *no* or the question is unsatisfactory; that is to say ambiguous or still complex. For some, this extreme simplification will be very unsettling, if not actually unacceptable. The "art of medicine" is replaced by a sequence of unemotional, uninteresting, and sometimes embarrassing questions. There is no doubt that an astute diagnostician is an artist who synthesizes a diagnosis taking into account an enormous amount of highly subjective data. He does it efficiently, often with apparent ease, drawing upon teaching and experience. Unfortunately, the number of such artists and the demands placed by modern medicine render the system incapable of meeting the demand. The only solution is to dissect portions of the art form, the laboratory for instance, and replace them with hard fact, basically an algorithm.

What Group Should Be Studied?

Clearly, practical considerations must be taken into account. But in light of the rudimentary state of our understanding of analytes such as serum proteins, one approach is to collect a total laboratory experience once a test has reached reasonable frequency of use and satisfactory precision. The latter presents an entirely different problem that will be addressed later.

Many laboratories have elected to use their own hospital staff as their reference population; certainly a practical start. Caution must be exercised. Hospital staffs are not representative of the general population. Their makeup is often skewed away from that of the population they serve. Racial, ethnic, socioeconomic, and sexual differences are often obvious to the casual observer and for this reason, the 50–100 samples collected from this group must be augmented by the patient sample stream to follow.

It is justifiable to include samples from clearly distressed individuals in this effort to describe a population. When a laboratory collects a suitably sized population from allegedly healthy persons, the distribution will initially appear to be narrow, expanding in the expected fashion as numbers increase. Simply stated, many individuals harbor some subclinical process manifesting as a nonnormal result for one or more analytes. Accepting the fact that apparently healthy individuals may have subclinical disease or a genetic make-up that will alter an analyte's concentration suggests that the converse is also true—that diseased individuals will often have individual analyte concentrations that appear "normal." The solution is to collect all data on an analyte as testing is performed and to include accurate demographics on important variables. What constitutes an important variable is indefinable and bears upon the interest of the laboratorian or clinician. Often the perception of the importance of a parameter appears late in the study, requiring tedious retrospective review or a new prospective study.

Establishing one's own clinical experience requires information not easily available to most laboratory personnel—clinical data. This does not mean admitting diagnosis or the diagnosis that appears on the request form but information obtained only from a professional review of the clinical record, a document with limited access that often appears disorganized and certainly difficult to read. It must be digested in its entirety before making a conclusion.

Further obstacles exist. Obtaining samples for studies of clinical relevance requires 1) that either volunteers be recruited and oriented to the purpose of the study who then ask patients to sign an informed consent sheet, or 2) that samples from the testing stream be selected for inclusion into the study after the identity of the individual is either carefully destroyed or coded so that the information cannot be used to the detriment of the patient. Legal implications thread through the entire process. Some of the parameters clearly needed to extract the proper information from a person's data are sensitive: racial and ethnic background, certain medications (e.g. antiepileptics, contraceptives, drugs for fun or abuse). Even if the information is presented, can it be believed? Drinking history? How much per day? Number of cigarettes? Number of cups of coffee per day, diet, etc.?

The construction of an algorithm for a complex subject, often composed of interdigitated parts, presents a bewildering task seemingly with no place to begin. As an example:

What is a normal total protein value?

The question is too complex and no answer is possible. To reduce this to a simpler form, a series of questions must be created such as:

What is the expected range for total protein in a population of
—nonobese?
—age 20–25 years?
—living in the northeastern United States?
—Caucasian males?

—without significant disease?

—with the subject having been ambulatory for
  at least 3 hours?

One may select total protein to illustrate a difficult but extremely common case. A great simplification would be to examine only albumin, which comprises 60–70% of the total protein. A narrower question is:

What is a normal serum albumin value?

However, it remains difficult to answer since the basic work has not been done to describe the subject indicated in the question. To restructure the question:

What is the "normal range" for albumin in Caucasian males?

—age 20–25 years?

—who are not obese?

—who live in the northeastern US?

—who are clinically well?

Further restraints that can be controlled:

—14-hour fast after a light meal and no
  alcohol?

—ambulatory for more than 3 hours?

To illustrate this approach briefly, I have selected the familiar analyte serum albumin because it may be the simplest of the proteins to examine. Its concentration is high and analysis is simple by a variety of methods. Reference preparations exist and are in general use. Genetic polymorphism plays no significant role in the evaluation of serum albumin, and analbuminemia is rare. Immunochemical quantification is not complicated by interfering substances; this is not true for a variety of chemical tests and age and sex differences are not considered important. Albumin, therefore, has been an uncomplicated analyte until a large population was examined by a relative precise method and the data stored in such a fashion as to allow efficient review of the whole as described below.

Some data pertaining to the list of qualifying statements about each sample as listed above are available, however, some of the most important are not included in the demographic information available to the investigator. Very often, the laboratory is not supplied with crucial information that will be required for the proper interpretation of a value. In the majority of instances, although by no means always, the laboratory knows the age and sex of the patient. These represent crucial parameters, without which interpretation, even for serum albumin, where sex and age has not been considered as important, is absolutely necessary. For example, in adults the distribution for serum albumin appears to be quite similar for males and females (Fig.

16) if the population is examined by serum concentration values alone. However, if the same population is examined by age (Fig. 17), it is clear that there are differences that significantly affect what is considered normal for each sex and age category. In general, median values for male and females change in concert over the years with the mean for the entire population differing by only 0.7%. Figure 16 shows clearly that between the ages of 17 and 33, the values for the two sexes diverge, so that at age 23 to 24, male albumin values are at their highest, being 8% above that for females of the same age. From the early teens to approximately age 50, female albumin values are consistently lower than that for males. However, beyond age 50, female values are higher than for males, reaching 4.5% above male values in the eighth decade (Fig. 18). The differences cannot be disregarded and at their maximum, significantly affect the interpretation of what is considered as "normal."

The question of which parameter to employ in describing a population experience has come under serious scrutiny. Means and medians are highly sensitive to the source of calibrators employed by a laboratoy. Medians for albumin that represent the central value fall above the mean since the dis-

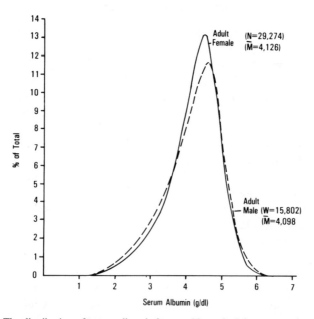

Fig. 16. The distribution of serum albumin by sex. Numerical data composing the raw curves were collected in steps of 0.2 g/dL.

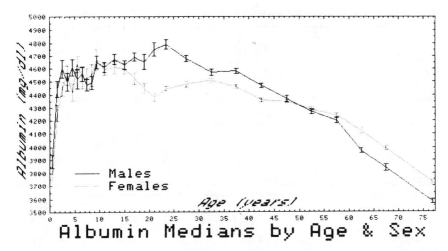

Fig. 17.   Distribution of serum albumin medians by sex. Numerical data were collected in one-year intervals up to age 9, two-year intervals up to age 24, and in five-year intervals above age 25.

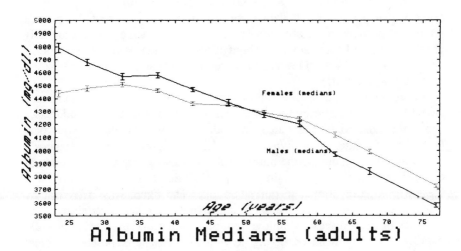

Fig. 18.   A more detailed illustration of the sexual difference in serum albumin values between ages 20 and 80.

TABLE II. Serum Albumin Values for Adults Older Than Age 22

	Male (mg/dL)	Female (mg/dL)
Mean	4098 (± 822)	4125 (± 735)
Median	4220	4230
Mode	4600	4400
N	15800	29271

TABLE III. Comparison of Albumin Values for Specific Groups

Class	Mean (mg/dL)	SD	CV
All albumin	4116	766	18.6
Male only	4098	822	20.1
Age 20–25 only	4620	750	16.2

tribution of all albumin values is skewed to the lower side, elevated values being rare. If, however, we examined only the total population of adults older than age 22, we see results reported in Table II.

It would be expected that as we insert further restrictions, the acceptable range would narrow. With data from our study, we find that the present interpretation may be in error by as much as 10%, which is considerably above the error of the method of about ±5%. In other words, methodology has surpassed our clinical information even for an analyte as well understood as albumin (Table III).

As presented in Table III a significant number of values from young men would be considered normal when in fact they are abnormal. This addresses one of the most troublesome areas of medicine: how to handle the equivocal or borderline value. As shown in Table II, refining population data goes a long way toward reducing the number of instances where interpretation is in doubt. For example, an albumin value of 3350 mg/dL is considered to be at the lower edge of normal in our laboratory. The figure was arrived at by examining a large number of individuals of both sexes who showed no evidence of overt disease. Employing our existing program, a value of 3400 mg/dL or even as much as 3500 mg/dL would be considered probably normal even if it were from a young man. The recent study of over 45,000 random cases, the value of 3350 mg/dL is exactly one standard deviation less than the population mean. With new insight, as illustrated in Table II, the value of 3500 would clearly be abnormal for males. The lower limit for this group is 3850 mg/dL, whereas for young women of the same age, the lower limit would be 3550 mg/dL. Interpretation, therefore, would be that a value is no longer equivocal, but clearly abnormal for a young male of the specified age.

Albumin has been selected here because it is a familiar analyte and as a result is usually treated in a cavalier manner. When other less familiar and

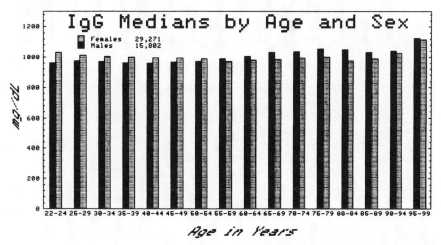

Fig. 19.   Immunoglobulin G values for adults.

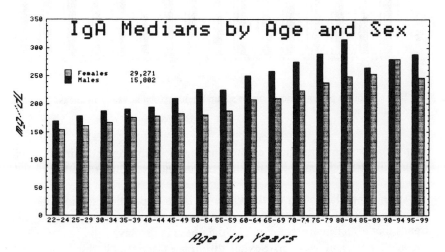

Fig. 20.   Immunoglobulin A values for adults.

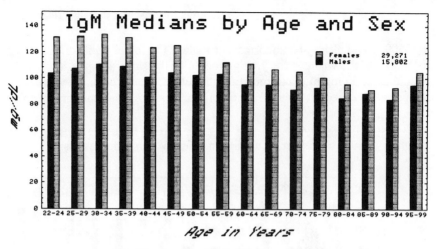

Fig. 21. Immunoglobulin M values for adults.

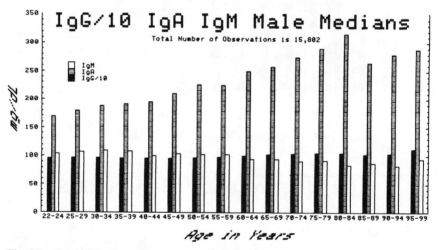

Fig. 22. Combined presentation of major serum immunoglobulin values in males. Note that the IgG values are divided by 10.

more complex analytes such as the immunoglobulins are examined, it will clearly illustrate the rudimentary state of our understanding of serum protein values.

As another illustration of the value of large population studies, the distribution of serum concentrations of the three major immunoglobulins reveal trends that affect interpretation. The data base is displayed in Figures 19–21 for adult men and women. Sexual differences are "negligible" for serum IgG, however, distinct and persistent differences for IgA and IgM are seen and are of such magnitude that these differences must be taken into account in clinical interpretation. When displayed as in Figures 22 and 23, the trends are more easily visualized. Unexpected shifts in IgA levels occur at age 80–85 for males and at age 90–95 for females. The overall curve for each sex is shown in Figure 12 and in detail for infants and children and young adults in Figure 24.

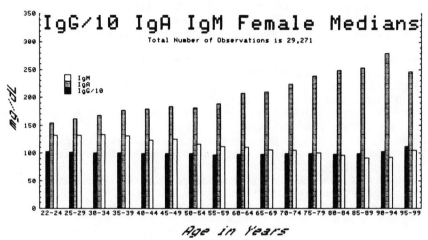

Fig. 23. Combined presentation of major serum immunoglobulin values in females. Note that the IgG values are divided by 10.

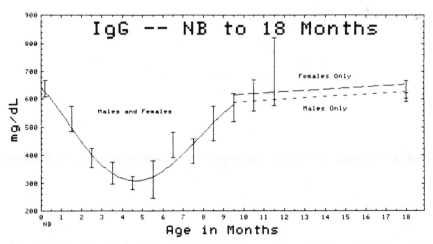

Fig. 24. Detailed representation of IgG values for newborns, infants and children. The equations represent formulae by which the plotted curve is generated.

REFERENCES

1. Dixon WJ, Brown MB (eds): "Biomedical Computer Programs." Berkeley: University of California Press, 1979.
2. College of American Pathologists: "College of American Pathologists Special Diagnostic Survey." Available from CAP, 7400 Skokie Boulevard, Skokie, IL 60077.
3. Nakamura RM, Hanson DJ, Keitges PW, et al.: Development of the CAP reference preparation for serum proteins. Pathologist 35:377, 1981.
4. Reimer CB, Smith SJ, Hannon WH, et al.: Progress towards an international reference standards for human serum proteins. J Biol Stand 6:133, 1978.
5. Reimer CB, Smith SJ, Wells TW, et al.: Collaborative calibration of the U.S. National and the College of American Pathologists reference preparations for specific serum proteins. Am J Clin Pathol 77:12, 1982.
6. Ritchie RF, Alper CA, Graves J, et al.: Automated quantitation of proteins in serum and other biological fluids. Am J Clin Pathol 59:151, 1973.
7. Ritchie RF, Automated precipitin analysis. In Ritchie RF (ed): "Automated Immunoanalysis," Vol. 1. New York: Dekker, 1978, pp 45–66.
8. Rowe VS, Anderson SG, Grab B: A research standard for human serum immunoglobulins IgG, IgA, and IgM. Bull WHO 42:535, 1970.
9. Smith DE, Ritchie RF: Acquisition and analyses of light scattering data under RTS-8. In "Proceedings of the Digital Equipment Corporation Users Society." Boston: Digital Equipment Corp., 1977, pp 1027–1031.
10. Sternberg J: A rate nephelometer for measuring specific proteins by immunoprecipitin reactions. Clin Chem 23:1456, 1977.
11. Thompson DK, Haddow JE, Smith DE, Ritchie RF: Serum protein changes in women with early breast cancer. Cancer 48:793, 1981.

PATHOPHYSIOLOGIC CONSIDERATIONS

Physiology of Immunoglobulins: Diagnostic and
Clinical Aspects, pages 193–304
© 1982 Alan R. Liss, Inc., 150 Fifth Avenue, New York, NY 10011

9

Antibody Structure, Function, and Active Sites

Gary S. Hahn, MD

INTRODUCTION

Immunoglobulins (antibodies) are members of a family of evolutionarily related molecules that constitute the "humoral" arm of the immune system. They are present in blood, most exocrine secretions, and in essentially every body compartment exposed to the lymphatic circulation. The term antibody originated from observations that certain serum proteins could specifically recognize and agglutinate substances previously injected into animals. It is now known that highly specific immunoglobulins (Igs) can be generated that will bind to antigenic determinants having virtually any molecular configuration. Once bound to antigen, Igs may trigger a wide range of host immune system functions which act through several mechanisms to kill foreign organisms. In addition, Igs present on the surfaces of certain lymphoid cells act as molecular sensors that can activate and regulate the differentiation of lymphoreticular cells. The ability of Igs to trigger cellular functions after sensing only a few molecules in the environment makes worthy the comparison of Igs to a transistor amplifier. In a junction transistor, a miniscule current applied to the base can trigger a huge current flow many thousands of times greater than the original signal. Similarly, when IgE molecules on the surface of mast cells bind to a single divalent antigen, the mast cells degranulate and release highly vasoactive substances into the surroundings. These substances are, in volume, millions of times greater than the antibody molecules that triggered the substances' release. Surrounding cells that sense the vasoactive compounds may be attracted to the site of release and, in turn, are stimulated to release different molecules which may then act as signals to recruit still other cells with destructive or regulatory abilities. This pattern in which small signals are amplified by a cascade of molecular events into a biologically meaningful end-point is a common theme throughout the immune system and in many unrelated metabolic pathways. Igs, serving as primary sensors for such cascades, are one of the major methods by which the immune system cells "see" the external milieu. Should this sensitive system become flawed through the presence of genetically "mutant" Igs or "fooled" into becoming activated when no actual invasive threat exists (as occurs in allergic disease), the destructive cascades may cause extensive inflammatory damage to the organism, which may even result in its death. Such inappropriate activation, largely mediated by Igs, forms the pathogenesis of many diseases such as rheumatoid arthritis, systemic lupus erythematosus, hemolytic anemias, serum sickness, and allergies. An understanding of the molecular mechanisms whereby Igs exert their many and varied bioactivities may lead to the development of new methods of diagnosis and treatment of a wide range of serious diseases.

IMMUNOGLOBULIN CHAIN STRUCTURE

All human Igs are divided into five major classes: IgG, IgA, IgM, IgD, and IgE. IgG, IgA, and possibly IgM are further divided into subclasses that result from minor amino acid sequence differences between each subclass [1]. Each Ig molecule consists of two pairs of identical polypeptide chains. The larger pair termed "heavy (H) chains" and designated γ, α, μ, δ, and ε, respectively, are unique for each class and are linked by disulfide bonds formed by homologous cysteine residues of each chain [2]. The smaller "light (L) chain" pair is common to all heavy chain classes and exists in two nonallelic forms, κ and λ [3]. A single pair of H chains always has two identical L chains. Within a single Ig class, however, molecules having either κ- or λ-L chains exist; the relative proportions in humans being approximately two thirds κ and one third λ [1,4].

Two classes of Igs, IgA and IgM, also exist in a polymeric form in which two IgA monomers or five IgM monomers are covalently linked by a 129 residue glycoprotein chain termed "joining chain" or "J chain" [5,6]. The pentameric form of IgM is normally the only one found in substantial quantities in plasma, whereas 85% of plasma IgA is monomeric [7,8]. The dimeric form of IgA is predominantly found in exocrine secretions and consists of two IgA molecules linked by a single J chain. In addition, secretory IgA has a second covalently linked polypeptide chain termed "secretory component" (SC), which makes the IgA dimer resistant to proteolysis from enzymes present in exocrine secretions [8].

Recent studies of Igs on the surface of B lymphocytes indicate that they have an additional peptide tailpiece of 30 to 40 residues that extends through the lymphocyte plasma membrane into the cell cytoplasm [9]. The tailpiece consists of a central stretch of predominantly hydrophobic (and hence lipophilic) amino acids, bounded at both ends by charged residues. The lipophilic residues are thought to form a helical structure that spans the lipid bilayer of the plasma membrane while the charged residues occur at the entrance and exit of the tailpiece through the membrane and thus serve as an anchor. Tailpiece residues extending into a cell's cytoplasm probably interact with the cellular cytoskeleton and with "transducer" molecules which convert the Ig's antigen-binding signal into appropriate biochemical changes within the lymphocyte. Although to date only IgM and IgD molecules have been observed to exist in both secreted and membrane (+ tailpiece) forms [9–11,355], it is probable that the other three Ig classes also have similar membrane versions [11].

SEQUENCE COMPARISONS OF IMMUNOGLOBULINS
Domain Homology

In 1969 Edelman first published the complete amino acid sequence of an intact myeloma protein IgG_1, Eu [12]. It was evident that both H and L chains were constructed from repeated homology units 105 ± 5 amino acid residues long. These observations prompted the suggestion that within the intact molecule, each homology unit formed a compact domain having a specific biologic function, e.g., antigen binding for variable (V) domains and effector functions such as complement binding for constant (C) domains. The amino acid homology further suggested that Igs had evolved by duplication of a single primordial gene coding for 100 to 110 amino acids, an idea earlier proposed by Hill et al. [13] and Singer and Doolittle in 1966 [14] on the basis of partial amino acid sequences. Figure 1 shows the four constant homology regions of IgG_1 Eu aligned with gaps inserted to maximize homology. It is evident that several amino acid positions are invariant and probably reflect residues that contribute to the structural stability of each domain. Of the eleven sequence positions that are invariant among the four domains, eight positions have hydrophobic or aromatic amino acids which would be expected to be shielded from solvent and to contribute to the stability of the hydrophobic core of each domain.

The domain structure of all L chains is identical regardless of the associated heavy chain class. Each L chain has two domains, one with constant amino acid sequence, termed C_L, and one antigen-binding domain with variable amino acid sequence, termed V_L [15].

H chains, by contrast, may have either three (IgG, IgA, IgD) or four (IgM, IgE) C domains [16,17], termed CH_1, CH_2, CH_3, and CH_4, and one variable domain, termed V_H. Alternatively, C domains may be designated according to their H chain class; thus Cε4 indicates the CH_4 domain of the ε H chain of IgE.

L chains are joined to H chains by a single disulfide bond between the C_L domain and the CH_1 domain of each H chain [17]. An exception to this

```
CL   (109-129)   T V A A P S V F I F P P S D E Q - - L K S G T
CH1  (119-139)   S T K G P S V F P L A P S S K S - - T S G G T
CH2  (234-256)   L L G G P S V F L F P P K P K D T L M I S R T
CH3  (342-362)   Q P R E P Q V Y T L P P S R E E - - M T K N Q


                                 *
CL   (130-150)   A S V V C L L N N F Y P R E A K V - - Q W K V
CH1  (140-160)   A A L G C L V K D Y F P E P V T V - - S W N S
CH2  (257-279)   P E V T C V V V D V S H E D P Q V K F N W Y V
CH3  (363-383)   V S L T C L V K G F Y P S D I A V - - E W E S


CL   (151-173)   D N A L Q S G N S Q E S V T E Q D S K D S T Y
CH1  (161-180)   - G A L T S G - V H T F P A V L Q S - S G L Y
CH2  (280-300)   D G - V Q V H N A K T K P R E Q Q Y - D S T Y
CH3  (384-404)   N D - G E P E N Y K T T P P V L D S - D G S F


                                                 *
CL   (174-196)   S L S S T L T L S K A D Y E K H K V Y A C E V
CH1  (181-202)   S L S S V V T V P S S S L G T Q - T Y I C N V
CH2  (301-323)   R V V S V L T V L H Q N W L D G K E Y K C K V
CH3  (405-427)   F L Y S K L T V D K S R W Q Q G N V F S C S V


CL   (197-214)   T H Q G L S S P V T - K S F - - N R G E C
CH1  (203-220)   N H K P S N T K V - D K R V - - E P K S C
CH2  (324-341)   S N K A L P A P I - E K T I S K A K G
CH3  (428-446)   M H E A L H N H Y T Q K S L S L S P G
```

Fig. 1. Alignment of the amino acid sequences of C_L, CH_1, CH_2, and CH_3 homology units (domains) from IgG_1 (Eu) (from [12]). Gaps, indicated by dashes, have been introduced to maximize homologies. Residues identical in three or more chains are boxed. The two stars represent the invariant cysteine residues which form the intradomain disulfide bonds. One-letter symbols for amino acid residues: A, alanine; C, cysteine; D, aspartic acid; E, glutamic acid; F, phenylalanine; G, glycine; H, histadine; I, isoleucine; K, lysine; L, leucine; M, methionine; N, asparagine; P, proline; Q, glutamine; R, arginine; S, serine; T, threonine; V, valine; W, tryptophan; Y, tyrosine.

rule exists in an allotypic variant of the IgA_2 subclass, $IgA_2m(1)$ in which no disulfide bond exists, and the two chains interact solely by noncovalent, predominantly hydrophobic interactions [18].

When domains from different Ig classes are aligned, similar homology is observed, suggesting that all Ig domains are evolutionarily related to a single primordial domain (Fig. 2). The highest degree of homology between heavy chain constant domains is approximately 50% between IgA, CH_3 and IgM, CH_4. Comparisons of other constant domains between different classes reveal homologies of about 20 to 30%. The two cysteine residues which form the intradomain disulfide bond of each domain occur in homologous positions in all domains and are separated by about 60 residues. In addition, two tryptophan residues located 14 to 16 residues after the first conserved cysteine and 8 residues before the second conserved cysteine are conserved in all domains with the exception of the second tryptophan in IgD, CH_3. Computer molecular modeling studies of IgG show that tryptophan side chains are buried in the interior of each domain [19] and contribute to each domain's structural stability [20].

The H chains of plasma IgA and IgM have a carboxy-terminal extension 18 and 19 residues longer than ε and γ, respectively, and 13 residues longer than IgD (Fig. 2). The single cysteine in each extension can form a disulfide bond with a cysteine of a J chain, thus producing the polymeric forms of IgA and IgM [8,7]. This 19 residue "tail" should be distinguished from the tailpiece of membrane Igs that are not found free in plasma.

Variable Domains

The antigen-binding capacity of Igs resides in the amino-terminal portions of both H and L chains. The molecular basis for the ability of Igs to specifically recognize and bind countless antigenic forms was first suggested in 1965 when Hilschmann and Craig [21] and Titani and Putnam [22] studied sequences of Bence Jones L chains. They observed that L chains from different patients had nearly identical sequences in the carboxy-terminal half but variable sequences in the amino-terminal 110 residues. In 1971, Wu and Kabat studied sequences of V domains from different L and H chains and observed that the sequence variation tended to occur in several discrete clusters, five to fifteen residues in length [23]. A graphical display of these "hypervariable" regions is shown in Figure 3, in which the degree of sequence variation is plotted as a function of each sequence position: a "Wu-Kabat plot." Using this technique Kabat and Wu found three hypervariable regions in both V_L and V_H domains, HV_1, HV_2, and HV_3 [24]. Shortly thereafter Capra and Kehoe found a fourth hypervariable region in V_H domains, HV He [25]. Through an affinity-labeling technique in which synthetic antigens covalently combine with amino acid residues at the antigen-binding site,

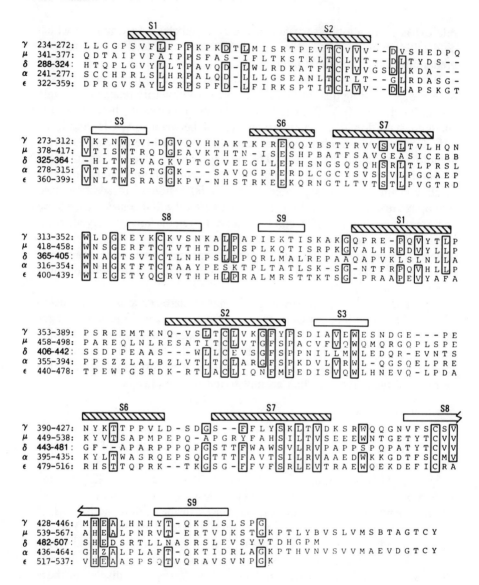

Fig. 2. Alignment of amino acid sequences of the Fc regions of human IgG (γ), IgA (α), IgM (μ), IgD (δ), and IgE (ϵ). Gaps have been inserted to maximize homologies. Residues identical in four or more chains are boxed. S1 through S9 represent segments of β-pleated sheet in IgG as determined by crystallographic refinement of a human IgG Fc fragment by Deisenhoffer [61]. The missing segments S4 and S5 represent the β strands that form the extra loop of V domains not present in C domains. The unshaded strands S3, S8, and S9 form each domain's "top" layer while the shaded strands S1, S2, S6, and S7 form the "bottom" layer. (IgD sequence numbers were derived from Putnam et al. [45] and Lin and Putnam [157]. Sequence alignments are from Lin and Putnam [157].)

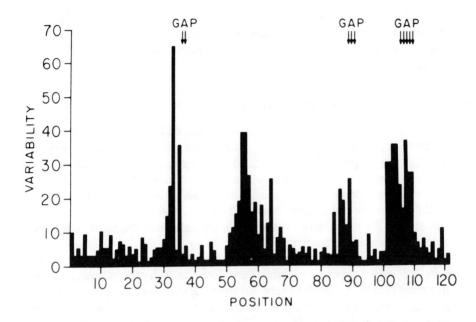

Fig. 3. "Wu-Kabat" variability plot from human V_H domains. The first, second, and fourth modes identify the three complementary-determining HV regions HV_1, HV_2, and HV_3. The third mode represents the extra noncomplementary-determining HV region, HV He, present in V_H domains but absent in V_L domains. Gaps represent positions where deletions or insertions have been introduced to maximize homology between domains. (Reproduced with permission [25].)

three of the four V_H HV regions and all three V_L HV regions were found to interact with antigen [26]. These antigen-binding HV regions were called complementary determining regions (CDRs) because in an intact V domain they form structures with three-dimensional complementarity to a specific antigen. X-ray crystallographic studies of variable domains revealed that the antigen binding site consists of CDR residues contributed from both V_H and V_L domains [27,28]. Isolated H or L chains, by contrast, have no affinity for antigen, demonstrating that CDR residues must have a specific spatial orientation relative to each other in order to "recognize" antigen [29]. Interestingly, this orientation can be experimentally achieved using isolated V_L domains that spontaneously associate to form V dimers [30]. Such dimers still exhibit antigen-binding activity and demonstrate that CH_1 and C_L domains are not required for proper V domain association. X-ray crystallographic analysis of a V_L dimer reveals that the CDR residues are indeed oriented as they are in natural molecules. These observations have prompted the suggestion that such V dimers may have formed, in ancient evolutionary history, primitive antibody molecules that were the ancestors of present day molecules [31].

IMMUNOGLOBULIN FRAGMENTS

A major advance in the understanding of the molecular basis of antibody structure occurred in 1959 when Porter digested rabbit IgG with the papaya-derived enzyme papain [32]. He found two fragments: one that retained the ability to combine with antigen while the other contained the majority of antigenic determinants recognized by antirabbit IgG antibody. The antigen-binding fragment, which he termed Fragment, antigen-binding (Fab), occurred in a 2:1 molar ratio to the easily crystallizable fragment, which he termed Fragment, crystalline (Fc).

Since then, many other fragments have been produced by enzymatic digestion; the most important of which are listed in Table I. Whereas papain treatment cleaves human IgG between amino acid sequence position (aa) 224 and 225 to produce two identical Fab fragments and one Fc fragment, pepsin digestion acts between aa 234 and 235, just on the carboxy-terminal side of the two intraheavy chain disulfide bonded cysteine residues at aa 226 and aa 229. The resultant Fab fragments therefore remain joined by the disulfide bonds and are termed $F(ab')_2$ fragments [36]. The fact the $F(ab')_2$ fragments are bivalent and can bind antigen but do not activate biological effector sites since they lack the Fc-fragment proved to be very important in studying the effect of "cross-linking" antigens on cellular surfaces [37].

Fragments in which entire domains have been enzymatically removed have proved to be very useful in studies to determine the domain locations of various Fc-effector sites. These fragments include Facb (fragment antigen and complement binding), which lacks both carboxy-terminal (CH_3 in IgG) [35] domains; $C\gamma2$ fragments, which consist of a single CH_2 domain and Fc at$C\gamma3$, tFc', and pFc' fragments, which consist of two noncovalently associated CH_3 domains [33,34].

IMMUNOGLOBULIN FRAGMENTS PRODUCED *IN VIVO*
Bence Jones Proteins

Bence Jones proteins (BJP) are fragments of Igs produced *in vivo* under pathological conditions that are usually dimers of two κ- or two λ-L chains. They frequently occur in urine of patients with multiple myeloma and represent excessive L chain synthesis by the proliferating clone of myeloma plasma cells [38].

TABLE I. IgG Fragments

Fragment	IgG treatment	Heavy chain sequence positions	Domain composition
Fv	(pepsin)	1–115	$V_H + V_L$
Fab	(papain)	1–224	V_H/C_H1 + light chain
F(ab')$_2$	(pepsin)	1–234	(V_H/C_H1 + light chain) dimer
Fd	(papain)	1–224	V_H/C_H1
Fc	(papain)	225–446	(C_H2/C_H3) dimer
Fc	(pepsin)	235–446	(C_H2/C_H3) dimer
Facb	(acid, plasmin)	1–326	$V_H/C_H1/C_H2$ + light chain
Cγ2	(acid, trypsin)	223–338	C_H2
(Cγ2)$_2$	(acid, trypsin)	223–338	(C_H2) dimer
pFc'	(pepsin)	334–446	(C_H3) dimer
Fc'	(papain)	342–433	(C_H3) dimer
tFc'	(pepsin, trypsin)	341–446	(C_H3) dimer
atCγ3	(acid, trypsin)	345–439	(C_H3) dimer

Heavy Chain Disease Proteins

The H chain counterparts of BJP are termed Heavy Chain Disease (HCD) proteins and consist of monoclonal H chains, which have partial deletions of domains or of the hinge region [39,40,41]. Such deletions may prevent the usual pairing of H and L chains and thus account for the synthesis and secretion of HCD proteins. HCD proteins occur as part of a rare lymphoma-like syndrome and have been reported for IgG, IgA, IgM, and IgD H chain classes, with IgA HCD being the most common [39,443].

Amyloid

Many types of amyloid protein have been shown to consist of fragments of Ig L chains that form the huge eosinophilic, macroscopically featureless aggregates characteristic of amyloidosis [42]. As L chain amyloidosis is a frequent accompaniment of multiple myeloma, it may be considered to be the tissue analog of Bence Jones proteinuria. Amyloidosis may also occur independently of an identifiable disorder, or may accompany chronic disease states such as a rheumatoid arthritis, ankylosing spondylitis, tuberculosis, leprosy, and osteomyelitis. Amyloidosis associated with infectious disease may result from the ineffective metabolism and clearing of Ig chronically deposited in antigen-laden tissues [43].

Hinge

The hinge region is a structurally important H chain sequence which separates the CH_1 and CH_2 domains in IgG, IgA, and IgD. It ranges in length from 12 residues in human IgG_2 to 64 residues in human IgD [44,45]. The two human IgA subclasses have hinges of intermediate length ($IgA_1 = 29$ residues and $IgA_2 = 16$ residues) [44]. Both IgM and IgE lack a hinge and have in its place an "extra" constant domain [44]. The hinge region in IgG, IgD and IgA contains the intra-H chain disulfide bonds that join both H chains. (IgA may contain a second intra-H chain disulfide bond in CH_2) [46]. Hinge regions are characteristically rich in proline residues that greatly restrict conformational mobility. Such restriction may contribute to the ability of the hinge to act as a swivel point about which the Fab arms move [189]. Electron micrographs of IgG antibodies show that the angle between Fab arms can vary from nearly 0° to 180° [48]. Yguerabide et al., have shown that the Fab arms of antibodies in solution normally move relative to the Fc through a 30° range within nanoseconds [47]. When Fab arms bind to antigen, and are thus restricted in their movement and fixed in position, resultant sheer forces may be transmitted through the relatively rigid hinge to effector structures in the Fc region [189]. Studies by Schlessinger et al., indicate that when bivalent antigen binds to IgG, tryptophan residues located in the Fc region experience a change in their chemical environment, as evidenced by changes in their circular polarization of luminescence (CPL) [49]. Exposure to univalent antigen does not produce similar Fc effects, while reduction and alkylation of the intraheavy chain disulfide bonds abolishes these CPL changes, indicating that the hinge region is critical for allosteric force transmission to Fc structures.

THREE-DIMENSIONAL STRUCTURE OF IMMUNOGLOBULINS

The Immunoglobulin Fold

Both L and H chains are composed of egg-shaped structural units termed domains which consist of a linear sequence of 100 to 110 amino acids internally stabilized by two disulfide-bonded cysteine residues [12]. The secondary and tertiary structures of both C and V domains has been termed the "Ig fold" and consists of seven polypeptide strands with antiparallel β-pleated sheet structure [50].

Variable domains have, in addition, two extra strands, S_4 and S_5, which form a loop between strands S_3 and S_6 (Fig. 4). The seven C domain strands form two layers that curve to form a slightly flattened cylinder. The "top" layer includes S_3, S_8, and S_9, which fold over the bottom layer formed by S_1, S_2, S_6, and S_7. Both layers are connected by the single disulfide bond formed by two noncontiguous cysteines located in S_2 and S_8.

Although C and V domains have a low degree of amino acid sequence homology, their tertiary structures are surprisingly similar. Comparisons of the relative spatial positions of 85 alpha-carbon atoms of a human C and V domain, for example, revealed a root-mean-square displacement of less than

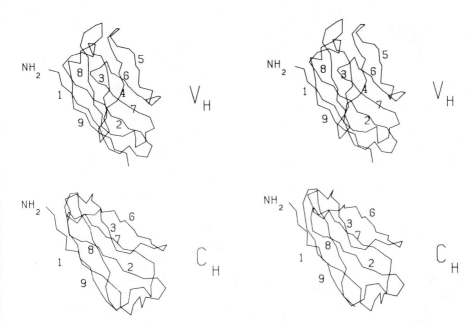

Fig. 4.   Stereo view of V_H and C_H domains to illustrate the immunoglobulin fold. The nine β-strands that characterize V domains are numbered sequentially beginning at the NH_2-terminal residue. The C_H domain has homologous β-strand structure, but lacks the extra loop of V domains formed by strands 4 and 5. With the exception of the extra loop, both V_H and C_H strands are nearly superimposable. Both V and C domain images represent the α-carbon polypeptide backbone of the V_H and CH_3 domains of IgG Dob. Atomic coordinates of IgG Dob were kindly provided by Dr. Enid Silverton [52]. Unless otherwise noted all computer-generated stereo images were produced using the molecular modeling system (MMS) in the UCSD Department of Chemistry's Research Resource Computer Facility. The MMS includes an Evans and Southerland Picture System controlled by a DEC PDP 11/40 computer, Zeta Model 3600 plotter, and MMS graphics software written by Steve Dempsey. Stereo images may be viewed using inexpensive stereo viewers, which may be purchased from Hubbard Scientific Company, P.O. Box 105, Northbrook, IL 60062; or from Abrams Instrument Corporation, 606 East Shiawasse Street, Lansing, MI 48901. Alternatively, it is easy to learn to "fuse" paired stereo images without optical aids by holding the images at arms length and staring at a distant object beyond the images. The viewer will perceive four out of focus images. The center two images must be superimposed to perceive the three-dimensional aspects of the image. With 15–30 minutes practice, most people will be capable "fusers."

1.5 Å [51]. Similar comparisons between domains from different species reveal the same degree of structural homology. Figure 5 shows the α-carbon backbone of V and C domains of the IgG_1 myeloma Dob. Except for the extra loop of the V domain, the β-strand structure of all four domains are superimposable. The variation between domains largely occurs in the bend regions which connect contiguous β-strands.

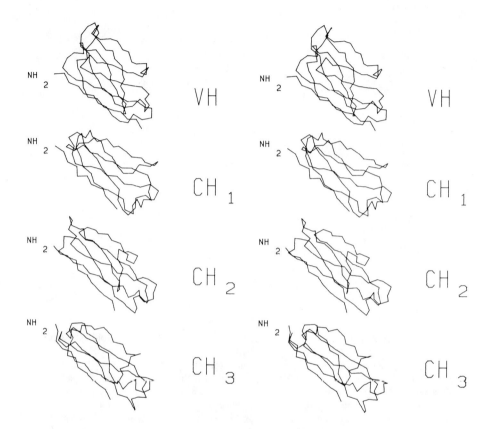

Fig. 5.   Stereo view of V_H, CH_1, CH_2, and CH_3 α-carbon backbones from IgG Dob. The β-pleated sheet structure of all four domains is seen to be highly conserved. Most of the structural variation occurs in the bends that connect contiguous β-strands.

Variable Domains

The hypervariable regions of V domains are located in areas of the Ig fold able to accommodate large changes in amino acid size and charge without significantly changing the domain's tertiary structure [29]. The three HV regions of V_L domains are loops 5 to 15 residues in length which connect strands S_2 and S_3 (HV_1), S_3 and S_6 (HV_2), and S_8 and S_9 (HV_3) [53]. HV regions of V_H domains occur at homologous loop regions and, in addition, include HV He, which exhibits less variability than the other three HV regions and connects S_7 and S_8 [54,55]. When V_L and V_H domains combine to form an intact antigen-binding unit, side chains of amino acids located within the CDR HV regions point towards the dimer interior and thus line the cleft that forms the antigen-combining site [27,28]. The depth of the cleft and therefore the size of the antigenic determinant which may be accommodated may vary depending on the length of the CDR regions [29,56]. Studies using synthetic antigens of known dimensions indicate that protein antigenic determinants (i.e., epitopes) are approximately three to six amino acid residues in length [57].

The three CDR HV regions are illustrated in Figure 6 in which the V_L/V_H dimer of the IgG_1 Kol myeloma is displayed. The amino acid side chains of the CDR HV region residues are visible, while the positions of the remaining polypeptide chains are shown by a line connecting the alpha carbons.

Figure 7 shows the HV region side chains as they exist in the intact $F(ab')_2$ fragment of IgG Kol. The side chains from the CDR HV region residues are seen to form a "patch" at the ends of both Fab arms. Only a few of the CDR residues visible directly interact with antigen while other CDR residues may themselves act as antigenic determinants of other antibodies and thus serve as idiotypic determinants.

Figure 8 shows the complete α-carbon backbone of the IgG_1 Dob myeloma protein. The two Fab arms are completely open and form an angle of about 180°. Since the Dob myeloma lacks the 15 residue hinge segment which normally separates the $C_\gamma 1$ and $C_\gamma 2$ domains, the molecule is shorter than normal IgG molecules [59].

Immunoglobulin Carbohydrates

All five classes of human Igs contain oligosaccharides covalently bonded to amino acids of the polypeptide chains [16,17]. In all instances, the oligosaccharides are linked to either asparagine (Asn), serine (Ser), or threonine (Thr) residues found in highly conserved carbohydrate "acceptor" sequences which have the form Asn-X-Ser/Thr, where X is any amino acid [60]. Most frequently the asparagine is linked by its amide nitrogen through an N-glycosidic bond to an N-acetylglucosamine residue of the oligosaccharide, although occasionally a serine hydroxyl group forms an O- glycosidic bond with galactosamine. The remainder of the oligosaccharide consists of several branched chains of N-acetylglucosamine, mannose, fucose, galactose, and N-acetylneuraminic acid (sialiac acid). The single oligosaccharide at aa 297 in IgG H chains, for example, consists of nine carbohydrate residues; four of N-acetylglucosamine, three of mannose, and one each of fucose and galactose, which form three branches (Fig. 9).

Oligosaccharides are thought to be coupled to Igs by site-specific transglycosylases located in the smooth endoplasmic reticulum and Golgi apparatus. Initial linkage of several carbohydrate residues may occur rapidly after polypeptide synthesis with additional residues being added during the final secretory steps within the Golgi apparatus [62].

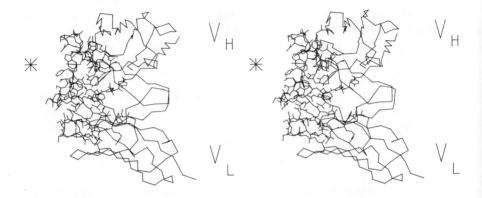

Fig. 6. Stereo view of the intact V_L/V_H dimer of IgG Kol. The amino acid side chains of the three complementary-determining HV regions are displayed, while the remainder of the residues are shown in α-carbon backbone form. The star marks the position of the putative hapten-binding site which is largely filled with aromatic amino acid side chains (tryptophan, tyrosine, and histadine). (Atomic coordinates of the IgG Kol F(ab')$_2$ fragment were kindly provided by Dr. Markus Marquart [58].)

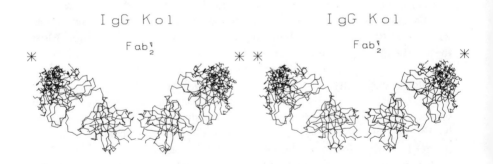

Fig. 7. Stereo view of the intact IgG Kol F(ab')$_2$ fragment. The amino acid side chains of the three complementary-determining HV regions are displayed while the remainder of the residues are shown in α-carbon backbone form. The star marks the position of the putative hapten-binding site. The CDR side chains form a diffuse "patch" at the ends of both Fab arms. The potential complexity of CDR-associated idiotypic determinants is illustrated by the relatively large surface area defined by CDR residues.

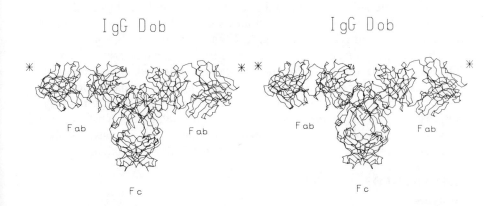

Fig. 8.   Stereo view of the intact IgG Dob α-carbon backbone. The fifteen residue hinge deletion in IgG Dob reduces the distance between the CH_1 and CH_2 domains, resulting in the inability of Dob to activate complement or bind to certain classes of macrophage Fc receptors. The star marks the position of the putative Dob hapten-binding site.

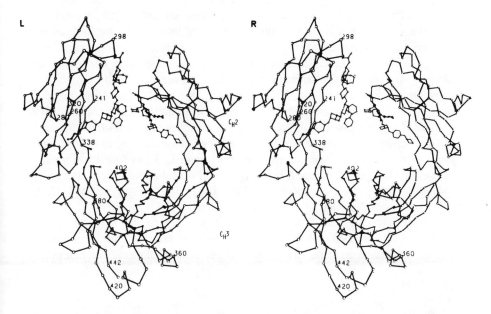

Fig. 9.   Stereo view of the α-carbon backbone of an intact human IgG Fc fragment. The branched oligosaccharide linked to both CH_2 domains at Asn 297 is visible and prevents direct CH_2/CH_2 contact. (Reproduced with permission from Deisenhofer [61].)

As illustrated in Figure 10, all five classes of Ig H-chains have oligosaccharide linkage sites, some of which occur in exactly homologous domain locations. Occasionally, oligosaccharides are found in the hinge regions as occurs in IgA_1 and IgD and, rarely, in H chain V domains [44–46].

The biological function of oligosaccharides in Igs is unknown. Oligosaccharides may be important for the intracellular transport and secretion of intact Igs. They may also act as bulky "spacers" to separate adjacent domains, as they do between the two CH_2 domains of IgG (Fig. 9). Alternatively, oligosaccharides may simply increase a protein's solubility. Whatever role oligosaccharides play, their high degree of conservation implies that they have an important, perhaps as yet undiscovered biologic function.

IMMUNOGLOBULIN GENETICS

Isotypes

Antisera directed against determinants of H and L chains have revealed that antigenic differences may exist within a particular class. Amino acid sequencing has demonstrated that many of these antigenic differences reflect the presence within each genome of closely related genes that code for similar gene products. L chains, for example, have separate gene loci in each haploid chromosome which code for κ and λ C_L domains [64]. The presence of multiple copies of related structural genes within a single haploid set of chromosomes is termed isotypy and the related gene products are called isotypes. Thus $C\kappa$ and $C\lambda$ domains are C_L domain isotypes. In humans, four isotypic subtypes of $C\lambda$ domains are known and are defined by amino and substitutions in the monoclonal L chains Oz, Kern, Mz, and Mcg, respectively [65]. Only one isotype of the human $C\kappa$ domain is known. Similarly, the five H chain classes γ, α, μ, δ, and ε are isotypes of each other. Several of the H chain classes have isotypic forms, called subclasses, to reflect their high degree of relatedness to each other. Human IgG has four known subclasses: IgG_1, IgG_2, IgG_3, and IgG_4. IgA has two subclasses: IgA_1 and IgA_2 [44]. IgM may have two isotypic variants [66] while no isotypes of IgD or IgE have been identified.

Characteristically, all isotypic forms of a molecule are simultaneously expressed in a particular individual, however the relative amounts of each isotype expressed may be subject to independent regulation. For example, polysaccharide antigens may preferentially elicit synthesis of the IgG_2 subclass [67].

Allotypes

Different structural forms of L and H chains also result from allotypic variation. Molecular allotypes result from the presence of multiple alleles which occur at single gene loci [1]. Two different allotypes may therefore

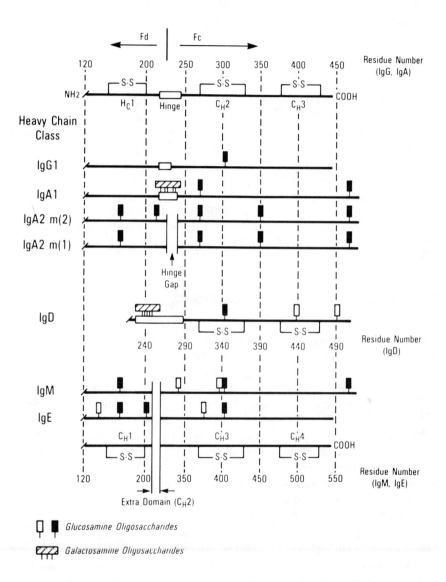

Fig. 10.   Carbohydrate locations in heavy chains of human IgG, IgA, IgM, IgD, and IgE. Vertical rectangles represent glucosamine oligosaccharides while horizontal rectangles represent multiple galactosamine oligosaccharides. Shaded vertical rectangles indicate oligosaccharides with homologous domain positions in two or more chains. The "extra" CH2 domains of IgM and IgE have been omitted to facilitate comparisons. (Redrawn after Torano et al. [60]. IgD data from Takayasu et al. [63], Lin and Putnam [157] and Shinoda et al. [155].)

exist in a normal diploid set of chromosomes. This implies that allotypic variants will be inherited in a codominant pattern when the gene loci occur on autosomal chromosomes. Many allotypic variants of human Igs are known. Those for which the amino acid substitutions are known are listed in Table II.

Idiotypes

When Igs directed against a single antigenic determinant are purified and injected into a different animal, antisera directed against V region determinants closely associated with the CDR HV regions may be generated. These determinants are associated with a particular V region specificity and are called idiotypic determinants or idiotypes [68]. They include amino acid residues in and surrounding the CDR HV regions [69]. Anti-idiotypic antisera have proved to be very useful in detecting T and B lymphocytes having antigen receptors for a specific antigen [70]. It must be emphasized, however, that such antigenic crossreactivity does not necessarily imply identity of the V regions used to generate the antisera with the antigen receptors on lymphocytes [71].

GENETIC BASIS FOR IMMUNE DIVERSITY

In an effort to explain the incredible diversity of Ig antigen specificities, three general mechanisms have been suggested. The first, termed the "germ line theory," holds that each antigen specificity is coded for by a separate V region gene [72]. This theory required the presence of thousands if not millions of separate V region genes to account for the observed diversity.

Two other "somatic generation" theories suggest that diverse V regions are generated, during embryogenesis and cellular differention, from a very small number of original germ line V genes. Two classes of mechanisms were proposed to somatically generate diversity. The "somatic mutation" theory proposed that a high rate of point mutations or recombinational events within V domains generated the sequence variation of the CDRs [73,74]. The observed clustering of variability in HV regions, however, could not be explained by this process alone. A second somatic mechanism, championed by Kabat, proposed that separate "minigenes" coded for HV regions and framework regions that were combined through a process of gene splicing to form an intact V region gene [75,76]. Both theories, germ line and somatic generation, now appear to partially explain V gene diversity.

The concept that V and C domains might be coded by separate genes was first proposed by Dreyer and Bennett in 1965 to explain how apparently identical V domains could occur simultaneously in several H chain classes [72]. It is now known that the structural genes for V and C domains are

TABLE II. Amino Acid Sequence Substitutions Associated with Human Immunoglobulin Allotypic Markers

Immuno-globulin chain	Domain	Allotype	Amino acid sequence				
γ_1	CH$_1$	G1m (3) or (f)	214 Arg				
		G1m (17) or (z)	214 Lys				
	CH$_3$	G1m (1) or (a)	355 Arg	356 Asp	357 Glu	358 Leu	
		G1m (1−) or (non-a)	355 Arg	356 Glu	357 Glu	358 Met	
γ_3	CH$_2$	G3m (21) or (g)	296 Tyr				
		G3m (21−) or (non-g)	296 Phe				
	CH$_3$	G3m (11) or (bO)	436 Phe				
		G3m (11−) or (non-bO)	436 Tyr				
γ_4	CH$_2$	[a]G4m (a)	309 Val	310 Leu	311 His		
		[a]G4m (b)	309 Val	310 ---	311 His		
	CH$_3$	[a]G4m (non-a)	355 Gln	356 Glu	357 Glu	358 Met	
α_2	CH$_1$	A2m (1)	212 Pro	221 Pro			
		A2m (2)	212 Ser	221 Arg			
			112	114	152	163	190
λ	C$_\lambda$	Kern (−), Oz (−), mcg (−)	Ala	Ser	Ser	Thr	Arg
		[b]Kern (+), Oz (−), mcg (−)	Ala	Ser	Gly	Thr	Arg
		[b]Kern (−), Oz (+), mcg (−)	Ala	Ser	Ser	Thr	Lys
		[b]Kern (+), Oz (−), mcg (+)	Asn	Thr	Gly	Lys	Arg
κ	C$_\kappa$	[c]Km (1 +, 2 −, 3 −)	153 Val				191 Leu
		[c]Km (1 +, 2 +, 3 −)	Ala				Leu
		[c]Km (1 −, 2 −, 3 +)	Ala				Val

[a]Isoallotypic determinant.
[b]Isotypic determinant.
[c]Formerly called Inv.

Allotypic markers in human immunoglobulins have been found in IgG, IgA, and κ-light chains. They result from amino acid substitutions which occur in allelic structural genes. In addition to allotypic markers which are restricted to a particular immunoglobulin subclass, isoallotypic markers act as allotypic markers within a single subclass and are present in all members of a different subclass. Allotypes are designated by their heavy (or light) chain class, e.g. G or K (for κ), followed by the subclass number, "m" (for "marker") and the numeric or letter designator in parentheses. Data taken from [1,44,65,326,444].

indeed separately coded and occur in three unlinked gene clusters in all mammals studied [77]. Each cluster contains both the V and C domain genes for either κ-, λ-, or H chain genes.

The nucleotide arrangement of a murine L chain gene was first reported by Brack in 1978 [87]. Examination of the germ line V_L gene revealed the existence of two distinct, separately coded gene segments. The first segment codes for aa 1–95 of the V_L domain (Kabat numbering system) [44] and therefore includes the first two CDR and two residues of the third CDR [44]. The second segment, termed J or joining segment, codes for 13 to 15 residues, which include the remainder of the third CDR [83].

Comparison between the germ line V_L gene and its form as expressed in a differentiated myeloma plasma cell revealed that in the plasma cell, the V and J segments were joined to form a continuous V gene.

The C_L gene, by contrast, remained separated from the V_{L1-95} and J genes in both the germ line and differented cells, implying that it must be joined to the V_L domain after the DNA had been transcribed into RNA. Subsequent gene cloning and sequencing of murine Ig genes have pieced together the sequence of events leading to intact V and C domain synthesis.

Light Chain Gene Assembly

It is now known that the κ- and λ-germline gene clusters have a very similar structure. In mice, the κ- and λ-clusters consist of multiple V region genes which code for aa 1–95, five J segment "minigenes," four of which are functional and multiple C genes which code for Cκ and Cλ isotypes [64,78,79]. Figure 11 shows these genes as they are linearly arranged in each cluster. Current evidence indicates that the murine κ-cluster contains up to 300 distinct V region genes [81] each of which is flanked by nontranscribed segments of DNA called intervening sequences or "introns," which contain specific sequences recognized by DNA "splicing" enzymes [82]. J segments [83] and C domains [84], which are coded by transcribed segments termed "exons," are similarly flanked by introns of varying length. Estimates of the number of human Vκ genes, by contrast, indicate that only 15 to 20 Vκ genes exist in each germline [85]. These findings are consistent with the suggestion that humans and mice use different mechanisms to generate antibody diversity. According to Burnet, small, short-lived animals like mice may rely on a large number of germline V genes with relatively limited somatic mutation while larger, long-lived animals like humans may have a small number of germline V genes that accumulate extensive somatic mutations and thereby generate diversity [86].

Two types of somatic recombination (gene splicing) are required to produce an intact L chain [87]. The first recombinational event occurs in embryogenesis during pre-B lymphocyte differentiation. This event, termed "V-

MURINE CHROMOSOME 6

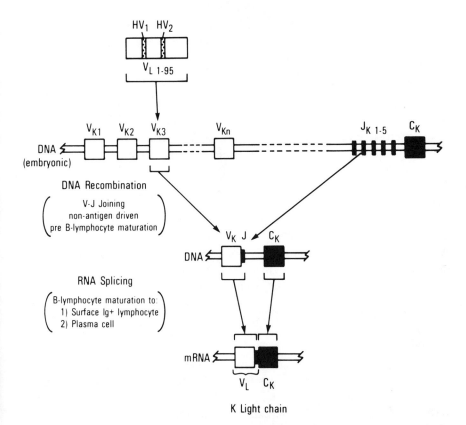

Fig. 11. Light chain gene assembly begins when embryonic DNA exons coding for a V region and J segment undergo random recombination producing a contiguous V-J DNA exon. DNA segments between the V and J segments are excised during the recombination. This first recombination event occurs independent of exposure to antigen during pre-B-lymphocyte maturation. The resultant V-J exon and J segment-associated C_κ or C_λ exons are then translated into RNA and subsequently joined by RNA splicing enzymes to form a continuous mRNA exon formed from the V, J, and C_L exons. The mRNA thus produced is continuously translated into an intact light chain. (Redrawn after Marx [80].)

J" joining, begins when site-specific DNA recombinases recognize small DNA sequences in the intron immediately adjacent to a single V and J gene. The recombinase then cuts the DNA adjacent to the recognition point and splices the V and J genes into a single continuous DNA strand. The selection of a particular V and J gene for splicing apparently occurs at random within a particular pre-B cell.

The second recombinational event leading to an intact L chain occurs after the V-J DNA segment is transcribed into RNA. Site-specific RNA splicing enzymes recognize intronic RNA sequences adjacent to the V-J segment and a $C\kappa$ or $C\lambda$ gene and splices them together to form a single messenger RNA which codes for an intact L chain [87].

Heavy Chain Gene Assembly

The events leading to the production of an intact H chain closely resemble those which produce L chains. V_H domains, in contrast to V_L domains, are constructed from three separate DNA exons: V_{H1-95}, which codes for V_H aa 1–95 [88]; a "D" or diversity-generating segment, which codes for 3–15 amino acids at the beginning of CDR 3 [89]; and a J segment, which codes for 13–15 residues and constitutes the remainder of CDR 3 and the V_H framework [90].

The first recombinational event of V_H genes results in the joining of a single V_{H1-95}, D and J segment into a single DNA transcript and thus resembles V_L joining [91,92]. (Fig. 12). After transcription, RNA splicing enzymes join the intact V_H segment with the first C domain group within the H chain cluster, which is the μ chain. The fact that IgM H chain genes are first in the cluster ensures that IgM is the first H chain class expressed by developing B lymphocytes [97].

Diversity of Antigen Specificity

Using current estimates of the number of exons which are assembled into intact V_L and V_H domains in mice, simple calculations can provide a minimum estimate of the number of Fab antigen specificities possible. Since approximately 300 $V_L\kappa_{1-95}$ and 4 functional J segment exons are thought to exist, $(4) \times (300) = 1200$ different $V_L\kappa$ domains are possible. If we assume that mice also have approximately 300 V_{H1-95} exons, then random combination with 4 J segments and 5 D segments produce $(300) \times (4) \times (5) = 6000$ different V_H domains. When 1200 possible $V_L\kappa$ domains from L chains combine with 6000 possible V_H domains to form a functional Fab arm, $(1200) \times (6000) = 7,200,000$ different antigen specificities may be produced. This number is probably a low estimate since mutations due to errors in V-J and V-D-J joining [98] and spontaneous point mutations of CDR and V framework residues [99,100] are known to contribute to diversity and have not been considered in these calculations.

An important as yet unanswered question concerns how the clusters of variability in the first two CDRs and HV He are produced. It is clear that variability in the third CDR derives from the J and D segments and their combination with V_{1-95} exons. The first two CDRs and HV He, however,

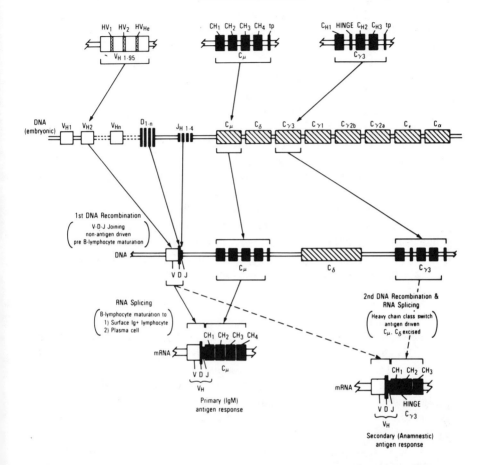

Fig. 12. Heavy chain gene assembly begins with the recombination of three embryonic DNA exons: a V region, D, and J segments. The V-D-J joining process is similar to light chain assembly in that intervening intronic DNA is excised to produce a continuous V/D/J exon adjacent to the J-segment-associated constant domain cluster. This process occurs during the maturation of all pre-B lymphocytes independent of antigen exposure. After transcription of pre-B lymphocyte DNA into RNA, heavy chain class-specific RNA splicing enzymes join the intact V region with the μ-constant domain cluster which is immediately 3′ or "downstream" from the J-segment cluster to form mRNA, which is subsequently translated. After exposure of the IgM-synthesizing B lymphocyte to antigen, a second DNA recombinational event may occur during which the intact V region exon is joined with one of the other heavy chain classes 3′ to the μ-cluster, e.g., Cγ3. Intervening DNA is excised with subsequent RNA splicing to produce an intact IgG₃ mRNA that lacks the exon which codes for the hydrophobic tailpiece (tp).

exist within germline DNA as an intact, linear DNA sequence of V_L and V_H exons. Kabat has suggested that minigenes may have indeed coded for CDR 1, CDR 2, and HV He at some time in the evolutionary past and subsequently became stabilized within the exons in reduplicated V domains [75,76]. This concept gains support from the finding of potential palindromic nucleotide sequences flanking CDRs 1 and 2 in a human $V\kappa$ domain [101]. Such palindromic sequences might act as sites for spontaneous recombination during meiosis [102]. Alternatively, there may exist an as yet uncharacterized localized mutational mechanism which produces mutational "hot spots" at CDR sites [64,81,99]. Finally, it has been suggested that the variability within V_{1-95} simply reflects the fact that CDR and HV He occur at domain locations which can accommodate amino acid variability without significantly distorting the basic polypeptide folding pattern of the domain [29,56]. Hypervariability may therefore reflect mutations accumulated over the evolutionary time span which proved to be "acceptable" to the domain's structure. The continued retention of CDR mutations in the germline would occur, according to this reasoning, because they allowed new antigens to be recognized by the immune system, thus giving an organism that retained such mutant V exons a selective advantage during evolution.

Heavy Chain Class Switch

Unlike L chains, whose differentiation within B lymphocytes is complete after the second recombinational event, a single B lymphocyte may express different H chain classes, each of which are associated with a single, identical V_H domain [103]. For example, a developing B lymphocyte first expresses the membrane form of IgM, followed by the simultaneous expression of IgM and IgD having identical V_H domains [104]. The final step of differentiation appears to involve the commitment of the cell to synthesis of one of the five H chain classes, again using the identical V_H domain. The mechanism producing the H chain class "switch recombination" involves a third recombinational event very similar to those which produce V-D-J joining. H chain class-specific DNA recombinases produce switching by joining the assembled V_H gene, located immediately 5' to the $C\mu$ gene cluster to the genes coding for γ-, ε- or α-H chains (105). The intervening DNA segments, including μ, δ, and exons 5' to the expressed class are deleted during the switch process [95]. A plasma cell that secretes IgE is therefore irreversibly committed to its synthesis since all other H chain genes have been deleted.

The switching mechanism that produces simultaneous expression of both IgM and IgD in immature B lymphocytes, by contrast, does not involve deletion of μ-exons. Instead, the DNA containing the assembled V_H gene, and μ- and δ-exons are continuously transcribed to produce a single precursor mRNA containing both μ- and δ-gene clusters [97]. Subsequent splicing by μ- and δ-specific RNA recombinases join the V_H gene to both the μ- and δ-genes to produce mRNA for each H chain class. Translation of both mRNAs produces the simultaneous expression of both IgM and IgD having identical antigen specificty.

Allelic Exclusion

Allelic exclusion is the phenomenon observed in Ig expression in which only one of a cell's homologous chromosomes express Ig structural genes [106]. This is in contrast to all other autosomal chromosomes that express both homologous gene products in a codominant fashion. Only the "X" sex-determining chromosomes demonstrate allelic exclusion, by a process known as Lyonization in which one of a cell's two X chromosomes becomes completely inactivated [107]. The inactivation process involves the physical condensation and repacking of the entire chromosome into nonfunctional "Barr bodies" and must be very different from Ig allelic exclusion, since condensation of autosomal chromosomes is not observed.

Studies of human B lymphocyte leukemia cells, by Heiter et al. indicate that isotypic (κ versus λ) and allelic (one κ-chromosome versus the homologous κ-chromosome) occur in the following manner [108]. The rearrangement of V_{L1-95} and J exons occurs in a hierarchical order in which Vκ precedes Vλ rearrangement. The order of rearrangements in both homologous chromosomes (CHR) is then: Vκ (CHR1) → Vκ (CHR2) → Vλ (CHR1) → Vλ (CHR2). If the first Vκ rearrangement (Vκ CHR1) produces a functional V gene, then further gene rearrangements cease and a complete light chain is synthesized. If a nonfunctional V gene is produced, however, then it is not transcribed and may be deleted, whereupon a second Vκ allele (Vκ CHR2) is rearranged. Rearrangement continues until either a functional V-J joining is achieved or all four chromosomal Vκ and Vλ sites have been exhausted, at which point the cell cannot synthesize L chains. The fate of such aberrant cells is unknown.

Unicellular Biclonal Gammopathies

In apparent violation of the rule of isotypic exclusion are those rare patients who simultaneously produce myeloma proteins belonging to two different H or L chain isotypes. Such "double myelomas" or "biclonal gammopathies" are exceedingly rare and usually represent synthesis by two distinct cellular clones. A statistical analysis of 6141 cases of productive myelomas by Bouvet et al. revealed that only 60 (0.98%) patients produced two distinct myeloma proteins [109]. A similar study by Bachmann identified only 7 out of 585 patients (1.20%) producing two myeloma components [110]. In a few instances, double myelomas have been observed to share antigenically identical idiotypes suggesting that the myeloma proteins originated from a single cellular clone. Double myelomas suspected of having a unicellular origin include IgM and IgG$_3$ [111]; IgG and IgA [112]; IgG$_1$ (κ) and IgG$_1$ (λ) [113]; and IgM and IgG$_2$ [114].

Extensive studies of murine myeloma cell lines also demonstrate the rare spontaneous development of double myelomas. Morse et al. examined 778 consecutive murine plasmacytomas and found 54 that produced multiple Ig classes. Of these 54, 52 represented simultaneously occurring independent myeloma clones while only two represented single clones producing two different paraproteins [115].

The genetic basis of double myeloma-producing plasma cell tumors is unclear. The observation that immature B lymphocytes simultaneously express two H chain isotypes on their plasma membrane offers a normal precedent for such double expression, however, and suggests that a defective class switch mechanism may be involved [103,104]. It is possible that mutations in the class switching-DNA recombinases or their intronic DNA recognition sites might prevent deletion of appropriate H chain exons. Transcription of such aberrant DNA might then produce a pre-mRNA transcript containing H chain genes of two classes, as has been proposed for simultaneous IgM and IgD expression [97]. Subsequent RNA splicing of the single V region with both H chain gene clusters would then produce the two different H chain classes which characterize double myelomas.

Alternatively, long-lived mRNA from a deleted H chain class may persist and be translated. This possibility seems unlikely, however, since double myelomas have been propagated through multiple generations and would be expected to lose such RNA during cytoplasmic dilution during cell division [97,116,117]. A third model proposes that one H chain gene on each of the two homologous chromosomes may become simultaneously expressed and may then be recombined with a single V region [116,117].

Mutant Immunoglobulins

In 1963 Franklin reported the first mutant Ig, a human IgG HCD protein [39]. Since that report, many human and animal Igs having mutations of both L and H chains have been characterized and sequenced. Several distinct mutational patterns have been observed and can be understood as errors of genetic recombination. Four major classes of Ig mutations include domain deletions, hinge deletions, point mutations, and intra-H chain recombination.

Domain Deletions

The most frequently detected mutant Igs are HCD proteins having internal deletions of part of the V$_H$ domain and all of the CH$_1$ domain [39]. The normal sequence of such mutants generally continues at the beginning of the hinge sequence at aa 216 in IgG [40]. Other human and murine mutant Igs lacking entire domains have deletions of all of V_H and CH_1 [41]; CH_1, CH_3, or the V_L domain [39]. All of these mutations are similar in that the deleted segment is identical to a separately coded domain exon or terminates at the end of an exon [84]. These mutations probably result from errors of exon recombination during RNA splicing. For example, a mutation in the intron adjacent to a heavy chain constant domain could destroy the recognition site for RNA splicing enzymes and thus prevent that domain from being incorporated into H chain mRNA.

Hinge Deletions

Several human Igs having deletions of the entire hinge region have been isolated and include IgG Dob, IgG Lec and IgG Mcg [59]. They all lack aa 216–230 of the H chain, which is identical to the hinge exon as defined by murine IgG gene mapping [84]. These deletions, like mutants with domain deletions, probably result from mutations of the intronic segments which flank the hinge and domain exons. The lack of a hinge region considerably restricts the conformational mobility of these molecules [118]. The resultant rigidity of one of these mutants (Dob) allowed the molecules to pack together to form a crystalline lattice sufficiently stable to produce a high resolution x-ray diffraction pattern. These data enabled Silverton et al. to produce the first molecular model of an intact IgG molecule at 6-Å resolution [53] (Fig. 8).

Molecules of the human IgG_3 subclass that normally represent about 4–8% of plasma IgG may be considered to be a mutant Ig that became fixed in the human genome. The normal IgG_3 hinge is a 62 residue segment which consists of a 17 residue segment followed by three identical 15 residue segments that are consecutively repeated [119]. The 17 residue segment is 67% homologous to the hinge of IgG_1 while each 15 residue reduplicated segment is 67% homologous to the IgG_1 hinge. It is probable that the IgG_3 hinge originated as a mutant in which tandem quadruplication of a 15 residue hinge segment occurred. Alternatively, the quadruplicated segment could have been formed by a series of unequal crossing over between normal IgG_1 hinge genes.

Point Mutations

Point mutations occur when one purine or pyrimidine base is substituted for another during DNA replication or transcription, and it may produce several types of mutations. A "silent" mutation having no amino acid change occurs when the base substitution results in a codon that still codes for the same amino acid [120].

The most frequent "visible" result of point mutations is a different amino acid at that position. Most of the variability of CDR_1 and CDR_2 in both V_L and V_H domains probably results from point mutations, possibly caused by an unknown mechanism to concentrate the mutations at the CDR sites [98–100]. Point mutations that result in a base deletion or insertion cause a "frameshift" mutation in which each codon reading frame 3' to the mutation is shifted, resulting in different amino acid residues at all shifted codon positions. Frameshift mutations are common at the junctions of V, J, and D segments and might substantially contribute to V region diversity [98]. Point mutations which generate so-called "nonsense" or "stop" codons terminate RNA translation and may result in an abnormally short polypeptide chain. Alternatively, if a point mutation occurs within a stop codon and results in a codon for an amino acid, the polypeptide chain will be elongated and will contain residues coded for in the adjacent intron. Several elongated Ig chains have been isolated that may represent such a mutation [39].

Intraheavy Chain Recombinants

The fourth class of defective Igs may be termed recombination mutants and have "hybrid" H chains constructed from domains of two H chain classes. These rare mutations have been observed in both human and murine Igs and usually involve the substitution of an entire "foreign" domain in place of the normal domain [121]. For example, Natvig and Kunkel described a hybrid human IgG_4/IgG_2 Ig in which a normal IgG_4 H chain had an IgG_2, CH_3 domain [122]. Such mutants probably result from a DNA crossover event between two Ig H chain genes at a site in the intron which separate domain exons [123,160].

Immunoglobulin Evolution

Ig-like molecules have been found in all vertebrate species [124]. Even the most primitive vertebrate fish, the lamprey and hagfish, synthesize antigen-inducible molecules directed towards a variety of complex antigens including sheep erythrocytes, keyhole limpet hemocyanin, Brucella abortus, and f-2 bacteriophages [125,126]. The hagfish antibody is a macroglobulin of about 10^6-dalton molecular weight composed of primarily 22,000-dalton L chain-like subunits [127]. Perhaps this molecule contains an analog of the V_L-V_L dimer, referred to earlier, which spontaneously forms from isolated human L chains. The antibody synthesized by the lamprey, by contrast, contains two 70,000-dalton H chains and two 25,000-dalton L chains and thus resembles modern Ig monomers [128]. Amino acid analysis of the lamprey antibody suggests that it is related to vertebrate H chains. According to these studies, the direct ancestors of the four-chain antibody may have evolved within primitive, jawless fish about 450 million years ago [128].

The cartilaginous fish, which include sharks, evolved about 350 million years ago and produce both monomeric and pentameric antibodies which closely resemble human IgM. Dogfish shark "IgM," for example, have molecular weights of 198,000 and 980,000 daltons, which dissociate after reduction and alkylation into 72,000-dalton heavy chains and 20,000-dalton L chains [128]. Nurse shark pentameric "IgM" proved to effectively activate bovine complement after binding to bacteria, indicating a high level of structural conservation with the region of bovine IgM that binds complement [129]. Shark pentameric IgM also contains a molecule resembling J chain that is absent in the monomeric form [130]. Partial amino acid sequence studies of shark antibody demonstrate significant homology with human V_L and V_H sequences and indicate that shark H chains are more closely related to mammalian H chains then they are to shark L chains [131]. This indicates that V_L and V_H domains must have diverged more than 400 million years ago.

The lungfish, an indirect ancestor of mammals, is the most primitive species having two distinct antibody classes: IgM and a smaller four-chain molecule with unique antigenic determinants [132]. Frogs, representing amphibians, also have an IgM-like molecule and, in addition, have two antigenically distinguishable classes of monomeric antibodies [133]. Salamanders, also members of the class amphibia, by contrast, have only a large molecular weight IgM antibody [134]. Reptiles, including turtles, evolved about 300 million years ago and have an IgM antibody and two low molecular weight antibody classes of 180,000 and 120,000 daltons [135]. The 120,000-dalton antibody appears to be antigenically related to the 180,000-dalton antibody but may lack two domains in its H chain.

Both birds and mammals evolved from reptiles about 180 million years ago and simultaneously developed a class of antibodies resembling IgA. Domestic chickens have an IgM that antigenically crossreacts with human IgM [136], an IgG-like antibody, and a secretory IgA-like antibody that combines with human secretory component [137]. Although antihuman IgA antiserum does not crossreact with chicken IgA, it does crossreact with IgA of over 90 mammalian species, indicating that it may be a characteristic mammalian antibody [138].

Antibodies mediating homocytotropic immediate-type hypersensitivity reactions are present in birds and in many mammals [138]. Because of the existence of homocytotropic IgG in many species, however, it is difficult to trace the evolutionary development of the IgE class without the benefit of amino acid sequence information. Pigeon homocytotropic antibody does resemble mammalian IgE, however, in its heat lability and long latency at passive cutaneous anaphylaxis (PCA) skin sites (14 days) and may represent avian IgE [139]. Antibodies having antigenic crossreactivity with human IgE exist in nearly all primates and in dogs [140] and rats [141].

IgD antibodies have been detected in all primates, mice, chickens, and possibly in the tortoise [105]. This indicates that IgD evolved shortly before the time that birds and mammals diverged from reptiles.

Evolutionary Relatedness From Amino Acid Homology

Estimates of the degree of relatedness of two proteins may be obtained by comparing their amino acid sequences. Such estimates are much more sensitive than serologic or functional analysis and allow detection of relatively distant evolutionary relationships. The likelihood that two proteins are evolutionarily related may be calculated by comparing the observed number of identical amino acids to the number of identities expected from chance matching alone based on each protein's amino acid composition [142]. More sensitive techniques developed by Fitch [143] and Barker and Dayhoff [144] detect relatedness by calculating the minimum number of mutations (Minimum Mutational Distance: MMD) required to convert one amino acid sequence to the other and comparing that number to the MMD observed between randomized sequences from both proteins.

These types of analysis led Hill et al. [13] and Singer and Doolittle [14], to propose that the most primitive evolutionary units of antibodies are 100 to 110 amino acid domains. Subsequent studies by many investigators have shown that Ig-type domains are evolutionary precursors of many immune system molecules, including all Ig H and L chains [144]; histocompatibility antigen H chain domains [147] and their L chain, β_2-microglobulin [148]; thy-1 antigen [149]; C-reactive protein [150]; thymopoietin [151] and the murine Qa antigens [152].

Some evidence exists suggesting that the basic Ig domain may, itself, be derived from precursor genes approximately one quarter to one half its size. Urbain was the first to demonstrate by statistical methods that Ig V and C domains contain internal repeated segments 20 to 30 residues long [153]. These findings were confirmed and extended by Wuilmart et al. using different statistical methods [154]. Recently, Shinoda et al. demonstrated that domains from all five human Ig classes can be divided into two segments that constitute the first and second half of each domain [155]. Both segments contain a half-cystine residue near the middle and are 50 to 60 residues in length. When both segments are aligned, 18–28% amino acid identities were observed, which is approximately equal to the homology observed when individual domains are compared. The authors concluded that Ig constant domains may have evolved from a primordial gene that coded for a segment about half of a domain in length. This conclusion is consistent with the observations of Hahn and Hamburger, who found that the 49 amino acid thymic hormone thymopoietin may be evolutionarily related to the carboxy-terminal half of rabbit $C\gamma3$, human $C\varepsilon4$ and HLA-B7 $\alpha3$, bovine β_2-microglobulin, and rat brain thy-1 antigen [151]. The gene for thymopoietin may represent a divergent evolutionary product of the putative half-domain Ig domain gene.

Using extensive computer analysis of Ig sequences, Barker et al. have proposed a likely series of evolutionary events that trace Ig development from single domains to intact H and L chains [156]. The recent availability of the human IgD sequence enabled Lin and Putnam to add IgD to this sequence [157]. In this model illustrated in Figure 13, a single primordial domain gene (which itself may be derived from a half domain gene) duplicates to form precursors of H and L chain constant domains. The H chain domain

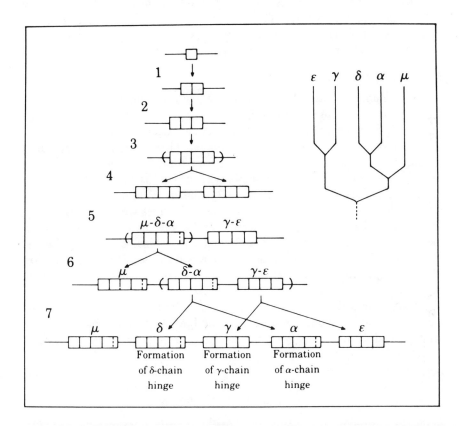

Fig. 13.   A hypothetical pathway depicting the possible evolutionary events which produced the five heavy chain classes. Each box represents a single immunoglobulin domain with intronic DNA segments being represented by a single line. In this scheme, the single primordial domain ancestor of immunoglobulins underwent a series of two equal and unequal duplications resulting in two ancestral chains; one common to μ-, δ-, and α-chains and the other common to γ- and ε-chains. Subsequent duplication and mutation led to the present five classes. (Reproduced from Lin and Putnam [157] with permission.)

gene then undergoes internal duplication producing a gene with two homologous domains. A partial internal duplication of the two domains produces a three-domain gene, followed by a second partial internal duplication which produces a four domain gene. A subsequent duplication produces two four domain genes; one of which evolves into the other μ-, δ-, and α-chains while the other evolves into γ- and ε-chains. The gene for the μ-, δ-, and α-chain then acquires a carboxy-terminal tailpiece, followed by its duplication to form the δ/α-ancestor. A complete duplication of the δ/α- and γ/ε-chains form the 5 H chain classes. The γ-, α-, and δ-genes next independently lose most of their second constant domain, leaving only a small hinge segment. The Ig "evolutionary tree" generated by Barker et al. (Fig. 14) summarizes both H and L chain development [156].

Evolution of the Hinge

The evolutionary origins of the Ig hinge have been unclear until recently. The obvious sequential relationship of the hinge to the "extra" domains of IgM and IgE prompted the suggestion by Putnam that the hinge may represent the evolutionary remnants of an ancient domain [158]. Recent evidence from the nucleotide sequence of murine Igs and from the recently sequenced human IgD hinge indicates that his hypothesis was correct. Tucker et al. compared the nucleotide sequences of murine IgG_{2b} and its 5' intron to a portion of the CH_1 domain and found that 38% of the nucleotides were identical [159]. This degree of homology is comparable to the 40% homology found when the nucleotide sequences of the CH_1 and CH_3 domains were compared. Yamawaki-Kataoka similarly found that the nucleotides of the hinge region of murine γ2a are homologous to those of the CH_2 domain of the murine μ-gene [160].

Putnam found that the human IgD hinge is homologous to a portion of the Cμ2 domain of human, mouse, and dog IgM. One 36 residue IgD hinge segment had 11 identities with human Cμ2, strongly implying a common evolutionary precursor [45]. On the basis of these data, it is likely that Ig hinge regions originated when an RNA splice-site adjacent to a primordial domain was shifted to a site within the domain, resulting in only a small fraction of the domain being translated [45,159,160].

BIOLOGICAL PROPERTIES OF IMMUNOGLOBULIN CLASSES
IgG Metabolism

IgG is the most plentiful antibody in humans, and it constitutes about 60 to 80% of the total Ig in plasma (Table III). The four subclasses of IgG have relative concentrations in adults as follows: IgG_1, 60%; IgG_2, 30%; IgG_3, 5% and IgG_4, 4% [165]. IgG has the distinction of having the longest half-

HEAVY CHAINS

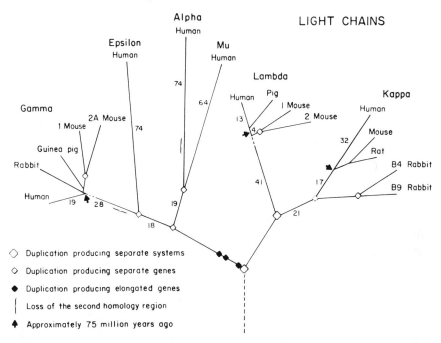

Fig. 14. Evolutionary tree of immunoglobulin C regions. The larger open diamonds on the tree represent duplications of entire genetic systems, which for the immunoglobulins includes V and C genes, a joining mechanism, and other control mechanisms. All of these components were present by the time of the divergence of heavy from light chains early in vertebrate evolution. Shortly after the heavy-light chain divergence, the heavy chain C-region gene underwent a series of internal duplications (represented by the solid diamonds) to produce a C gene four times the length of the light chain C gene. Duplications that produced C-region genes located on the same chromosome are indicated by the smaller open diamonds. Four of the five known classes of human heavy chains are represented here. All four, as well as both types of light chains were present well before the mammalian radiation about 75 million years ago. Most likely the alpha and gamma chain C genes have undergone a shortening by way of unequal crossing-over independently after their respective divergences from the mu and epsilon chains. Sequence data from nonmammalian vertebrates are needed to characterize these events more precisely. The position of the divergence of the rabbit kappa chains from the others is much earlier than expected and, therefore, it is postulated that it represents a gene duplication rather than a species divergence. Branch lengths are given in accepted point mutations per 100 residues. This tree is based on a matrix of estimated accepted point mutations between the sequences, derived from an alignment in which the human light chain C regions were repeated three times and aligned with the heavy chain C regions excluding the extra domains of mu and epsilon, the hinge regions of gamma and alpha, and the extra carboxyl-terminal piece of alpha and mu. The branches leading to the gamma and lambda subtrees are dashed because there were additional solutions almost as good as the minimal topologies shown. (Reproduced from Barker et al. [156] with permission.)

TABLE III. Normal Human Serum Immunoglobulin Concentrations

Age	IgG (mg/dL)	IgA (mg/dL)	IgM (mg/dL)	IgD (mg/mL)	IgE (IU/mL)
Neonates	1,004	<5	9	0.20	0.22
(cord blood)	(598–1,672)	(0–<5)	(6–15)	(0.13–0.31)	(0.04–1.28)
1–3 mo	365	32	24		0.69
	(218–610)	(20–53)	(11–51)		(0.08–6.12)
4–6 mo	381	44	38		2.68
	(228–636)	(27–72)	(25–60)		(0.44–16)
7–9 mo	488	44	47		2.36
	(292–816)	(27–73)	(12–124)		(0.76–7.3)
10–18 mo	640	67	56		3.49
	(383–1,070)	(27–169)	(28–113)		(0.80–15)
2 yr	780	89	65		3.03
	(423–1,184)	(35–222)	(32–131)		(0.31–29)
3 yr	798	100	57		1.80
	(477–1,334)	(40–251)	(28–116)		(0.19–17)
4 yr	906	120	41		8.58
	(542–1,515)	(48–301)	(20–82)		(1.07–69)
7	1,006	223	48		12.89
	(638–1,783)	(89–559)	(24–98)		(1.03–161)
10 yr	991	188	60		23.66
	(593–1,657)	(75–472)	(29–120)		(0.98–571)
14 yr	940	217	67	19[a]	20.1
	(562–1,571)	(86–544)	(33–135)	(0.76–479)	(2.1–195)
Adult	1,061	226	76	17[a]	13.2
	(635–1,775)	(106–668)	(37–154)	(1.02–274)	(1.53–114)

Because of the non-Gaussian distribution of serum immunoglobulin concentrations in humans, all means are calculated as geometric means. Bracketed numbers are 95% confidence intervals for the population concentrations. Data for IgG, IgA, and IgM taken from Buckley et al. [161], IgD from Josephs and Buckley [162], IgE (ages 0–14 yr) from Kjellman et al. [163], and IgE (adult) from Zetterström and Johansson [164].
[a]IgD concentrations are for ages 1–20 yr and 21–70 yr, respectively.

life of any plasma protein, approximately 21 to 24 days. Among subclasses, IgG_1, IgG_2, and IgG_4 have approximately equal half-lives of 21 to 24 days, while that of IgG_3 is considerably shorter at 9 days [166] (Table IV). The relatively rapid degradation of IgG_3 is probably due to its extended hinge, which renders the molecule very susceptible to enzymatic degradation by plasma proteases [167]. The distribution of IgG in body compartments is divided approximately equal between plasma and extravascular space. Its synthetic rate is 35 mg/kg/d (normal range = 20–60 mg/kg/d) which is equivalent to about 2.5 g/d for a 70-kg human [166]. Recent studies of the IgG synthetic rate of human lymphoblastoid cells indicate that each cell can synthesize and secrete about 10^5 IgG molecules per hour or 2.4×10^6 molecules per day [168].

TABLE IV. Biological and Physical Properties of Human Immunoglobulins

Property	IgG	IgA	IgM	IgD	IgE
Serum half-life (days)	$\gamma_1, \gamma_2, \gamma_4 = 22$ $\gamma_3 = 9$	$\alpha_1 = 5.9$ $\alpha_2 = 4.5$	5.1	2.8	2.7
Fractional turnover rate (% day)	$\gamma_1 = 8.0, \gamma_2 = 6.9$ $\gamma_3 = 16.8, \gamma_4 = 6.9$	$\alpha_1 = 24$ $\alpha_2 = 34$	10.6	37.0	94.3
Distribution ratio (intravascular)/(extravascular)	$\gamma_1 = 0.51, \gamma_2 = 0.53$ $\gamma_3 = 0.64, \gamma_4 = 0.54$	0.54	0.74	0.75	0.41
Molecular weight	$\gamma_1, \gamma_2, \gamma_4 = 146,000$ $\gamma_3 = 165,000$	160,000 (monomer) 400,000 (secretory)	900,000	170,000	190,000
Sedimentation coefficient	6–7	7 (monomer) 15 (secretory)	19	7	8
Percent carbohydrate	2.9	7.5	11.8	12.3	12
Domains in heavy chain	4	4	5	4	5
J-chain polymerization	no	yes: dimers trimers	yes: pentamers	no	no

The rate at which plasma IgG is catabolized is proportional to its concentration in plasma. In conditions accompanied by elevated IgG levels such as myeloma or chronic infections the catabolic rate may more than double from its normal rate of 7% of the plasma pool per day to 16–18%. By contrast, low plasma IgG levels found in hypogammaglobulinemia are accompanied by catabolic rates as low as 2% [166]. The sites of catabolism of human Igs is not known. Recent evidence using radiolabeled rat IgG_{2a} indicates that the liver, spleen, and lymph nodes are the primary catabolic sites in the rat [169]. This view is consistent with the known function of these organs as primary "filters" of blood and lymph, respectively.

IgG is the only Ig that crosses the placenta from the maternal to fetal circulation and thus serves as an important source of immunity for the newborn infant [170]. Although the fetus may secrete IgG as early as 20 weeks [170], IgG is not synthesized by the neonate in appreciable amounts until about six months after birth [171]. Maternal IgG appears to be transmitted across the placenta by an IgG-specific transport mechanism and by passive means [172,173]. At abnormally high maternal IgG concentrations, the neonatal IgG levels reflect the elevated maternal levels, implying a predominantly passive transfer [174]. When maternal IgG levels are normal or low, however, fetal concentrations just prior to birth are usually higher than the mother's, indicating that IgG-specific transport must be occurring. The IgG transport mechanism employs a placental IgG receptor which binds a site in the Fc portion of IgG [175]. Over two thirds of maternal to fetal IgG transfer occurs after the 28th week of gestation. Premature infants therefore usually have a hypogammaglobulinemia whose severity is related to the degree of prematurity [176]. Because the neonate does not begin to synthesize adequate quantities of IgG until six months of age, a normal infant has a four-to-six-month period after birth during which its IgG levels are extremely low (Table III). This "physiologic hypogammaglobulinemia of infancy" is explained by the fact that maternal IgG, having an average half-life in the infant of 30 days, is degraded to one eighth of its original concentration about 90 days after birth, during which time the infant's own IgG synthesis is rapidly increasing.

Synthesis

Upon the first exposure to an antigen, the usual antibody produced is of the IgM class and is termed the "primary" response. The second exposure to the same antigen elicits the secondary or anamnestic response, which usually consists of predominantly IgG antibodies. In contrast to the IgM generated during the primary response, which has a relatively low affinity for the antigen, IgG produced during a secondary or subsequent response has relatively high antigen affinity [177]. This class switch from IgM to IgG production is regulated by lymphocytes and macrophages located in lymphoid organs where antigens are recognized by "memory" lymphocytes [178]. In humans and animals whose spleens have been removed, the IgM and IgG class switch may be significantly impaired for blood-born antigens [179]. Such individuals are at increased risk for fatal septicemia, especially from diplococcus pneumoniae, Haemophilus influenzae, staphylococcus aureus, group A streptococcus and Neisseria meningitidis [180]. By contrast, the IgM to IgG class switch elicited by a subcutaneously administered antigen is essentially normal in splenectomized patients, indicating that significant "partitioning" of the IgG immune response occurs within lymphoid organs and depends upon the route of antigen exposure [179].

IgG Subclasses

The four human IgG subclasses were originally defined by antigenic differences between IgG myeloma protein H chains. Interestingly, these antigenic differences are so slight that rabbit antiserum is unable to differentiate them. Monkey antiserum, by contrast, is reported to produce the best serologic means of distinguishing the subclasses [181].

IgG Subclass Structural Differences

The amino acid sequences of myeloma proteins from all four IgG subclasses are known [44,182]. Sequence comparisons among the subclasses reveal a very high degree of homology between all constant domains. The carboxy-terminal CH_3 domain shows the highest degree of homology ranging from 96–99%, while homologies between CH_1 and CH_2 domains range from 89–93% and 92–97%, respectively [183]. By contrast, sequence comparisons of the hinge regions of the four subclasses reveal much lower homologies of approximately 50–60% [144]. The length of the hinges among subclasses varies significantly, having 12 residues in IgG_2 and IgG_4, 15 residues in IgG_1 and 62 residues in IgG_3 [44]. As previously mentioned, the extremely long IgG_3 hinge evolved from a quadruplicated 15 residue hinge segment resembling that of IgG_1 [119]. In addition to the differences in length, significant differences exist in the positions of the inter-H chain and H/L chain disulfide bonds. In both IgG_1 and IgG_4, for example, each H chain contains two inter-H chain disulfide bonds while IgG_2 and IgG_3 have 4 and 11 disulfide bonds, respectively [44].

As shown in Figure 15, the pattern of disulfide bonds connecting the H and L chains also differ between the subclasses. In IgG_1, the H/L chain cysteines (Cys) are located at aa 214 and aa 213, respectively. In the other three sublcasses, the H/L chain link occurs between Cys 214 and Cys 131. The proline (Pro) content also varies among the similarly sized hinges of IgG_1, IgG_2, and IgG_4 and may further influence the relative rigidity of the

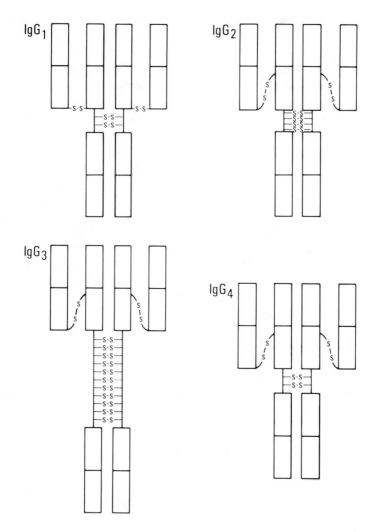

Fig. 15. Schematic hinge region disulfide bonding pattern in human IgG subclasses. The extended 62 residue hinge of IgG$_3$ results from quadruplication of a 15 residue hinge segment resembling that of IgG$_1$.

hinge region. These three subclasses have an identical sequence Cys-Pro-Pro-Cys-Pro in which the two Cys residues form two inter-H chain disulfide bonds. IgG$_4$, by contrast, has two additional proline residues immediately preceding the first Cys which may considerably restrict mobility of this region.

The observed structural variability of the subclass hinges, coupled with the high degree of homology between the remainder of the H chains has led to the notion that the different biological and physicochemical properties exhibited by the subclasses are due, in part, to the hinge differences. This concept is strongly supported by studies in which the activity of intact IgG molecules are compared to their Fc fragments which lack the hinge segments and Fab arms.

The ability to activate the complement cascade via the "classical" pathway, for example, is highly dependent on the particular IgG subclass, the relative order of activity being $IgG_3 > IgG_1, \gg IgG_2$, with IgG_4 being essentially inactive [184]. When Isenman et al. tested the activity of the Fc fragments of IgG_1 and IgG_4, however, both were equally active in activating complement [185]. Isenman suggested that the short, proline-rich IgG_4 hinge reduces Fab mobility which sterically hinders the complement Fc binding site within IgG_4 Fc and thus prevents activation.

A similar phenomenon was observed by McNabb et al. who found that intact IgG_2 did not bind to the placental IgG Fc receptor involved in maternal/fetal IgG transport, while the IgG_2 Fc fragment had an affinity equal to IgG_1 [186]. Similarly, the variation in plasma half-life observed among the IgG subclasses are due to differences in the hinge/Fab region, since Fc fragments from the four subclasses are catabolized at the same rate [187]. Other biophysical properties of IgG subclasses correlate with the Fab mobility and include the sensitivity of the hinge region to papain digestion [167] and the tendency for IgG to aggregate when heated; a property which primarily depends on the ability of the Fab arms to noncovalently associate [188]. Both properties have a similar activity pattern: $IgG_3 > IgG_1 \gg IgG_4 > IgG_2$ [187,188]. The extended hinge of IgG_3 and the resultant mobility of the Fab arms are probably responsible for the high degree of spontaneous aggregation exhibited by this subclass. Cebra and Kunkel reported a striking concentration-dependent aggregation of IgG_3, which is thought to be responsible for a number of clinically significant hyperviscosity states associated with elevated plasma IgG_3 concentrations. In patients having IgG_1 or IgG_3 myeloma, the hyperviscosity syndrome occurred when plasma concentrations of IgG_3 were as low as 4.2 g/dL, while patients with IgG_1 myeloma did not exhibit hyperviscosity until IgG_1 levels reached 15 g/dL [190].

REGULATION OF IgG SUBCLASSES
Genetic Influences

The levels of IgG subclasses found in blood are influenced by both genetic factors and by environmental exposure to specific classes of antigens. IgG_3 levels in individuals homozygous for the $G_3m(b)$ allotypic determinant, for example, are twice that found in individuals homozygous for the $G_3m(g)$ allotype. Heterozygotes display an IgG_3 level intermediate between that of both homozygotes. Similarly, individuals homozygous for the $G_2m(n)$ allotype have higher levels of IgG_2 than do homozygotes for $G_2m(n-)$. IgG_3 and IgG_4 levels are similarly correlated with the presence of various Gm allotypes [165].

The distribution of IgG subclasses on human peripheral blood lymphocytes (PBL) varies as a function of subclass and does not reflect serum concentrations. About 15% of normal human PBL have membrane-bound Ig in amounts sufficient to be visually detectable by fluorescent anti-Ig antisera ("B lymphocytes"). By this technique, about 50% of these lymphocytes stain for IgM while 5–10% stain for IgG. Of these 5–10%, Simmons found the following proportions of IgG subclasses: IgG_1, 28%; IgG_2, 43%; IgG_3, 12%; and IgG_4, 34%. This distribution is in sharp contrast to the observed percentage of cells containing cytoplasmic IgG: IgG_1, 30%; IgG_2, 2%; IgG_3, 61%; and IgG_4, 7% [191]. Such asymmetry of surface IgG distribution is particularly interesting since IgG_2 and IgG_4 constitute only 30% and 4% of circulating IgG, respectively [165]. Furthermore, native IgG_2 and IgG_4 have little affinity for lymphocyte Fc receptors [184], suggesting the possibility that these subclasses may have an IgM-type membrane tailpiece when expressed on lymphocyte surfaces.

The fact that IgG_2 is the predominant IgG subclass expressed on lymphocytes may be related to the observation that IgG_2 is, antigenically speaking, the most primitive of the four human subclasses. IgG_2-specific antigenic determinants exist in nearly all nonhuman primates while determinants specific to IgG_1, IgG_3, and IgG_4 first appeared at the time when Old World monkeys diverged from New World monkeys about ten million years ago [192].

IgG Subclass Response to Antigens

The response of the IgG subclasses to antigenic exposure is highly heterogeneous and dependent upon the type of antigen. IgG antibodies directed toward polysaccharide carbohydrates including dextran, levan, and teichoic acid are largely restricted to the IgG_2 subclass [67]. It is for this reason that antibodies to pneumococci are said to not activate the classical complement pathway, since the predominant antibody to the polysaccharide pneumococcal capsule is IgG_2, which is a poor activator of C_1 [193]. Similar subclass restriction has been observed in IgG antibodies elicited by hemophilic factor VIII (IgG_4) [194], and Rhesus (Rh) human erythrocyte antigen (predominantly IgG_1, IgG_3) [1,195]. By contrast, the IgG response to tetanus toxoid, diphtheria toxoid, and thyroglobulin are distributed among the four subclasses in quantities roughly proportional to their normal serum concentrations [184].

Rheumatoid Factors

IgG molecules may themselves serve as antigens and elicit a predominantly IgM and IgG antibody response to determinants in the Fc region. Such anti-Ig autoantibodies are termed rheumatoid factors [196] and are present in very small quantities in normal individuals [197,198]. An elevated level of rheumatoid factors accompanies many autoimmune diseases, including rheumatoid arthritis, systemic lupus erythematosus, Sjögren's syndrome, and vasculitis [197,199,200]. The sites in IgG Fc which serve as antigens for rheumatoid factors include allotypic determinants and as yet uncharacterized determinants located in both the CH_2 and CH_3 domains [201,202]. Natvig has suggested that a minimum of four separate Fc sites are reactive with rheumatoid factors; three in $C\gamma2$ and one in $C\gamma3$ [202]. A particularly common rheumatoid factor determinant is termed the Ga antigen and is believed to be located near the carboxy-terminus of $C\gamma2$. It is present in only IgG_1, IgG_2 and IgG_4 [202] and may thus be spatially related to the staphylococcal protein A (SPA) Fc binding site, which is partly located in the carboxy-terminal portion of CH_2 and is also restricted to the IgG_1, IgG_2, and IgG_4 subclasses [203].

Reagenic IgG: Homocytotropism and Heterocytotropism

Antibodies cytophilic for basophils and mast cells and able to release histamine are termed homocytotropic if both antibodies and cells are from the same species, and heterocytotropic if the cells and antibodies are from different species [184]. Besides IgE, which Ishizaka has shown to be the heat-sensitive homocytotropic antibody associated with allergies [204], many species also have a homocytotropic IgG subclass. In rats, for example, IgGa is homocytotropic, and it has been shown to bind to rat IgE Fc receptors [205].

In humans, evidence exists that IgG may also have homocytotropic activity. Among the four IgG subclasses, IgG_4 has been primarily implicated. Homocytotropism in humans has been clinically assessed by injecting serum containing antibodies to defined antigens intradermally and subsequently challenging the site with antigen 24 hours later. This method is termed passive cutaneous anaphylaxis (PCA) or, in humans, the Prausnitz-Küstner (P-K) reaction after the two investigators who first described the procedure in 1921 [206]. Because of the risk of disease transmission among humans, PCA studies of human IgE and IgG have been usually done *in vitro* or in non-humans. Although human IgE has a high degree of species specificity for binding to cellular Fc receptors, Ishizaka demonstrated that monkey skin can be sensitized for PCA by human IgE [207]. Stanworth subsequently confirmed that human IgE could elicit PCA reactions in monkeys and baboons and demonstrated that human IgG_4, but not IgG_1, IgG_2, or IgG_3, could inhibit the IgE-mediated reaction [208]. Nakagawa et al. [209] and Vijay and Perl-mutter [210] demonstrated that human leukocytes release histamine after sensitization *in vitro* with human IgG_4 and subsequent exposure to anti-IgG_4 antisera. Leukocytes similarly exposed to human IgG_1 and IgG_3 and challenged with anti-IgG_1 and anti-IgG_3 antisera, by contrast, produced no histamine release. To confirm that IgE-contamination of the IgG preparations did not contribute to the observed histamine release, human atopic serum was heated at 56°C for two hours to destroy the sensitizing capacity of any IgE present. Anti-IgE treatment of the cells caused no histamine release, whereas anti-IgG_4 released a significant amount of histamine [210]. The failure of earlier investigators [211] to demonstrate human IgG homocyto-tropic activity has been attributed to the use of antisera to pooled human IgG, which has very low histamine releasing activity, rather than IgG_4-specific antisera [210].

Studies of the skin-sensitizing kinetics of homocytotropic IgG indicate that the duration of its sensitizing ability is much shorter than that of IgE which persists for several weeks. In a study of serum from asthmatic patients with known antigen sensitivity, Bryant et al. found that fractions containing IgG produced maximum skin sensitization at 2 hours after injection that was not detectable at 12 hours. The IgE-enriched fraction, by contrast, produced maximum sensitization 24 hours after injection and could be detected many days later. Exposing both IgE and IgG-enriched fractions to procedures known to inactivate IgE-sensitizing activity, such as heating at 56°C for 4 hours, reduction and alkylation or passing the sera through an anti-IgE immunoab-sorbent column completely removed the PCA activity from the IgE fraction, but did not affect the IgG fraction. By contrast, passing both fractions over an anti-IgG immunoabsorbent column abolished the sensitizing activity of the IgG-enriched fraction but was without effect on the IgE-enriched fraction [212]. These data are consistent with studies of homocytotropic IgG in mice for which the maximal level of PCA sensitization occurs at 1 to 2 hours after injection. Maximum sensitization by murine IgE, by contrast, occurs at 48 hours [213].

While the existence of human homocytotropic IgG seems well established, its degree of participation in the production of clinical allergic disease symptoms is controversial. In a study of sera from 310 allergic patients, Stanworth found no correlation between allergen-specific IgG_4 antibodies and positive skin-test reactivity [214]. Recently, however, Kimura provided evidence that basophils from patients with atopic asthma having low (< 100 IU) IgE levels had more degranulation when exposed to anti-IgG antisera than anti-IgE antisera while those patients with IgE levels above 1000 IU showed the reverse pattern. They concluded that IgG may play a role in the allergic sensitization of low IgE asthmatic patients [215]. Clearly, more research is needed to clarify the role of IgG_4 in human allergic disease.

IgG IMMUNOLOGICAL ACTIVITIES: LOCALIZATION OF ACTIVE SITES

Complement Activation

The classical pathway for complement activation consists of 11 proteins that are activated to form a biochemical cascade beginning with the first complement component, C_1 and ending with a cellular "attack complex" consisting of C_5, C_6, C_7, C_8, and C_9. The pattern of activation is highly specific and begins when C_1 binds to antibody-antigen complexes of either IgG or IgM [216]. The C_1 molecule consists of three subunits, designated C_1q, C_1r and C_1s. C_1q is a 400,000-dalton molecule, approximately 300 × 375 Å, and contains six identical 65-Å diameter receptors for the Fc portion of IgG and IgM. In electron micrographs, these six receptors are clustered at one end of the molecule and connected by six 120-Å long collagen-like strands to a central 50 × 100-Å "stalk" which contains the C_1r and C_1s subunits [217]. The entire C_1 complex strikingly resembles a bunch of tulips. Upon binding to antigen-antibody complexes, C_1r is cleaved and gains serine esterase activity which, in turn, cleaves C_1s, which also gains esterase activity and subsequently activates C_4, which continues the cascade [216]. The six C_1q Fc receptors have been enzymatically isolated as 37,000-dalton subunits that have a binding affinity for IgG of 1.8–5.8×10^4 L/mol, which is similar to the measured affinity of intact C_1q for IgG monomers of 5×10^4 L/mol [218]. These affinities are in contrast to that measured between intact C_1q and IgG aggregates, which is 10^7–10^8 L/mol, indicating that significant binding cooperativity occurs when multiple C_1q receptor subunits bind to multiple Fc sites [216]. The site in IgG to which the C_1q receptor binds has been localized to the CH_2 domain [219]. Kehoe and Fougereau were the first investigators to further localize the binding site to a 62 aa CH_2 fragment [aa 253–314] isolated from a murine IgG_{2a} Ig that could activate the classical pathway when adsorbed to latex beads [220]. Subsequent studies by Johnson and Thames [221] and later by Boackle et al. [222] demonstrated that peptides with sequences derived from CH_2 at aa 274 to 281 were approximately as effective in activating complement as heat aggregated IgG. Lukas et al. recently showed that a peptide from the adjacent CH_2 region at aa 281–292 was able to inhibit C_1-mediated immune hemolysis. This 12 residue peptide was half as effective as monomeric IgG in inhibiting hemolysis and equally effective when chemically dimerized by a cross-linking reagent [223]. These data are consistent with previous reports that chemical modification of lysine, arginine, aspartic acid, glutamic acid, tyrosine, or tryptophan residues of IgG, which are present in this region, inhibit C_1 activation [221,224–226]. As shown in Figure 16, the region 274 to 292 is entirely exposed and constitutes the "top" of the CH_2 domain as it exists in the IgG H chain. Figure 17 shows this region as it exists within the intact Fc fragment.

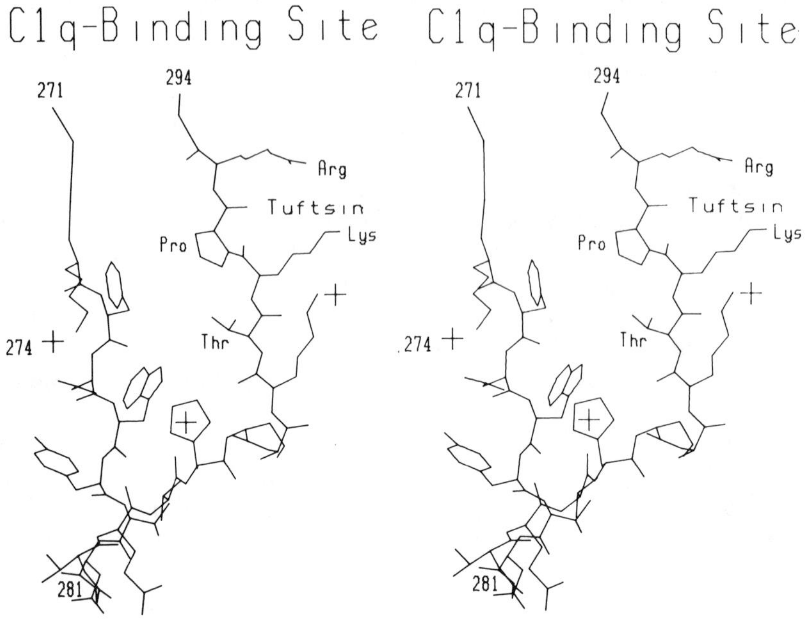

Fig. 16. Stereo view of IgG, CH_2 amino acid residues which interact with the C_1q subunit of the first complement component C_1. Positively charged amino acid side chains thought to be important for C_1q binding include Lys 274, His 285, Lys 288 (the former three residues are identified with a "+") and Lys 290 and Arg 292. The indole nucleus of Trp 277, whose chemical modification prevents C_1 activation, points to the interior of the domain. A synthetic peptide identical to aa 274–281 was reported to be nearly as active as IgG aggregates in activating C_1. Conversely, a synthetic peptide identical to aa 281–292 was reported to be 50% as active on a molar basis as monomeric IgG in inhibiting C_1-mediated hemolysis. The tuftsin peptide (aa 289–292) inhibits C_1-mediated hemolysis with one tenth the activity of aggregated IgG.

It is particularly interesting that residues included in the C_1q-binding region have been shown by Deisenhoffer to be mobile and disordered in crystal complexes of IgG Fc and the SPA Fb fragment. These mobile residues at aa 266–287 and aa 295–302, flank a stable segment, aa 288–294 [203]. It is also in this region that conformational changes occur when bivalent antigen binds to intact IgG, as evidenced by changes in the circular polarization of luminescence of tryptophan [49,288]. It is possible that conformational changes within this region are induced by antigen and cause a similar conformational change within C_1q which results in C_1 activation. In order to bind this region,

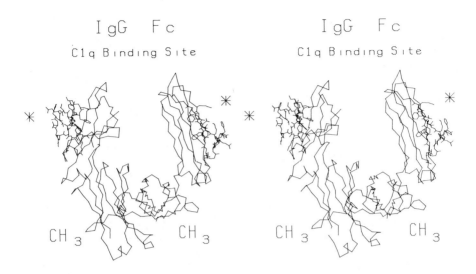

Fig. 17.   Stereo view of an intact human IgG Fc fragment. Amino acid side chains of aa 274–292 are displayed while the remaining residues are represented as their α-carbon backbone. The star represents the presumed position of the C_1q binding head when bound to CH_2. (Atomic coordinates of the Fc fragment were kindly provided by Dr. Johann Deisenhofer [288].)

a single 60-Å in diameter C_1q receptor must completely envelop the 25 × 25 × 40-Å CH_2 domain. Furthermore, since this region of the CH_2 domain occurs on opposite sides of the intact IgG molecule, it is apparent that a single monomeric IgG could not simultaneously bind to two C_1q Fc receptors located in the same C_1q molecule; hence the observed requirement for two adjacent IgG molecules for complement activation [227].

Phagocytosis

A major defense function of IgG is to bind to the surface of a cellular or molecular antigen and thus coat its surface with exposed Fc regions. When granulocytes, monocytes, or macrophages encounter such a coated structure, IgG-specific Fc receptors bind to the Fc region and stimulate the cell to ingest or phagocytize (from the Greek *phagein*—"to eat") the particle [228,229]. IgG performing this function is said to be an opsonin (from the Greek *opson*, roughly meaning "food seasoning"). Other opsonins exist and include the proteolytic fragments of the third and fourth complement components, C_3b and C_4b [228]. Opsonin-stimulated phagocytosis is particularly important for defense against bacteria having thick polysaccharide capsules such as pneumococci and Klebsiella. In the absence of opsonic IgG, these organisms are very poorly phagocytized and may rapidly kill the host in diseases such as pneumococcal or Klebsiella pneumonia. Opsonic IgG, however, overcomes the antiphagocytic properties of the capsular material and stimulates rapid phagocytosis of the organisms. The appearance of substantial titers of IgG antipneumococci in a host with pneumococcal pneumonia coincides with the classical "crisis" phase of the disease, after which clinical resolution usually occurs rapidly [229].

Evidence that IgG subclasses differ in their ability to stimulate phago-cytosis exists but is somewhat conflicting. Messner and Jelinek found that IgG_1 and IgG_3 effectively inhibited phagocytosis of IgG-coated erythrocytes, whereas IgG_2 and IgG_4 were not inhibitory [230]. Henson et al., by contrast, did not find clear differences between the subclasses when the ability of aggregated IgG to release neutrophil lysosomal enzymes was measured. Phagocytosis by monocytes, however, showed strong subclass specificity in that tanned erythrocytes coated with IgG_1 and IgG_3 were actively phagocy-tized, while those coated with IgG_2 were not significantly ingested [231].

Recent studies by Schanfield indicate that IgG_3 is more effective than IgG_1 in promoting phagocytosis by neutrophils. He found that IgG_3 directed against human erythrocyte blood group alloantigens was over 2.5 times more active in stimulating neutrophil phagocytosis than were similarly directed IgG_1 antibodies [232]. Similar subclass differences were observed in patients with hemolytic anemia who had more severe hemolysis with IgG_3 autoantibodies than with IgG_1 antibodies [233].

The submolecular site in IgG Fc recognized by phagocytosis-stimulating Fc receptors of granulocytes may require an intact Fc fragment since the Facb fragment (Fab_2 + 2 CH_2) from rabbit IgG could not inhibit phagocytosis [234] nor could isolated CH_2 domains, pFc', or atCγ3 fragments inhibit granulocyte IgG binding [235]. This is consistent with the observation that staphylococcal protein A, which inhibits IgG-stimulated phagocytosis [236], only binds to intact Fc fragments. It is possible, however, that small phago-cytosis-stimulating "active" sites may be distorted or masked when isolated domains are used as probes. The importance of domain quaternary structure for Fc fragment phagocytosis stimulation is illustrated by studies showing that reduction and alkylation of IgG intra-H chain disulfide bonds greatly reduce granulocyte phagocytosis [235]. Nevertheless, it may be possible to isolate the critical regions responsible for phagocytosis stimulation as active peptides much smaller than an intact domain. Expression of the biological activity of such peptides would be unhindered by adjacent mobile domain regions that are stabilized in the intact Fc fragment by interaction with the remainder of the molecule. Two peptides with phagocytosis-stimulating ability, tuftsin and rigin, have been isolated from IgG, and they may represent such biologically active sites expressed by intact IgG.

Tuftsin

Tuftsin is a tetrapeptide, with sequence Thr-Lys-Pro-Arg; it is present in the second constant domain of all human IgG subclasses and in guinea pig IgG_2 at aa 289–292 [44]. It was originally isolated from proteolytic digests of IgG by Najjar, who found it to stimulate phagocytosis of granulocytes, monocytes and macrophages *in vitro*. Subsequent studies have shown tuftsin to be active in nanomolar concentrations in many species, including humans, cows, dogs, rabbits, guinea pigs, and mice. In addition to its phagocytosis-stimulating ability, tuftsin has been shown to stimulate antibody-dependent cell-mediated cytotoxicity (ADCC), Natural Killer (NK) cell activity, macrophage-dependent T-cell education, and antibody synthesis to T-cell-dependent and independent antigens *in vitro* and *in vivo* [240,243]. Stereospecific receptors for tuftsin are known to exist on granulocytes, macrophages, and lymphocytes [244–246]. Scatchard analysis of tuftsin receptors on macrophages revealed 72,000 receptors having a dissociation constant of 5×10^8 L/mol [246]; a value comparable to the affinity of intact IgG for Fc receptors [247]. Whether tuftsin binds to IgG Fc receptors or to a distinct receptor remains to be determined.

Analysis of the tuftsin sequence within an intact IgG Fc fragment indicates that residues of tuftsin are exposed to the exterior and could bind to the cellular tuftsin receptor as an intact sequence within the IgG H chain. Figure 16 depicts the tuftsin sequence as it exists in $C\gamma2$. It is observed that the threonine and proline side chains of tuftsin point toward the opposite β-strand and are exposed to the "top" of the domain while the two positively charged lysine and arginine side chains are parallel and point away from the domain. The latter observation is best illustrated in Figure 18, which shows the orientation of the tuftsin side chains as they exist in an intact IgG Fc fragment. It is also observed that the tuftsin sequence is contained within the complement blocking peptide (aa 281–292) and is therefore part of the putative C_1q binding site. The potential interaction of the tuftsin sequence with C_1q was recently confirmed by Lukas et al., who showed that tuftsin was one tenth as active as intact monomeric IgG in blocking C_1-mediated hemolysis [223]. This surprising finding indicates that biologically active sites of Ig domains have been conserved for use by several different immune system receptors.

Rigin

Rigin is also a phagocytosis-stimulating tetrapeptide derived from human IgG [268]. Its sequence at aa 341–344 (Fig. 19) is located within the IgG

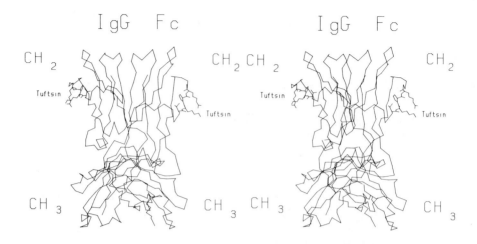

Fig. 18.   Stereo view of the α-carbon backbone of an intact human IgG Fc fragment. The amino acid side chains of the tuftsin site, aa 289–292, are displayed. The exposed nature of the tuftsin residues may allow them to bind to cellular tuftsin receptors as an intact sequence within the IgG heavy chain.

"switch region" that connects the CH₂ and CH₃ domains and has the sequence Gly-Gln-Pro-Arg, which is structurally similar to tuftsin. This H chain site is particularly interesting since the SPA Fb fragment is known to block the degree of conformational mobility [203,249] and is in an exposed portion of the Fc region, directly adjacent to the SPA Fc binding site [61,249]. This is particularly interesting since the SPa Fb fragment is known to block the binding of intact IgG to granulocyte Fc receptors [250].

If rigin does represent a biologically active site of IgG, its location in the switch region may enable it to respond to conformational changes induced by antigen binding or IgG aggregation; conditions known to stimulate phagocytosis.

Antibody-Dependent Cell-Mediated Cytotoxicity (ADCC)

ADCC may be mediated by lymphocytes [251]. granulocytes [252], monocytes, macrophages [253], and eosinophils [254] and occurs when Fc receptors on these cells bind to antigen-bound IgG. Upon binding to an IgG-coated cell, the ADCC cell may kill the target cell within several hours. This process does not involve phagocytosis or activation of the complement system. ADCC is thought to be particularly important in the killing of neoplastic or virus-infected cells. The importance of ADCC relative to other defense systems in humans is, however, unclear. *In vitro,* human blood mononuclear

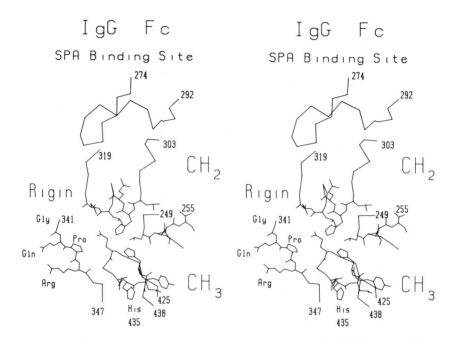

Fig. 19.   Stereo view of the staphylococcal protein A (SPA) Fc binding site of human IgG. The SPA Fc contact residues are displayed and include aa 251–254, aa 309–315 in CH_2, and aa 430–436 in CH_3. In addition, the amino acid side chains of the immunologically active tetrapeptide rigin at aa 341–344 (Gly-Gln-Pro-Arg) are displayed. The close proximity of rigin residues to the SPA-binding site, which is spatially related to the neutrophil and ADCC Fc receptor-binding sites, suggests that intact rigin residues may interact with these Fc receptors. α-Carbon backbones of aa 274–292 (the C_1q binding site), aa 303–308, aa 316–319, and aa 343–347 are displayed for visual orientation.

cells have been shown to kill herpes simplex virus (HSV)-infected cells within three hours of infection; long before release of newly replicated infectious viruses [253]. *In vivo* studies similarly show decreased mortality of HSV-infected mice through ADCC killing [255].

Whereas all monocytes, macrophages, neutrophils, and eosinophils may mediate ADCC, only 4% of human T lymphocytes have ADCC activity [256], a value consistent with the observed frequency of human peripheral blood T lymphocytes bearing IgG Fc receptors, 5–15% [257]. IgG subclass specificity in ADCC killing has the frequently observed hierarchy: monomeric $IgG_1 = IgG_3 >$ aggregated $IgG_2 \gg$ aggregated IgG_4; monomeric IgG_2 and IgG_4 having no inhibitory activity [258]. The portion of the IgG molecule to which ADCC receptors bind is located in the Fc region, since Fc fragments inhibit ADCC killing [258]. Attempts to localize the ADCC Fc binding site further have produced conflicting results. Wisloff found that paired CH_3

domains (pFc' fragment) from human IgG were unable to inhibit ADCC killing, whereas an Fc fragment from human IgG_3 with an extended amino terminus had even greater inhibitory capacity than intact Fc fragments, indicating that CH_2 may contain ADCC binding sites [258]. MacLennan, by contrast, found that the Facb fragment [Fab_2 + 2 CH_2] had no ADCC-inhibitory ability [259]. The submolecular site in IgG Fc recognized by ADCC Fc receptors may be spatially related to the SPA Fc binding site, since SPA can substantially (> 90%) inhibit ADCC killing [260].

The inconclusive results of ADCC inhibition by Fc subfragments may indicate that the ADCC receptor binds to an Fc site that may become conformationally unstable after enzymatic fragmentation. An ADCC site spatially related to the SPA Fc binding site might have such properties, since the SPA site includes residues in the CH_2/CH_3 contact region that are stabilized by interdomain contacts [61,249].

QUELLUNG REACTION

The word *Quellung,* which means "swelling" in German, is associated with the reaction which takes place when bacterial type-specific antibody (predominantly IgG) combines with the polysaccharide capsule that surrounds virulent strains of *Diplococcus pneumoniae* (pneumococci) or other bacteria or fungi with capsules [229]. First described by Neufeld in 1902, the quellung reaction refers to the dramatic swelling and increased refractivity of the capsular material. Electron microscopic studies by Baker of the quellung reaction in type I pneumococci show that exposure to type-specific antiserum causes the capsule to swell 10–12-fold, from a thickness of 450–550 Å to 4500–5000 Å [261]. The swelling is thought to arise from hydration of the capsular polysaccharide matrix after mechanical disruption caused by the simple act of Fab cross-linking of polysaccharide. Although the quellung reaction is not usually classed as an antibody "effector" mechanism, it does illustrate that the mere act of an antibody binding to a cell can cause profound alterations in a cell's architecture, independent of other effector systems such as complement or ADCC. The role, if any, that the quellung reaction plays in immune defense is unknown.

IgG directed against other surface components of bacteria, such as the adherence-mediating pili of *Escherichia coli,* does play a significant defense role. IgG directed against pili-resident structures that bind to host cells can prevent bacterial attachment by sterically blocking the pili receptors. Such physical blockade of adherence is thought to be important for immunity against many pathogenic enteric bacteria [229].

T LYMPHOCYTE Fc-RECEPTOR INDUCTION

Studies of mice [262] and humans [263] with myeloma have shown that their circulating T cells have a three- to fourfold increase in the number of Fc receptors specific for the myeloma isotype. These T cells are not derivatives of the neoplastic clone and appear to be normal except for their increased expression of Fc receptors. Hoover et al. recently demonstrated that it is the plasma concentration of the myeloma protein which seems to determine the level of T-cell Fc expression. They found that mice injected with purified myeloma protein developed large numbers of T cells with Fc receptors specific for the myeloma isotype. Similar increases in Fc receptor-bearing cells were observed after *in vitro* administration of myeloma protein [264].

The T-cell subset responsible for the elevated Fc receptor expression in mice proved to have the Lyt $1-2+$ antigenic phenotype which has been linked with suppressor and cytotoxic T lymphocytes [265]. This finding suggested that the myeloma protein might be triggering a normal negative feedback regulatory circuit in which T-suppressor cells sense elevated antibody levels by binding their Fc portion and proliferate to suppress synthesis of the elevated isotype. This concept is consistent with observations by Moretta et al., who found that IgG immune complexes can activate T lymphocytes bearing IgG Fc receptors to develop suppressor activity for B lymphocyte differentiation into antibody-secreting plasma cells [266]. The portion of the myeloma protein sensed by the lymphocyte was presumed to be within the Fc region; however, studies with Ig fragments were not performed.

IgG-DERIVED CHEMOTACTIC FACTORS

Neutrophil Chemotactic Factors

Proteolytic digestion of IgG from animals and humans produces fragments with chemotactic activity for neutrophils. Hayashi isolated a 14,000-dalton thiol-dependent protease from rabbit neutrophils that produce limited proteolytic cleavage of rabbit and human IgG [267]. After one-hour digestion, dialyzable peptides were released; however, Fab or Fc fragments were not produced even after 24 hours of digestion. The released peptides were very small in size since the molecular weight of the partially digested IgG was not distinguishable from that of the native molecule [268]. Furthermore, the structural changes experienced by the digested IgG must have been very minor, since the IgG could still mediate PCA and RPCA reactions in guinea pigs [268].

The partially cleaved IgG was chemotactic for rabbit, guinea pig, rat, and mouse neutrophils (human cells were not tested), but was inactive for macrophages or lymphocytes. By contrast, the dialyzable peptides, native IgG, and papain-produced Fab and Fc fragments had no neutrophil chemotactic activity [267]. Although all four human IgG subclasses showed chemotactic activity when treated with the protease, both IgG_2 and IgG_4 were more active than IgG_1 or IgG_3; a reversal of the usual pattern of biologic activity [167]. Interestingly, very limited papain digestion of IgG_2 and IgG_4 but not IgG_1 or IgG_3 also produced chemotactically active molecules. This pattern of activity is probably related to the increased sensitivity of both IgG_1 and IgG_3 to papain digestion, which apparently destroys the chemotactic site(s) in the molecules more readily than in IgG_2 or IgG_4 [267].

Lymphocyte Chemotactic Factors

When the same investigators tested the neutrophil-inactive dialyzable peptides for chemotactic activity in cells other than neutrophils, they found that rat thoracic duct and splenic lymphocytes became chemotactically activated [269]. The partially cleaved parent IgG, by contrast, had no chemotactic activity. The peptides originated from the Fc portion of IgG, since protease-treated Fc fragments, but not Fab fragments, released the active peptides. Intact IgG, or papain-derived Fc and Fab fragments, showed no chemotactic activity. The chemotactically activated lymphocytes were probably B cells, since they were adherent to nylon wool columns and had surface Igs. By contrast, lymphocytes freely passing through the column (presumably T lymphocytes and null cells) had no chemotactic activation [269].

It is intriguing that the time course of the generation of neutrophil and lymphocyte chemotactic factors from IgG parallels the order of appearance of inflammatory cells at an infected site. Neutrophils are normally the first cells to arrive while lymphocytes later repopulate the site [229]. In these studies, IgG digestion similarly produces neutrophil chemotactic activity maximally at the beginning of digestion. Continued digestion decreases chemotactic activity for neutrophils while simultaneously increasing lymphocyte chemotactic activity [269].

Macrophage Chemotactic Factor

Limited enzymatic digestion of guinea pig IgG by a neutrophil-derived serine-dependent protease also produced a partially digested IgG molecule with chemotactic activity for macrophages, but not neutrophils or lymphocytes [270]. In a manner similar to the partially digested IgG chemotactic for neutrophils, the serine-protease digestion also produced dialyzable peptides without measurably altering the molecular weight of the IgG. Intact IgG, Fc, or Fab fragments had no chemotactic activity.

IgG Binding Factor

T lymphocytes that have been "activated" by antigenic or mitogenic exposure spontaneously secrete a glycoprotein that specifically binds to the Fc portion of IgG. Fridman, who first isolated the protein and named it IgG binding factor (IBF), found that it suppresses IgG synthesis to both T-dependent and T-independent antigens [271]. IBF also suppresses IgM responses to a lesser extent than IgG responses. Although IBF does not inhibit B-cell proliferation, it does inhibit B-cell differentiation into antibody-secreting plasma cells. Physicochemical studies indicate that IBF has two subunits, 38,000 and 60,000 daltons in size, which contain Ia antigens and probably represent a soluble form of the T-cell IgG Fc receptor [272]. Binding studies show that IBF binds with high affinity to human IgG_1, IgG_2, and IgG_3, murine IgG_1 and IgG_{2a}, and rabbit IgG, but not to human IgG_4, murine IgG_{2b}, β_2-microglobulin, IgM, or IgA from either species. The site in IgG to which IFB binds is located within the Fc portion, since Fc fragments, but not $F(ab')_2$ fragments, bind IBF. Within the Fc fragment, IBF probably binds predominantly to the CH_3 domain, since both isolated human and rabbit CH_3 domains, but not CH_2 domains, inhibit IBF binding. A secondary binding site in the CH_2 domain cannot be excluded, however, since C_1q binding to CH_2 domains is inhibited by IBF [271].

Fc-Derived T-cell-replacing Factor

In 1979 Berman et al. found that papain-generated Fc fragments of murine and human IgG, IgA, IgM, and IgD stimulated DNA synthesis of murine B lymphocytes as measured by tritiated-thymidine incorporation [273]. This mitogenic stimulation was also produced by isolated IgG and pFc' fragments, but not by intact antibody or Fab fragments. Subsequent studies by Morgan, Thoman, and Weigle have shown that Fc fragments and their proteolytic digestion products also stimulate human T lymphocytes to secrete a soluble T-cell-replacing factor, which, in combination with an Fc subfragment, stimulates B lymphocytes to differentiate into Ig-secreting plasma cells [274]. In addition, they found that Fc subfragments act as adjuvants for antigen-specific Ig synthesis and can potentiate allogenic mixed lymphocyte culture (MLC) responses [275]. The active Fc subfragment involved appears to be produced by macrophage digestion of the Fc fragment and probably represents a 23 residue peptide from the CH_3 domain.

Placental Transfer of IgG

The transfer of passive immunity from the mother to her young occurs when maternal antibodies, primarily IgG, are passed prenatally via the placenta or yolk sac and/or postnatally through the gastrointestinal tract [170]. In humans, rabbits, and guinea pigs, IgG transfer takes place prenatally when

IgG-specific Fc receptors bind maternal IgG and release it into the fetal circulation [170,172]. Studies of human placental tissue indicate that both IgG_1 and IgG_3 bind with an affinity at 4×10^6 L/mol, while IgG_4 has less affinity and IgG_2 shows very little binding [175,186]. By contrast, neither IgA nor IgM showed any binding. The Fc fragment of IgG_2, however, binds with an affinity equal to intact IgG_1 and its Fc fragment, indicating that the Fab and hinge structure significantly modulate binding affinity [186]. Ig carbohydrate does not participate in binding since enzymatic carbohydrate removal does not affect transport [276].

The placental and yolk-sac Fc receptors appear to bind primarily to a site in the CH_2 domain of IgG. CH_3 domains isolated as pFc' fragments demonstrated no yolk-sac Fc binding while Facb fragments containing CH_2 domains had 60% greater binding affinity than did native IgG [277].

Plasma Half-Life-Determining Fc Receptor

The observation that human IgG_1, IgG_2, and IgG_4 have a plasma half-life longer than other proteins prompted investigators to search for structures within IgG that protect it from proteolytic degradation [166]. Fragmentation of IgG revealed that such half-life-extending structures did exist within the Fc fragments, since they were catabolized at a rate similar to intact IgG, while Fab fragments were rapidly removed from circulation [187]. Furthermore, the relatively short half-life of IgG_3 (9 days versus 23 days for IgG_1, IgG_2, and IgG_4) is probably explained by its extended protease-sensitive hinge, since the isolated IgG_3 Fc fragment has a half-life similar to that of the other IgG subclasses [167,187]. Since the identity of the cells responsible for Ig catabolism is unknown, traditional Fc receptor binding studies have not been possible. Studies of the rate of elimination from plasma of Fc fragments, however, indicate that the CH_2 domain contains the sites recognized by IgG "protecting" receptors. Yasmeen studied isolated CH_2 and paired CH_3 domains (pFc') in rabbits and found that CH_2 domains had a half-life comparable to that of native IgG. By contrast, pFc' and β_2-microglobulin, which is similar in size to isolated CH_2, were eliminated much more rapidly [219]. Since the CH_2 fragment used in these studies had a molecular weight of 16,600 daltons, it should have been freely filtered through the kidney glomeruli. The extended half-life observed for CH_2, however, indicates that it must be selectively recognized and protected from filtration and degradation. Similar findings by Arend using rat IgG_2 fragments also indicate that structures within the CH_2 domain control the rate of IgG catabolism [279].

The CH_2 structure(s) recognized by the putative catabolic receptor do not include the CH_2 carbohydrate chains, since mutant Igs lacking carbohydrates or normal Igs from which carbohydrate has been enzymatically removed have normal half-lives [187,279].

Staphylococcal Protein A Binding Site

The ability of SPA to bind to the Fc fragment of IgG from many species is well documented [280]. In humans, SPA binds to all IgG subclasses except IgG_3 [280] with an affinity constant of 10^8 L/mol [281]. In addition, SPA has been reported to bind to the Fc fragment of IgA, IgM, and to the Fab fragment of IgG and IgE [282–285]. The intact SPA molecule has a molecular weight of 42,000 daltons and contains four highly homologous Fc binding structures that can be isolated by tryptic digestion to form four active fragments of about 7,000 daltons each [286]. SPA binds only to intact IgG Fc fragments and displays no affinity for isolated CH_2 or CH_3 domains, suggesting that the H chain binding site consists of residues at the CH_2/CH_3 junction [237]. An active SPA fragment (designated SPA Fb) is reported not to block C_1q binding to CH_2, suggesting that the "top" of CH_2, which contains the C_1q blocking peptides (aa 274–292), is not involved [203] (Fig. 16, 17). Recent x-ray crystallographic analysis by Deisenhoffer of the SPA Fb fragment bound to an intact IgG Fc fragment confirmed that SPA binds to two identical CH_2/CH_3 junctional sites located in both H chains. SPA contacts CH_2 in two locations at aa 251–254 and aa 309–315 and in CH_3 at aa 430–436 [61] (Figs. 19, 20). It is at aa 435 that IgG_3 has an arginine instead of the histadine present in the other three subclasses that bind SPA [44]. Deisenhoffer has suggested that the increased size and charge of Arg 435 prevents IgG_3 from binding to SPA [203]. This idea is supported by the recent observation that an IgG_3 myeloma protein having a histidine at aa 435 binds to SPA with high affinity [287].

The interaction of SPA with Ig appears to have been highly conserved in mammalian evolution. Kronvall examined antibodies from 62 mammalian species and found that SPA reacted with antibodies from all species except the oppossum. In addition, one bird species, the primitive flightless *Rhea Americana,* had antibodies reactive with SPA [280].

It seems surprising that the amino acid sequence of the Fc portion of mammalian Igs would have been sufficiently conserved through evolution to allow a bacterial protein to maintain a high binding affinity for the site. The degree of conservation of the Fc site must indeed be high, since only a single amino acid subsitution in IgG_3 prevents SPA binding. Furthermore, the three loop regions in Fc that form the SPA binding site are not important for stabilization of domain tertiary structure and should therefore accommodate amino acid substitutions freely without regard for size, charge, or polarity [16,53,288]. It is unlikely that a mammalian host derives a survival benefit by maintaining such a bacterial interaction site, since SPA can subvert the phagocytic and ADCC defense mechanisms used by the host immune system to destroy staphylococcal bacteria [236,250,260].

It is possible, instead, that the Fc site used by SPA has been conserved to interact with another highly conserved host molecule, perhaps a cellular

L   R

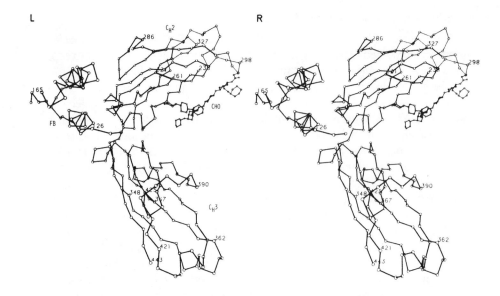

Fig. 20.   Stereo view of the staphylococcal protein A (SPA) Fb fragment bound to the CH$_2$/CH$_3$ domains of an IgG Fc fragment. Both SPA Fb fragment and the CH$_2$ and CH$_3$ domains are displayed as α-carbon backbones. The compact pair of parallel helicies which produce the Fb binding structure are clearly visible. The oligosaccharide attached to CH$_2$ at Asn 297 is also displayed. (Reproduced from Deisenhofer [61] with permission.)

Fc receptor? If so, cellular Fc receptors and SPA may have structural similarity, since they would both bind to the same Fc site. An intriguing study by Biguzzi provides support for this concept [289]. He found that antiserum from chickens and rabbits specific for purified SPA crossreacts with human lymphocyte Fc receptors for aggregated IgG. When human lymphocytes were preexposed to the anti-SPA chicken IgG and rabbit F(ab')$_2$ fragments, IgG erythrocyte rosettes were strongly inhibited. The antiserum was shown to specifically react with only the IgG-rosette forming lymphocyte subset since fluorescence-conjugated anti-SPA antiserum stained only the population of lymphocytes that could also be separated by rosette centrifugation. Double fluorescent staining for surface Ig and the structure detected by the anti-SPA antiserum revealed that two thirds of the lymphocytes had no detectable surface immunoglobulin, indicating that the cells were predominantly T lymphocytes or null cells. Biguzzi concluded that the SPA combining site for IgG was structurally similar to the lymphocyte Fc receptor for aggregated IgG.

Platelet IgG Fc Receptors

Platelets from humans and other mammalian species have been shown to specifically bind to aggregated IgG, but not to IgA, IgM, IgD, or IgE [290,291]. Upon binding to IgG-antigen complexes, platelets release vasoactive substances, including serotonin, and experience accelerated uptake by reticuloendothelial cells [290–292]. Although one study by Pfueller and Lüscher reported that aggregated IgG_1 and IgG_3 had a higher affinity for platelets than IgG_2 and IgG_4 [290], a larger study by Henson and Spiegelberg found no difference among human IgG subclasses [291]. The platelet Fc receptor has recently been isolated as a 255,000-dalton glycoprotein that contains a 50,000-dalton subunit that specifically binds to immobilized IgG Fc fragments [292].

IgG CYTOPHILIA

Many investigators have studied cytophilic properties of IgG using relatively pure preparations of various cell types. Many studies were initially performed using antibody-coated erythrocytes which bind to cellular Fc receptors through the exposed Fc on the erythrocyte surface. Cells binding such "indicator" erythrocytes look like flower bunches and are termed rosettes [293]. Later studies have detected cellular Fc receptors using radiolabeled (usually ^{125}I) antibodies which are detected as cellularly adherent radioactivity. Scatchard analysis of such binding can then determine the amount of Fc-specific binding and can produce estimates of receptor number and binding affinity [294].

Granulocyte IgG Cytophilia

All three classes of human granulocytes—neutrophils [230], eosinophils [295], and basophils [209]—have Fc receptors for IgG. Neutrophil Fcγ receptors mediate ADCC, phagocytosis, and lysosomal enzyme release [184]. Fcγ receptors of eosinophils have similar functions except they do not release lysosomal enzymes [296–298]. The only known function for basophil Fcγ receptors is to cause release of histamine upon exposure to antigen [209,212].

Lawrence et al. found that neutrophils can bind IgG_1 and IgG_3 with equal affinity in their monomeric form, but can bind all four subclasses when aggregated [294]. This supports earlier observations that all four aggregated IgG subclasses caused release of neutrophil lysosomal enzymes [231]. The intact IgG Fc fragment binds to neutrophils with affinity equal to intact IgG, whereas reduced and alkylated IgG or Fc loses most of its binding capacity, indicating the importance of the molecule's quaternary structure for binding [235]. The importance of quaternary structure is also illustrated by the failure of isolated Facb, CH_2, or CH_3 domains (pFc′ and atCγ3) to inhibit Fc binding by neutrophils [234,235]. The apparent sensitivity of the IgG-Fc binding site to proper CH_2/CH_3 spatial orientation is reminiscent of studies of SPA, which has similar Fc binding characteristics and suggests that both Fc sites might be spatially related. This concept is supported by the recent observation by Barnett-Foster that the isolated SPA Fb fragment strongly inhibits IgG binding to neutrophils [250]. Teleologically speaking, it would be logical for staphylococcal bacteria to develop a molecule able to block the phagocytic process which would otherwise destroy them.

Cytophilic Studies for Heterocytotropic and Homocytotropic IgG

Attempts to isolate an IgG fragment capable of blocking an IgG-induced PCA reaction indicate that an intact Fc region is the smallest active fragment [300]. Minta and Painter are the only investigators to have reported that CH_3 domains (pFc′ and Fc′) could inhibit extravasation of radioactive albumin induced by an IgG PCA reaction [299]. These fragments were not able to inhibit PCA-induced extravasation of previously injected Evans blue dye, however, indicating that the previous results may have been artifactual [300].

Lymphocyte IgG Cytophilia

IgG Fc receptors present on T and B lymphocytes have both effector and regulatory functions [184,274]. Like neutrophils, lymphocytes can significantly bind only monomeric IgG_1 and IgG_3, but can bind all four IgG subclasses when aggregated [294]. Studies of human IgG subclass binding to murine T lymphocytes indicate that monomeric IgG_1, IgG_2, and IgG_3 all have significant affinity. Binding by IgG_4 and its Fc fragment, by contrast, was not observed. Isolated CH_2 and CH_3 domains both showed significant binding to murine T lymphocytes, albeit with less affinity than intact IgG. The isolated pFc′ fragment had about one tenth the affinity of monomeric IgG, while the CH_2 domain was one one hundredth as active. These results suggest that both domains probably contribute to an Fc binding site, with the CH_3 domain providing the large contribution [301]. Immunofluorescent analysis of IgG present on human B lymphocytes also suggests that the CH_3 domain may interact with membrane surface molecules. Froland and Natvig found that antiserum specific for intact IgG Fc could easily detect surface IgG. Fluorescent antiserum specific for antigens located in the CH_3 domain (pFc′), however, were only rarely detected, suggesting that they were not exposed [302]. It must be noted, however, that the IgG detected on B lymphocytes may be anchored either by Fc receptor interaction or by a carboxy-terminal hydrophobic tailpiece characteristic of the membrane forms of Igs [11,303]. Differences in the relative surface orientation of these two forms of Igs are unknown and therefore complicate the interpretation of such immunofluorescent studies.

Monocyte IgG Cytophilia

IgG Fc receptors present on monocytes are known to mediate effector functions such as phagocytosis and ADCC killing [253,304]. Huber et al. and Hay et al. found that the monocyte IgG receptor has a substantial subclass specificity and binds IgG_1 and IgG_3, but not IgG_2 and IgG_4 [304,305]. Scatchard analysis by Alexander et al. revealed that human monocytes have 20,000–100,000 IgG receptors per cell and confirmed that IgG_1 and IgG_3 had the highest binding affinities, with equilibrium Ka values of 1.1×10^8 and 8×10^7 L/mol, respectively. The Ka of IgG_4 and IgG_2 was substantially lower at 4.4×10^7 and 2×10^6 L/mol, respectively [306]. Analysis of IgG subfragments revealed that paired CH_3 domains (pFc' and atCγ3) significantly inhibit IgG binding by monocytes while CH_2 domains were inactive. Surprisingly, the pFc' fragments were reported to preserve the hierarchy of monocyte subclass affinities; pFc' $_{(1)}$ = pFc' $_{(3)}$ $\gg$ pFc' $_{(2)}$ = pFc' $_{(4)}$ [307]. The amino acid differences between the CH_3 domains of the four subclasses are minor [44] and together with possible subclass allotypic differences (Table II) must be responsible for the differing affinities of the pFc' fragments.

Further localization of amino acid residues critical to IgG monocyte binding was achieved by Ciccimarra et al., who isolated a decapeptide able to block IgG binding to monocytes. This peptide is derived from the CH_3 domain of IgG at aa 407–416. When present in nanomolar concentrations, the peptide was shown to block monocyte binding of IgG/erythrocyte rosettes by 90% [308]. In contrast to the conclusions by Dorrington that the decapeptide is completely buried in the interior of the Fc [309], we observe that four of its ten residues are completely exposed. Figures 21 and 22 show that the four carboxy-terminal residues of the peptide are exposed in intact IgG pFc' and are probably responsible for the peptide's blocking activity.

Macrophage IgG Cytophilia

Macrophage IgG Fc receptors are known to function in both phagocytosis of IgG complexes and in ADCC [309]. Cultured human macrophages and human macrophage cell lines (U-937) were shown to have 80,000 and 14,000 IgG Fc receptors per cell respectively, the latter receptors having an equilibrium dissociation constant (Kd) of 5×10^9 mol/L (310). IgG Fc receptors of the promyelocytic cell line HL-60, which differentiates into macrophages under appropriate conditions, show the highest affinity for IgG_1 and IgG_3, moderate affinity for IgG_4, and minimal affinity for IgG_4 [311,314].

The majority of the work characterizing macrophage Fc receptors has used macrophages derived from animals, mostly mice. Fortunately, human IgG has functional crossreactivity with murine IgG subclasses so that binding of human IgG to murine macrophages is probably reflective of binding to human macrophages.

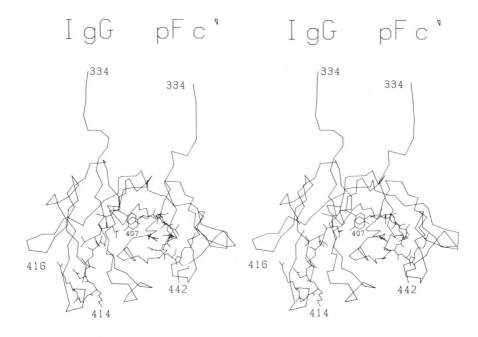

Fig. 21. Stereo view of amino acid residues within an intact IgG Fc fragment that produce a pFc' fragment (dimer of aa 334–446). The orientation of the two CH_3 domains is similar to that seen in Figure 18. The amino acid side chains of the decapeptide isolated by Ciccimarra et al., able to block IgG binding to monocytes, are displayed (aa 407–416). The remainder of the pFc' fragment is shown in its α-carbon backbone form. The four carboxy-terminal residues of the decapeptide (aa 413–416) are clearly exposed to the molecule's exterior. This view was prepared using atomic coordinates from an intact IgG Fc fragment [61]. An isolated pFc' fragment may therefore have a more compact tertiary structure (e.g., the amino-terminal extension from aa 334–340 would probably fold back upon the paired CH_3 domains). The four carboxy-terminal residues of the IgG Fc fragment (aa 443–446) did not produce a recognizable diffraction pattern and are therefore not displayed.

Recent studies have shown that mouse macrophages have two distinct Fc receptors for IgG. The first receptor is trypsin-sensitive and binds both monomeric and aggregated murine IgG_{2a}. The second receptor, which is trypsin-resistant and phospholipase-sensitive, binds only the aggregated forms of murine IgG_1, IgG_{2a}, and IgG_{2b} [312]. Walker has shown that different murine IgG subclasses may preferentially mediate phagocytosis and ADCC. He found that aggregated IgG_{2a} inhibited IgG-induced phagocytosis by 52% compared to 13% inhibition by IgG_{2b}. By contrast, aggregated IgG_{2b} inhibited ADCC by 93%, compared to 17% inhibition by IgG_{2a} [313].

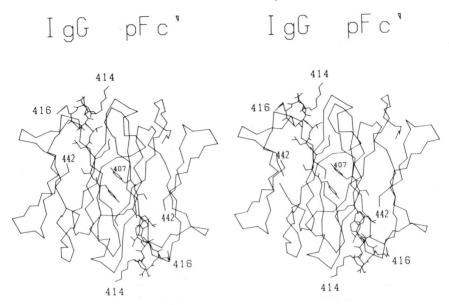

Fig. 22. Stereo view of the "bottom" of the pFc′ fragment depicted in Fig. 21. The six amino-terminal residues of the cytophilia-blocking decapeptide (Tyr 407—Val 412) are seen to be buried in the molecule's interior while the four carboxy-terminal residues (Asp 413— Arg 416) are seen to be fully exposed. The side chain to Trp 417 is also displayed in one of the CH₃ domains.

Human IgG is also recognized by two distinct murine macrophage Fc receptors. Haeffner-Cavaillon and Dorrington reported that SPA could prevent the binding of IgG_1 and its Fc fragment to murine $P388D_1$ macrophages but could not inhibit IgG_3 [315]. In the human HL-60 cell line, approximately one half of the Fc receptors can bind an IgG-SPA complex, whereas the binding to the other half is inhibited indicating that two receptor populations exist [311].

Studies of the Dob and Lec IgG_1 myeloma proteins that have hinge deletions show that both are able to inhibit IgG_{2b} binding to $P388D_1$ receptors, but cannot inhibit IgG_{2a} binding. Normal human IgG can, however, inhibit both murine IgG classes [118]. These findings suggest that the murine IgG_{2a} and IgG_{2b} receptors recognize structurally distinct regions of the immunoglobulin heavy chains. The structural basis of the Lec and Dob inhibitory patterns are related to their hinge deletions, which result in an abnormally close contact between the CH_1 domains in the Fab arms and the CH_2 domains [52]. The resulting steric hindrance of portions of the CH_2 domain prevents these proteins from binding to C_1q and apparently to the IgG_{2a} Fc receptor [118]. These results, suggesting that one of the Fc binding sites occurs primarily in the CH_2 domain, are supported by observations that the Facb fragments can bind to macrophage Fc receptors [300]. In addition, a mutant murine IgG$_{2b}$ (M311) lacking both CH$_3$ domains, can effectively bind to macrophages. Other investigators have shown that paired CH$_3$ domain (pFc') fragments can bind to macrophages, and may therefore contain all or part of a second Fc receptor binding site [219,316,317].

IgA

IgA is the predominant Ig of external secretions, including colostrum, breast milk, tears, saliva, nasal fluid, pulmonary fluid, intestinal fluid, and bile. It is present at all mucosal surfaces and thus forms a molecular "first line of defense" against invasion of foreign organisms. For this reason, Tomasi has likened IgA to an "immunological paint" which coats the surface of fragile mucous membranes [318,319].

Two different structural forms of IgA exist: monomeric "serum" IgA and polymeric "secretory" (sIgA) IgA. Monomeric IgA is the predominant form present intravascularly and makes up 85% of total plasma IgA. The majority of the remaining plasma IgA exists as dimers with higher polymers occurring in very small amounts. IgA of external secretions, by contrast, predominantly exists as dimers with smaller amounts existing as higher polymers. IgA has two subclasses termed IgA$_1$ and IgA$_2$ [46,327]. Approximately 90% of serum IgA is IgA$_1$, while 60% of sIgA is IgA$_2$ [8].

IgA Metabolism

Serum IgA is synthesized at a rate roughly equivalent to that of IgG, approximately 24 mg/kg/day for IgA$_1$ and 21 mg/kg/day for IgA$_2$. The serum half-life of both subclasses is substantially less than IgG, however (IgA$_1$ T$^{1/2}$ = 5.9 days, IgA$_2$ T$^{1/2}$ = 4.5 days), which results in a substantially lower steady state serum concentration of 180 mg/dL and 22 mg/dL, respectively [166] (Table IV). Unlike IgG, the rate of IgA catabolism is independent of its plasma concentration. Serum IgA is primarily synthesized by submucosal plasma cells that secrete J-chain dimerized IgA that is subsequently transported into secretory fluids. Fluorescent anti-IgA staining of ileal Peyer's patches and the lamina propria of the human gastrointestinal tract reveals a great preponderance of IgA-containing plasma cells, approximately 25 for each IgG-staining cell. It appears that the secretory IgA system is especially organized to locally synthesize sIgA in response to antigenic challenge [320,321]. Local synthesis by gut-associated lymphoid tissue (GALT) appears to be a major source of both secretory and serum IgA in animals [322,324]. Studies of rats and dogs indicate that over 80% of lymphatic IgA is produced by GALT plasma cells [324]. In humans, by contrast, most sIgA is probably derived from the bone marrow [323]. Oral antigen challenge of the gut produces both circulating and secreted antibodies that are predominantly IgA [324,325], whereas parenteral immunization produces a predominantly IgM or IgG response [179].

Secretory IgA Structure

Secretory IgA dimers are composed of two molecules of IgA monomer (mol wt = 150,000 daltons), containing 7–8% carbohydrate, one molecule of secretory component (SC) (mol wt = 70,000) and one J chain (mol wt = 16,422) [6,8] (Table IV). The H chain of IgA, like IgM, has a carboxy-terminal extension about 18 residues long (Fig. 2) and contains a cysteine residue that bonds to J chain and other IgA molecules. The J chain is a glycoprotein composed of 129 amino acids and a single oligosaccharide linked to asparagine 43 [6].

Polymeric forms of IgA and IgM are formed when a single cyteine residue within a J chain binds to the penultimate carboxy-terminal cysteine residue of two monomeric IgA or IgM H chains [7,8,331]. Recent ultrastructural localization of J chains in human plasma cells indicates that J chains combine with nascent Ig within the cell's endoplasmic reticulum [328]. Dimerized IgA or IgM may then serve as a "nucleus" about which further polymerization of antibody monomers occurs [329,331]. During further polymerization, monomers do not bind to the dimer's J chain, however, but instead form disulfide bonds between homologous penultimate cysteine residues of one of the dimer H chains. Although the precise mechanism of J chain-induced polymerization is unknown, it is thought that initial dimerization causes a conformational change within the antibody monomer that facilitates close contact by free monomers and subsequent polymerization [329,331]. J chains are synthesized by antibody-secreting plasma cells in parallel with antibody synthesis. It appears that the relative synthetic rates of antibody and J chain determine what fraction of secreted antibody will be polymerized [329]. Surprisingly, J chain is also synthesized by myeloma plasma cells secreting only IgG and IgD, neither of which can be polymerized [330]. The functional significance of this finding is unclear.

Secretory component interacts with dimeric or polymeric IgA, primarily via the Fc regions, and acts to reduce the susceptibility of the complex to proteolytic digestion. This protective action is thought to be particularly important for the survival of IgA in enzyme rich secretions, especially in the gastrointestinal tract [8]. Structural studies indicate that SC is disulfide bonded to only one of the two monomer IgA subunits of dimeric IgA, but confers protection against enzymatic attack to both subunits [327]. It has been suggested that SC forms a coil around both dimerized Fc regions that extends to both hinges [8,327]. Figure 23 shows a model of the proposed structure of secretory IgA. In it, the two IgA subunits are stacked end to end with Fab regions facing in opposite directions.

SC is synthesized by cells of the mucosal epithelium, where it serves as a surface receptor for J-chain-polymerized IgA or IgM. The SC-antibody complex is then transported from the lamina propria across the epithelial barrier into external excretions where the intact complex is released [332]. Rare patients having normal IgA synthesis but lacking SC fail to transport IgA into secretions and thus have a selective sIgA deficiency [333]. Recent evidence indicates that SC also serves as a receptor for IgA on hepatocytes which transport the complex into the biliary tract [334].

As in the IgG subclasses, major structural differences exist in the hinges of the two IgA subclasses. In IgA_1 at aa 223–237, there is a tandem duplication of an octapeptide sequence containing three oligosaccharide chains that is deleted in IgA_2 [46,326]. The comparable region of IgA_2 has, instead, an unusual sequence of five proline residues, which must greatly restrict conformational flexibility [326]. These structural differences are directly reflected in the susceptibility of the two subclasses to digestion by an IgA-specific protease produced by Neisseria gonorrhea, Neisseria meningitides and streptococcal bacteria in human saliva and colonic fluid. The protease readily cleaves IgA into Fab and Fc fragments by attacking a proline-threonine bond in the duplicated octapeptide sequence in the IgA_1 hinge [335]. The enzyme is inactive toward IgA_2 molecules, however, which lack the cleavage site [326,335]. It seems likely that the IgA_2 hinge deletion represents an evolutionary adaption that permits IgA_2, the predominant form of secretory IgA, to resist destruction by bacteria which regularly colonize human secretions.

Two allotypes of IgA_2 exist and are termed $IgA_2m(1)$ and $IgA_2m(2)$. They have significantly different frequencies in various human races, $IgA_2m(1)$ being prevalent in Caucasians and $IgA_2m(2)$ being prevalent in Mongoloid and black people [18]. The determinant(s) which distinguish the two allotypes are associated with the absence of H chain/L chain disulfide bonds in $IgA_2m(2)$ [18].

IgA IMMUNOLOGICAL ACTIVITIES: LOCALIZATION OF ACTIVE SITES

Secretory IgA exerts a major protective function when it binds to bacteria or viruses and thereby prevents their adherence to mucosal cells. Such nonadherent organisms are swept along by epithelial cilia and normal fluid currents present at mucosal surfaces and are therefore prevented from adhering and forming colonies [336,337]. The bacterial or viral determinants recog-

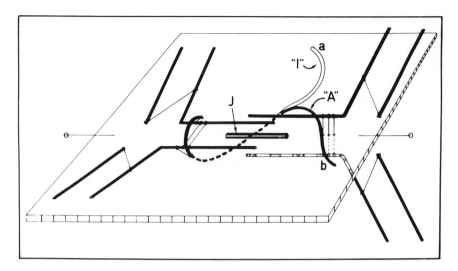

Fig. 23. Schematic model of secretory IgA. The planes containing the Fab arms of both IgA monomers are at right angles to each other. The J chain (J) is assumed to be in a largely concealed central position within the complex as suggested by chemical and antigenic analysis. Upon contacting an IgA dimer, the secretory piece ("A") may change conformation (from a to b) and coil around the two Fc regions, thus shielding some secretory piece antigens ("I"). The secretory piece is shown coiled around the two Fc portions and extends to the hinge of both IgA molecules, thus providing protection from proteolytic attack. (Reproduced from Heremans [8] with permission.)

nized by such adherence-preventing sIgA include bacterial pili and viral receptors that bind to specific structures on epithelial cell surfaces and thus serve as anchors for the organisms. Inhibition of bacterial adherence and colonization by sIgA has been experimentally observed for many pathogenic bacteria including *E. coli* to urinary tract and gut epithelium, *Neisseria gonorrhea* to cervical and vaginal cells, *Shigella* and *Vibrio colerae* to gut epithelium and *Streptococcus mutans* to cariogenic polysaccharides in dental plaque [229]. sIgA similarly prevents adsorption and colonization of many viruses including rhinovirus, influenza, myxovirus, and polio virus. sIgA exerts an additional protective effect when it binds to exotoxins elaborated by pathogenic bacteria and thereby prevents interaction of the toxin with cellular receptors. Cholera toxin, for example, is completely inactivated by interaction with IgA [229,338].

sIgA is also important in preventing absorption of potentially antigenic molecules by the gut and lung epithelium. The consequences of the lack of such "immune exclusion" is observed in patients with selective IgA deficiency. This condition is present in one person in 500–700 and is clinically defined when the serum IgA concentration is less than 5 mg/dL [339]. These patients usually have high titers of IgG antibodies directed toward many commonly ingested foods including milk proteins (casein, bovine serum albumin) and animal and vegetable proteins [340]. Such IgA-deficient patients may have detectable circulating immune complexes containing milk proteins one hour after drinking a single glass of milk [341]. The relatively high incidence of atopic allergy and autoimmune disease in selective IgA-deficient patients may also be related to a reduction in immune exclusion. Inhaled or ingested antigens crossreactive with "self" molecules, if presented to the systemic immune system at a sufficient dose, may overcome self-tolerance and thus induce autoimmune reactivity [342]. Similarly, excessive absorption of potentially atopic allergens in early life may stimulate abnormally high levels of IgE synthesis resulting in allergic disease [339].

Patients having selective IgA deficiency who have received transfusions of human blood or its fractions are at risk of developing IgE sensitization directed against IgA determinants. Retransfusion of such patients may produce an anaphylactic response [343].

Complement Activation

Native IgA does not activate the complement system by the classical pathway, although it can activate the alternative pathway upon binding antigen [184]. The biological importance of alternative-pathway activation by IgA is, however, unknown, since complement is present in very low concentrations in external secretions.

Interestingly, several investigators have reported that isolated IgA Fc fragments are nearly as effective as IgG in activating the classical complement pathway [344,345]. These observations imply that the C_1q binding site of IgA Fc is sterically hindered or modified by the Fab arms as occurs in human IgG_4.

ADCC

IgA appears to be incapable of mediating ADCC by either granulocytes, monocytes, macrophages, or lymphocytes [346]. Recent studies by Shen and Fanger indicate, however, that sIgA may enhance ADCC killing by IgG, possibly by increasing adherence of the ADCC cell to the target cell through IgA Fc receptor binding [346].

Fc RECEPTORS FOR IgA
Staphylococcal Protein A

Although it is usually stated that IgA does not bind to SPA, numerous studies have shown that certain human IgA molecules have significant SPA-binding ability [282,347]. The site in the IgA Fc region to which SPA binds is probably similar to the IgG Fc site, since IgG_1 and IgA_1 can both inhibit

SPA binding to the other [282]. The possibility exists, however, that the four distinct Fc binding subunits within SPA may exhibit some degree of selectivity for H chain classes, since inhibition of SPA binding to radiolabeled proteins was greatest for the homologous inhibitor.

Various investigators have reported that IgA binding by SPA has [348] or does not have [282] subclass specificity. It does seem clear, however, that within a subclass, significant SPA binding heterogeneity exists.

Cellular IgA Fc Receptors

IgA-specific Fc receptors have been found on human granulocytes [349], monocytes [349], and lymphocytes [349,350,351]. Lawrence et al. first demonstrated that both aggregated and monomeric IgA bound to Fc receptors on human neutrophils. Both subclasses of aggregated IgA had a greater affinity than monomeric IgA [294] and caused release of lysosomal enzymes and phagocytosis of insoluble IgA complexes [231]. Fanger et al. using IgA-sensitized ox erythrocytes, found that 35% (range 24–40%) of human granulocytes have IgA Fc receptors, which showed little specificity for a particular subclass or state of aggregation. Approximately 37% (range 27–46%) of human monocytes also display subclass-nonspecific IgA Fc receptors. In both monocytes and granulocytes, neither J chain nor SC significantly influence binding [349]. Unlike granulocytes or monocytes, lymphocyte Fc receptors seem to have a higher affinity for the IgA_2 subclass.

The submolecular region(s) in IgA Fc that are recognized by Fcα receptors include a site in the CH_2 domain, since the IgA_1 myeloma (Wal) which lacks the CH_3 domain could block IgA rosette formation. For granulocytes and monocytes, IgA Wal was a more effective inhibitor than intact IgA_1. Since IgA Wal exists only as a half molecule, the CH_2 site must not depend on trans interactions with the second H chain [352].

IgM

IgM is the largest Ig, having a molecular weight of about 960,000 daltons, of which 12% is carbohydrate (Table IV). Sometimes referred to as a "macroglobulin," it consists of five covalently bonded IgM monomers, each having two H and L chains and one J chain. In addition, IgM found in secretions may also contain secretory piece [7].

IgM is the most primitive of the Ig classes. Molecules structurally similar to human IgM are present in sharks and other primitive vertebrate fish [128]. In Ig ontogeny, IgM is the first antibody class detectable in the liver of the developing fetus at about nine weeks of gestation [353]. It is also the first antibody class synthesized after primary antigen challenge and may be induced by thymus-independent antigens with minimal regulation by T-helper cells [177].

IgM Metabolism

● The serum IgM concentration in adults is approximately 75 mg/dL or 5% of total circulating Igs. Its plasma half-life of five days is similar to that of IgA. IgM is synthesized at a rate of 2.2 mg/kg/d or 154 mg/70 kg human, of which 74% remains in the intravascular pool (Table IV). The catabolic rate of IgM is 11% of the plasma pool per day and, like IgA, the rate is independent of its serum concentration [166]. Approximately 7.5% of normal human peripheral blood lymphocytes have detectable surface IgM [191].

IgM Subclasses

Two subclasses of IgM have been distinguished on the basis of their ability to activate the classical complement system [66]. The structural or antigenic basis for this division is, however, unclear, and may reflect allotypic or mutational differences in the IgM myeloma proteins examined.

IgM Structure

The pentameric form of IgM resembles a star in electron micrographs and is shown schematically in Figure 24 [354]. The H chain of each IgM monomer has five domains instead of the four present in IgG, IgA, and IgD. The "extra" domain is located at the site of the hinge in IgG, IgA, and IgD, and is designated $C\mu2$ [16,158].

In addition, the monomeric membrane form of IgM has a polypeptide tailpiece with a 26 residue hydrophobic core that spans the lymphocyte plasma membrane [9]. The tailpiece derives from a separately coded DNA exon that exists immediately 3' to the $C\mu4$ domain. The 41 residues that comprise the tailpiece replace the 20 residue carboxyterminal segment of secreted IgM and allow IgM to act as a lymphocyte antigen receptor, along with a similar membrane form of IgD and possibly other Ig classes [10,97,355].

The mechanism of polymerization of IgM resembles that of IgA and involves initial J-chain-induced dimerization followed by disulfide bonding between penultimate cysteine residues (aa 575) of IgM monomers [330,331].

Normal serum may also contain small amounts of IgM monomers that are structurally intact. The functional significance of this secreted form of IgM is unknown. Large amounts of monomeric IgM frequently accompany diseases with abnormally high rates of IgM synthesis, such as chronic infections, IgM monoclonal gammopathy, rheumatoid arthritis, systemic lupus erythrematosus, and ataxia-telangiectasia [7,357].

IgM has two inter-H chain disulfide bonds, one of which immediately precedes the beginning of $C\mu3$ and therefore resembles the IgG hinge disulfides. The second inter-H chain disulfide bond occurs within $C\mu3$ at aa

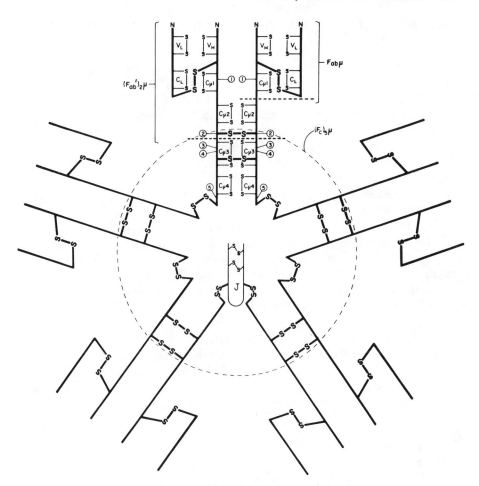

Fig. 24. Schematic model of mammalian IgM. The five IgM monomers are covalently linked to each other or, in the case of two of the monomers, to a single J chain. The five oligosaccharide attachment sites are indicated by circled numbers (see also Fig. 10). The dashed line separating oligosaccharides 2 and 3 indicate the site of cleavage to produce the two domain Fcμ fragment, which consists of Cμ3 and Cμ4. When pentameric IgM is cleaved in this manner, the $(Fc)_5$ μ fragment is produced (indicated by dashed circle). (Reproduced from Cathou [354] with permission.)

414, 12 residues before the second intradomain cysteine [158,358,359]. This unusual arrangement must result in a unique quaternary structure of IgM and its Fc fragment which, like IgG, consists of the two carboxy-terminal H chain domains [158,356].

IgM IMMUNOLOGICAL ACTIVITIES: LOCALIZATION OF ACTIVE SITES

The multivalency of pentameric IgM makes it a very efficient agglutinator. Its ten antigen-binding arms are able to bridge adjacent cells and are responsible for the isohemagglutination reaction of type A and B human erythrocytes [360]. The term "complete antibody" was coined to represent this agglutinating ability of IgM when compared to "incomplete" antibodies of the IgG class [361]. When bound to antigens on a single surface such as a bacterial flagella, electron micrographs reveal that IgM resembles a staple in which the Fab arms point downward [362]. This demonstrates that significant segmental flexibility between Fab and Fc regions exists even though IgM lacks a hinge.

The ability of IgM to aggregate bacteria and viruses is probably important for the clearance of these organisms by the reticuloendothelial system. In addition, IgM is much more efficient than IgG in activating complement and is therefore a "logical" first antibody to respond to the initial stages of a bacterial or viral infection [363]. The importance of IgM as an antibody "first line of defense" is well illustrated by humans who lack IgM. They are very susceptible to rapid and fatal bacterial sepsis [364].

A number of antigens elicit an antibody response that is predominantly IgM, even upon repeated immunization, which usually triggers a switch from IgM to other classes. These antigens include gram-negative bacterial endotoxins, rheumatoid factors, erythrocyte A and B polysaccharides, and the infectious mononucleosis heterophile antigen [442].

IgM EFFECTOR FUNCTIONS

Complement Activation

IgM is the most active antibody in its ability to activate the classical complement pathway. This ability is related to the pentameric structure of IgM which contains five Fc regions, each of which contains C_1q binding sites [184,363]. Hurst found that an isolated IgM Fc fragment has about 1/40 the complement activity of pentameric IgM, which demonstrates the cooperative effect of the pentameric structure [366]. A fragment consisting of paired $C\mu3$ domains and the amino-terminal portion of $C\mu4$ had 1/20 the activity of pentameric IgM; even higher activity than the Fc fragment. Other fragments from the $C\mu4$ domain consisting of a 24 residue peptide (aa 468–491) linked by the $C\mu4$ intradomain disulfide bond to a 32 residue peptide (aa 515–546) had 1/46 the activity of pentameric IgM; about equal to the activity of the Fc fragment [367]. The activity of this peptide suggested that the $C\mu4$ domain contains the C_1q binding site of IgM. It must be noted, however, that $C\mu3$ domains have not been isolated and tested for complement activating ability. A synthetic pentapeptide that mimics the sequence of $C\mu4$ at aa 487–491 was shown by Johnson and Thames to have about 1/200 the ability of human IgG_1 in activating complement [221]. This peptide and the carboxy-terminal portion of the 24 residue peptide mentioned previously are homologous to the region of IgG, CH_2, implicated as the C_1q binding site. This implies that the same domain region of nonhomologous domains ($C\gamma2$ and $C\mu4$) have similar effector sites.

ADCC

The ability of IgM to mediate ADCC killing is controversial. The unequivocal demonstration of IgM-mediated ADCC killing is difficult because even trace IgG contamination of the IgM preparation will produce measurable killing of targets [368]. Studies using hybridoma-derived IgM have failed to demonstrate ADCC killing [368]. Structural analysis of these hybridomas to prove that they have a normal amino acid sequence, however, has not been done. Other investigators, taking extreme precautions to exclude contaminating IgG, have found significant IgM ADCC killing by human PBLs [369,370]. Shen et al., while failing to find ADCC killing by monoclonal IgM, found that IgM could synergize with IgG to increase IgG-mediated ADCC killing [368].

IgM LEUKOCYTE CHEMOTACTIC FACTOR

Aoki et al. has reported that a 12,000-dalton tryptic fragment from human IgM exhibits a strong chemotactic activity towards rabbit peritoneal neutrophils. This chemotactic fragment is derived from the Fc portion of IgM; however, its location has not been further characterized [371]. Its chemotactic activity is reminiscent of the activity found in enzymatic digests of IgG discussed earlier.

Fc RECEPTORS FOR IgM
Staphylococcal Protein A

IgM from both normal serum and monoclonal sources has been shown to bind to SPA [283]. All sources of IgM, however, do not have SPA-binding ability, suggesting that IgM structural heterogeneity exists. This observation has prompted the suggestion that two IgM subclasses exist, an idea previously proposed on the basis of IgM complement activation studies [66]. In support of this concept, Grov has shown that some IgM macroglobulins have SPA reactivity that is associated with the presence of unique IgM antigenic determinants [365]. SPA can bind to both monomeric and pentameric forms of IgM. The structure of the binding site in IgM is probably similar to that of IgG, since both antibodies can reciprocally inhibit the binding of the other [283].

CELLULAR IgM Fc RECEPTORS

Fc receptors specific for IgM have been demonstrated on T [372] and B [373] lymphocytes but not on neutrophils, monocytes, or macrophages [294,374,375]. Approximately 60% of human peripheral blood T lymphocytes have Fc receptors for IgM [372]. These receptors have the highest affinity for monomeric IgM, but have significant affinity for pentameric IgM as well [372]. Moretta first reported that T lymphocytes with Fcμ receptors function as T-helper cells [376]; however, further analysis has revealed that helper activity also occurs in other cell types [377]. The B lymphocyte Fcμ receptor is similar to the T lymphocyte Fcμ receptor in its preference for monomeric IgM, although it too binds pentameric IgM [373]. The Cμ4 domain has affinity for lymphocyte Fcμ receptors. Conradie and Bub showed that the enzymatically isolated Cμ4 domain (cleaved at Lys 445) could inhibit IgM/erythrocyte rosette formation with human PBLs as effectively as the intact Fcμ fragment. A Cμ4 domain with its normally present carbohydrate chain at Asn 563 had less inhibitory capacity than did the Cμ4 domain lacking the carbohydrate, indicating that oligosaccharide structures do not form part of the Fc binding site [378].

IgD

IgD was discovered in 1965 by Rowe and Fahey in the serum of a patient with a previously unrecognized myeloma protein [379]. It is present in very low concentrations in normal adult serum at approximately 17 μg/mL [162] (Table III). For many years the function of IgD remained enigmatic because it could not be shown to have a distinct biologic role in the immune system. A clue to its function came in 1972 when Van Boxel found that IgD was a major surface antibody of lymphocytes [380]. The discovery by Rowe in 1973 that both IgD and IgM exist simultaneously on lymphocytes prompted the suggestion that IgD may act in concert with IgM as membrane-bound antigen receptors, an idea that has received considerable experimental support [381].

IgD Metabolism

IgD is synthesized at a rate of 0.4 mg/kg/d (28 mg/70 kg human) and has an unusually short half-life of 2.8 days in human plasma [166] (Table IV). This is probably due to the unusual sensitivity of its hinge to proteolysis by plasma proteases [17,45]. IgD, like IgM, exists predominantly in the intravascular space (75%) with about 37% of this pool being degraded per day. IgD is unusual in that its plasma half-life is inversely proportional to its plasma concentration; a low concentration being associated with a rapid rate of degradation and vice versa [166]. Analysis of the IgD concentration in 112 normal sera revealed a trimodal distribution with modes at 0.35 μg/mL, 7 μg/mL, and 49 μg/mL. Such a distribution is consistent with a monogenic inheritance mechanism in which serum IgD levels are controlled by single high and low IgD alleles at one gene locus [382]. Approximately 3–5% of normal human peripheral blood lymphocytes have detectable surface IgD [380].

IgD STRUCTURE

Serum IgD has a molecular weight of about 170,000 dalton and contains 12.3% carbohydrate. It has a four-chain structure of two H chains, each having one V and three C domains, and two L chains (Fig. 25) [17]. The proportion of myeloma IgD molecules having λ L chains is greater than 90%, compared to all other H chain classes, which have 40% λ L chains [383]. The primary structure of IgD was deduced in 1981 and was found to be unusual in several respects [17,34,155,157]. IgD has an extended hinge of 64 residues with only a single inter-H chain disulfide bond, making it unique among human Igs [45]. Only one hydrophobic residue and three or four proline residues occur in the hinge which suggest that it is probably open and very flexible. The amino-terminal half of the hinge contains four or five oligosaccharide chains within a 20 residue stretch. The carboxy-terminal half, by contrast, has no carbohydrate but contains a highly charged 24 residue segment containing 10 negatively charged glutamic acid residues and 10 positively charged residues; 7 lysines and 3 arginines. It is this 24 residue charged hinge segment that is highly sensitive to tryptic digestion and yields small peptides, which, according to Lin and Putnam, may have immunoregulatory activity [17,157]. The Fcδ fragment, by contrast, is very resistant to proteolysis and has 226 residues with an unremarkable sequence distribution except for two nearly identical 8 residue segments in Cδ3, each of which contain 5 prolines [155].

In contrast to human lymphocytes, murine B lymphocytes have two molecular forms of surface IgD; the usual four-chain monomeric IgD structure, murine IgD_I and a unique two-chain half-molecule IgD consisting only of a single disulfide-bonded H and L chain (IgD_{II}) [384,385]. The amount of IgD_{II} expressed appears to be genetically linked to a murine H chain allotype locus and is present in many normal mouse strains [386]. The IgD_{II} H chain appears to be normal except for the absence of inter-H chain cysteine residues. The functional significance of IgD_{II} in mice is unclear. Whether similar half-molecular forms of IgD exist in animals other than mice is unknown.

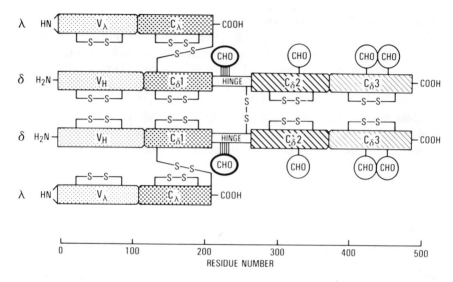

Fig. 25. Schematic model of human IgD. IgD has a four-domain heavy chain structure and an extended 64 residue hinge with multiple oligosaccharide (galactosamine) attachment sites indicated by the oval CHO symbol. Glucosamine-containing oligosaccharides are indicated by circular CHO symbols. A single disulfide bond connects the two heavy chains which, together with the extended hinge, must provide considerable segmental flexibility between Fab arms and the Fc portion. (Redrawn after Lin and Putnam [17].)

IgD IMMUNOLOGICAL ACTIVITIES: LOCALIZATION OF ACTIVE SITES

IgD exists together with IgM on the surface of a majority of circulating B lymphocytes and serves as a membrane-bound antigen receptor. In this form, membrane-bound IgD (mIgD) probably has a hydrophobic tailpiece that spans the plasma membrane, similar to that demonstrated for mIgM [10,355].

IgM is the first class of antibodies detected on cells early in mammalian development, followed by IgD. In newborn mice, over 90% of B lymphocytes have only IgM on the cell surface [385]. At this time, B lymphocytes are very easily tolerized by exposure to thymus-dependent (TD) antigens. (Exposure to thymus-independent [TI] antigens at this time, by contrast, may elicit an antibody response.)

The mIgM antigen receptor, upon binding a TD antigen, appears to deliver a tolerizing signal to the lymphocyte that renders it unresponsive to a subsequent exposure to antigen. During the first week of life, B lymphocytes mature and begin to express mIgD. At this point, antigen-induced tolerance becomes very difficult to induce. Exposure to antigen can then trigger antibody synthesis, isotype switch and generation of memory B lymphocytes [388]. Antigen binding by mIgD, therefore, appears to act as a nonspecific signal necessary for B lymphocytes to respond for the first time to TD antigens [389]. If mIgD is removed from B lymphocytes, either enzymatically or by anti-IgD treatment, tolerance to TD antigens once again becomes easy to induce. Removal of mIgM, by contrast, abolishes antibody responses to both TD and TI antigens, indicating the importance of IgM for a TI antigen response [390].

After an mIgM[+], mIgD[+] B lymphocyte is first exposed to antigen, some cells of the proliferating clone lose their mIgM and become mIgD[+] memory B lymphocytes. A subsequent encounter with antigen triggers memory cells to rapidly develop into plasma cells secreting high-affinity IgG, IgA, or IgE. This differentiation process is illustrated schematically in Figure 26, which traces the development of a pre-B lymphocyte into a plasma cell [389].

IgD Effector Functions

IgD appears to be devoid of recognized effector activities, including complement activation, ADCC, or phagocytosis stimulation [391,392]. In addition, its low serum concentration would appear to make IgD relatively ineffective in opsonization or excluding antigen from body compartments.

Fc RECEPTORS FOR IgD
SPA-Like Bacterial Receptors for IgD

Although SPA does not bind to IgD, many bacterial strains have receptors that can bind to human IgD. Forsgren and Grubb found that 44 bacterial strains belonging to 19 bacterial species have IgD binding capacity. The highest level of IgD binding was observed in *Neisseria catarrhalis* and *Hemophilus influenzae* with moderate binding being observed in groups A, C, and G *Streptococci*. The site in IgD to which the bacteria bind appears to be in the Fab fragment, although a lower degree of binding was also observed in the Fc fragment [393]. This pattern of binding activity is reminiscent of SPA, which also binds to IgG and IgE Fab fragments in addition to Fc [285]. Whether bacterial IgD binding has any functional importance in regulating antibody responses to bacteria is unknown.

Cellular IgD Receptors

IgD Fc receptors have been detected on granulocytes, monocytes, and macrophages. Recently, Sjöberg found that 2.2% of human PBLs express IgD-specific Fc receptors. T lymphocytes had 1.2–2.6% Fcδ receptors, whereas

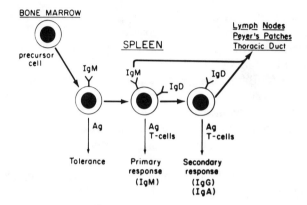

Fig. 26. Schematic model of B lymphocyte differentiation. Immature pre-B lymphocytes express only IgM on their surface, and are readily tolerized by exposure to antigen. Mature B lymphocytes express both surface IgM and IgD and may be triggered by antigen exposure to synthesize IgM (primary response). Memory B lymphocytes bearing only surface IgD (possibly in conjunction with a second heavy chain isotype) are triggered by antigen exposure to synthesize high-affinity IgG, IgA, or IgE directed toward the stimulating antigen (secondary anamnestic response). (Reproduced from Kettmen et al. [389] with permission.)

5.7–11.6% of non-T lymphocytes had Fcδ receptors [394]. Since IgD has no known cell-killing function, it is probable that Fcδ receptors help to regulate IgD synthesis or metabolism.

IgE

IgE is the most recently discovered class of Igs first characterized by Ishizaka in 1966, and independently described in a myeloma IgE by Johansson. Ishizaka called the new antibody "gamma E globulin" because it produced experimental erythema [204]. It proved to be the long-sought-after "reagenic" antibody first described by Prausnitz and Küstner, who in 1921 showed that fish-allergen sensitivity could be transferred by the serum from an allergic person to a nonallergic individual [206].

IgE Metabolism

The concentration of IgE in serum is the lowest of all the immunoglobulin classes at 50 ng/mL in nonallergic adults, about 1/20,000 the concentration of IgG. It has the shortest half-life (2.7 days) and highest fractional turnover rate (94% of plasma IgE/day) of any Ig (Table IV). Of the 4 µg/kg/day synthesized, approximately 40% remains within the intravascular pool. The catabolic rate of IgE is independent of its serum concentration, except at extremely elevated levels, as may occur in myeloma when the half-life may be doubled [395].

IgE plasma cells are found in large numbers in the lamina propria of mucous membranes, especially in the respiratory and gastrointestinal tracts. The tonsils and adenoids in particular have the highest concentration of IgE plasma cells of any lymphoid organs. By contrast, systemic lymphoid organs, including spleen and lymph nodes, have few IgE plasma cells [396]. This plasma cell distribution closely resembles that of IgA and [320,321] suggests that IgE also plays an important role as an antibody of secretions. It is interesting in this regard that the structural genes for the IgE and IgA H chains in mice are the last two in the murine H chain gene cluster, respectively [96] (Fig. 12).

IgE synthesis in mice and humans appears to be significantly regulated by suppressor T lymphocytes. Treatment of mice with procedures known to eliminate T lymphocytes such as thymectomy, sublethal whole body irradiation, antithymocyte serum, and cyclophosphamide all cause long-term enhancement of IgE production. Subsequent injection of syngeneic hyperimmunized T lymphocytes into treated mice causes the elevated IgE levels to rapidly return to normal [397,398]. Diseases in humans accompanied by abnormal T-cell function frequently have high serum IgE levels. Notable among these are Wiskott-Aldrich, Nezelof, and Di George syndromes, Hodgkin's lymphoma, hyper IgE-syndrome, atopic dermatitis, and occasionally selective IgA deficiency. Other immunodeficiency diseases, however, may be accompanied by a deficiency of IgE and include ataxia-telangiectasia and Bruton's hypogammaglobulinemia [399].

Certain parasitic diseases produce extremely high elevations of IgE and have prompted the suggestion that IgE may act as an antiparasitic antibody. Intestinal helminths and bronchopulmonary aspergillosis, in particular, produce strikingly elevated serum IgE concentrations [400].

Hamburger and associates first demonstrated that the total IgE level in humans is strongly influenced by genetic factors and suggested that two alleles at a single genetic locus may regulate total synthesis [401]. Subsequent work by Marsh provided evidence that a single autosomal gene locus with a dominant low IgE level allele (R) and recessive high level allele (r) could adequately explain observed IgE inheritance patterns [402]. This IgE regulator gene is not linked to HLA or H chain Gm alotype loci. Other genes linked to HLA loci appear to independently regulate antigen-specific IgE responses.

The ability to make an IgE response to the ragweed-derived allergen Ra5, for example, is strongly linked to the HLA-B7 locus regardless of total IgE levels. Thus, persons having a low total IgE level (genotype R/R or R/r) may yet make a clinically significant IgE response to allergen if they possess the appropriate antigen-specific immune response genes [403].

The combined action of serum IgE regulator genes and immune response genes are responsible for the significant familial association of IgE-mediated (atopic) allergies including asthma, allergic rhinitis, urticaria, and anaphylactic reactions to insect bites. This familial tendency may be approximately quantified as follows: The probability that a child will have allergic disease is about 50% if both parents are allergic, 30% if one parent is allergic, and 13% if neither parent has allergic disease [404]. If both parents are allergic and have the same allergic disease, the probability of an allergic child climbs to about 70%.

IgE Structure

IgE has a molecular weight of about 190,000 daltons, of which 12% is carbohydrate. It has two L chains and two H chains, each with a molecular weight of about 72,000 daltons. The IgE H chain, like IgM, has four constant domains and lacks a distinct hinge region. The two inter-H chain disulfide bonds occur at aa 231 and aa 318, and flank the "extra" $C\epsilon_2$ domain [405]. (Fig. 27). This IgM-like inter-H chain bonding pattern and lack of hinge are probably responsible for the relative rigidity of intact IgE when compared to IgG using fluorescence polarization and spin-labels [406]. Papain digestion splits IgE into two Fab fragments and one three-domain Fc fragment that contains two class-specific antigenic determinants, $D\epsilon_1$ and $D\epsilon_2$. Combined papain and pepsin treatment produces stable $C\epsilon_2$ domains that contain the $D\epsilon_1$ determinant and conformationally unstable $C\epsilon_3$ and $C\epsilon_4$ domains that contain the $D\epsilon_2$ determinant [407]. IgE is unique among the five Ig classes in its heat sensitivity. Heating at 56°C for 30 minutes causes irreversible thermal denaturation with parallel loss of both the $D\epsilon_2$ determinant and cytophilic binding activity for mast cells and basophils. Dorrington and Bennich found that the $C\epsilon_3$ and $C\epsilon_4$ domains contain the heat sensitive structures of Fcϵ. Heating Fcϵ fragments produced irreversible changes in the circular dichroism spectrum from the $C\epsilon_3/C\epsilon_4$ region and caused exposure of buried tryptophan and tyrosine residues [408]. The Fcϵ fragment is also sensitive to reduction and alkylation of disulfide bonds which similarly causes loss of cytophilic activity [409]. Removal of carbohydrate residues does not affect cytophilia of rat IgE, indicating that the cytophilic structures are protein in nature and do not depend on carbohydrate for stability [410].

IgE IMMUNOLOGICAL ACTIVITIES: LOCALIZATION OF ACTIVE SITES

The great majority of the symptoms associated with IgE-mediated allergic diseases are caused by substances released from circulating basophils and tissue mast cells. Both cell types contain surface Fc receptors with high

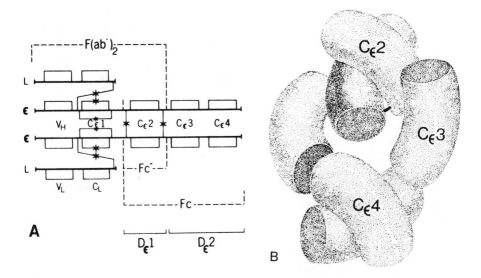

Fig. 27. (A)Schematic structure of human IgE. The heavy chain consists of five domains, one V domain and four C domains. Unlike other immunoglobulin classes, the IgE Fc fragment contains three C domains per heavy chain fragment (Cε2, Cε3, and Cε4). The thin lines represent disulfide bonds. Those disulfide bonds marked with a star are relatively labile and are reduced by mild chemical treatment. Dε1 and Dε2 are the two major class-specific antigens located in the FCε fragment. (B) Hypothetical molecular model of the Fc region of human IgE. The two Cε4 domains are shown to have extensive noncovalent interactions that resemble those of the Cγ3 domain of IgG. The Cε3 domains, by contrast, do not interact and are held apart by the "extra" Cε2 domains. The proposed spatial separation of the Cε3 domains resembles that observed in Cγ2 domains which are separated by bulky oligosaccharide chains contributed by both Cγ2 domains. (Reproduced with permission from Dorrington and Bennich [408].)

affinity for monomeric IgE ($Ka = 10^9$ L/mol). Human basophils were estimated to have 40,000 to 100,000 Fcε receptors, while rat mast cells have considerably more, from 300,000 to 1,400,000. Even with the high affinity of IgE for its Fc receptor, the extraordinarily low levels of IgE in plasma result in only partial saturation of Fc receptors [411].

To provide perspective to the number of molecules and sizes of cells involved, one can imagine a 15-μ diameter basophil at a scale of 3 Å/mm. At this scale, a hydrogen atom is 0.33 mm in diameter, an IgE molecule is about 1.6 inch high and 1.2 inch wide, an erythrocyte is 83 ft in diameter and a basophil is 164 ft in diameter. A basophil with 100,000 Fcε receptors would have one receptor per 11 × 11-inch square; at 1,000,000 receptors, one receptor per 3.5 × 3.5-inch square.

An observer viewing the IgE/Fcε receptor complexes would see them "floating" in the fluid lipid bilayer of the cell's plasma membrane. Recent estimates of the lateral mobility of Fc receptors in the plasma membrane suggest that each Fc receptor may randomly contact other receptors about 65 times per second [412]. In order for IgE to trigger degranulation, a divalent antigen must simultaneously bind to two adjacent IgE molecules and thus "bridge" them. This bridging reaction may occur in a stepwise manner in which a single IgE Fab arm binds to an antigen and "floats" in the plasma membrane until it encounters another IgE molecule having the same antigen specificity. IgE bridging may also be mimicked by anti-IgE antibody which also cross-links adjacent IgE molecules and by anti-Fcε receptor antibody which directly cross-links the Fcε receptor. These physical events result in calcium influx, methylation of Fcε-receptor-associated membrane proteins and ultimate degranulation and release of vasoactive substances including histamine, leukotriene C (formerly called slow-reacting substance of anaphylaxis, SRS-A), platelet activating factor (PAF), eosinophil chemotactic factors, and a variety of other substances [407]. Because of the requirement for antigen bridging, the probability of an antigen encountering two IgE molecules with V regions directed toward the antigen is proportional to the fraction of the total cell-bound IgE that is directed toward the particular antigen [408]. In other words, the likelihood of an antigen causing degranulation of a basophil with 10,000 IgE molecules, 1,000 of which are antigen reactive, is the same as for a cell having 100,000 IgE molecules, 10,000 of which are antigen reactive. This fact explains how persons with a low total serum IgE level may be allergic to a particular allergen if a high proportion of their IgE is directed toward the allergen. Conversely, a person having a high total IgE level may have no allergic disease if no single clone of IgE predominates.

The degranulation event causes a rapid increase in vascular permeability, which produces extravasation of plasma, causing edema and the typical wheal and flare of cutaneous anaphylaxis. Chemotactic substances released also attract eosinophils and other leukocytes that contribute to the general inflammatory response. Such an immediate, large-scale response to a potentially minute amount of antigen may be considered as an early warning "first line of defense" which rapidly recruits large numbers of cytotoxic cells and antibodies (IgG and IgM) [413]. The high concentrations of IgE elicited by parasitic invasion has prompted the suggestion that IgE might be important in controlling such infection. Experimental infection of animals with intestinal helminths do support such a role since the local anaphylactic response and diarrhea elicited by gut invasion causes worms to be expelled [414].

ADCC

Recent evidence indicates that both eosinophils and macrophages are able to kill microfilaria and *Schistosoma mansoni* by an IgE-mediated ADCC-like mechanism. Both cell types bind to antigen-bound IgE by its Fc portion and appear to kill by direct cell contact [415].

COMPLEMENT ACTIVATION

IgE is incapable of activating the classical complement system. Aggregated IgE can activate the alternative complement pathway; however, the biological significance of this observation is unknown [411].

SPA BINDING

Although SPA does not bind to the Fc fragment of IgE, it does bind to sites in the $F(ab')_2$ portion of IgE. These sites, unlike those responsible for cytophilic binding, are heat-stable and may include portions of $C\epsilon_2$, $C\epsilon_1$, or the V_H domain [284].

CELLULAR IgE Fc RECEPTORS

In addition to mast cells and basophils, Fc receptors for IgE have been demonstrated on lymphocytes [417], monocytes [417], macrophages [418], and eosinophils [415]. Lawrence et al. first demonstrated that normal human peripheral lymphocytes bound aggregated human IgE myeloma proteins [294]. Further studies by Gonzalez-Molina and Spiegelberg demonstrated that about 1–2% of normal human B lymphocytes have $Fc\epsilon$ receptors [416]. Fewer normal T lymphocytes proved to have $Fc\epsilon$ receptors (less than 0.5%); however, approximately 20% of human monocytes were found to have $Fc\epsilon$ receptors [417]. The binding affinity of IgE for $Fc\epsilon$ receptors in both T and B lymphocytes and monocytes is about 1×10^6 to 7.5×10^7 L/mol; less than 1/100 the affinity of $Fc\epsilon$ receptors on human mast cells or basophils. Both lymphocyte and monocyte $Fc\epsilon$ receptors bind only to native IgE or its Fc fragment and show no affinity for reduced and alkylated IgE.

The function of lymphocyte $Fc\epsilon$ receptors is unknown. Recent studies of allergic humans show that the expression of lymphocyte $Fc\epsilon$ receptors more than doubled during clinical exacerbation of allergic rhinitis, but returned to normal when the patients became asymptomatic [419]. Severely allergic patients, by contrast, had a continuous five- to sixfold elevation of $Fc\epsilon$-

bearing lymphocytes. As in the nonallergic controls, about 90% of these cells were B lymphocytes. No correlation between elevated Fcε expression and IgE levels was found indicating that the IgE alone was not enhancing Fcε expression. These Fcε-bearing lymphocytes are presumably involved in the regulation of IgE synthesis.

IgE BINDING FACTORS

A subpopulation of T lymphocytes expressing Fc receptors has been recently shown to secrete soluble glycoprotein "factors" which can either stimulate or inhibit IgE synthesis in vitro. These factors have a molecular weight of 10,000–20,000 daltons and have either stimulatory or inhibitory activity depending on whether they bind or do not bind to lentil lectin, respectively. These factors are optimally generated under conditions which favor an IgE response and include helminth infection (Nippostrongylus brasiliensis) or injection of complete Freund's adjuvant. After release, the factors appear to bind to IgE present on B lymphocytes and subsequently regulate B cell differentiation and IgE synthesis. These factors, like cellular receptors for IgE, only bind to native IgE or its Fc fragment [420,421].

BIOLOGICALLY ACTIVE PEPTIDES FROM IgE
Human IgE Pentapeptide (HEPP)

In 1975, Hamburger reported that a pentapeptide, L-Asp-Ser-Asp-Pro-Arg, with sequence identical to aa 320 to 324 of the human IgE H chain [405] could inhibit the human P-K response by up to 89% [422]. Since the peptide did not inhibit either codeine-induced degranulation or histamine wheal and flare reactions, Hamburger suggested that the peptide might bind to the Fcε receptor and thus block IgE cytophilia for mast cells and basophils. Although early attempts to replicate these findings failed [423], other investigators confirmed the peptide's ability to inhibit IgE-mediated degranulation [424,425]. Later studies by Hamburger suggested that HEPP may have an affinity for the Fcε receptor, although with an affinity constant at least 1 million-fold less than intact IgE [426]. Studies by Tzehoval et al. found that HEPP also has tuftsin-like activity in its ability to stimulate macrophage-dependent T-cell education [243]. The therapeutic implications for allergy treatment of a small peptide able to block IgE cytophilia are obvious. In addition, if peptides from IgE could be found that selectively block binding of regulatory IgE binding factors, IgE levels could be regulated.

IgE HISTAMINE-RELEASING PEPTIDES

Certain peptides with sequences derived from human IgE have been reported by Stanworth to stimulate histamine release by rat mast cells. These peptides are all highly charged and have sequences identical to aa 486–496: and smaller fragments thereof. The action of these peptides seems to be related to their amino-terminal cluster of positive charges (Arg-Lys-Thr-Lys) and may thus resemble the chemical releasing action of other degranulating agents such as bee venom melittin and compound 48/80 [427].

THEORETICAL ANALYSIS OF CONSTANT DOMAIN ACTIVE SITES: A GENERAL THEORY

The locations and organization of constant domain "active sites" remains a major unsolved question in immunology. Amino acid residues within active sites bind to third-party Fc receptors and thus directly mediate the many biologic activities characteristic of antibodies.

Edelman was the first to provide a theoretical framework that attempted to organize observations of Ig structure/function relationships. His "domain hypothesis" proposed that each Ig homology unit is folded into similarly shaped compact domains that have evolved to perform specific biologic functions. He envisioned that each constant domain contained residues which contribute to at least one active site that would mediate a function characteristic of a particular Ig class [12]. This concept has been confirmed by the many investigators who have demonstrated that isolated domains and their peptide fragments can mimic or inhibit biologic activities of intact Igs. The precise location of these active site residues, however, and their organization within the constant domains remain a mystery for most antibody functions.

To this end, we have recently proposed a general theory that predicts the location of biologically active sites within the constant domains of Igs and other molecules having an Ig-fold domain structure. [428,429]. These molecules include HLA and H-2 histocompatibility antigens, β_2-microglobulin, C-reactive protein, Thy-1, and Qa antigens. According to our theory, these active sites, termed binding regions (BRs), are located at positions spatially homologous to the four HV regions 1, 2, He, and 3 in the V_H domain of Ig H chains, and occupy similar positions in each domain when viewed in three dimensions. The four BRs of each domain are numbered according to the corresponding HV regions and are BR1, BR2, BRHe, and BR3.

The locations of the four BRs in each constant domain of human IgG were identified by producing computer-generated stereo images of an intact human IgG Fc fragment from x-ray diffraction-derived atomic coordinates kindly provided by Johann Deisenhofer [288].

If BRs contain immunologically active sites as this theory predicts, we reasoned that peptides derived from them might cause either inhibition or activation of the event normally triggered by the BR site from which the peptide was derived. Some examples of molecules found to use BRs as active sites are presented in the following sections.

Complement-Activating/Inhibiting Peptides

The CH_2 domain of IgG contains a binding site for the C_1q Fc receptor. IgG residues critical for this interaction have been identified through the use of synthetic peptides identical with sequences in CH_2. The octapeptide described by Boackle et al. identical to aa 274–281 is only slightly less active than intact, heat-aggregated IgG in activating the classical complement pathway [222]. The 12 residue peptide identical to aa 281–292 was shown by Lukas et al. to be one half as effective as monomeric IgG in inhibiting C_1q-mediated hemolysis. Both these peptides have residues located within BR2 of CH_2, which includes aa 275 to 290.

Tuftsin

The tetrapeptide tuftsin is also located within human IgG CH_2 at aa 289–292. It displays a wide range of immunological activities, including the ability to stimulate phagocytosis, ADCC, and macrophage-dependent T cell education [238–243]. We observe that one half of the tuftsin site is located within BR2.

Staphylococcal Protein A IgG Binding Site

In humans, SPA binds to the Fc fragment of all IgG subclasses except IgG_3 [280]. SPA binds only to intact IgG Fc fragments and displays no affinity for isolated CH_2 or CH_3 domains, which suggests that the H chain binding site includes residues at the CH_2/CH_3 junction [237]. The active SPA Fb fragment is reported not to block C_1q binding, therefore eliminating the C_1q binding site [203]. If the SPA Fc binding site includes CH_2/CH_3 junction, our theory predicts that the SPA-binding residues should be located in Brs in that vicinity. The only two BRs fulfilling this requirement are BRHe, CH_2 at aa 307–317 and BR3, CH_3 at aa 428–437. X-ray crystallographic analysis by Deisenhofer of the SPA fragment bound to an intact IgG Fc fragment revealed that 15 residues of the Fc fragment bind to SPA Fb. Of these 15, 5 are in BRHe, CH_2 (aa 309, 310, 311, 314, 315), 6 are in BR3, CH_3 (430, 432, 433, 434, 435, 436), and 4 are in a loop which is adjacent to and contacts BRHe, CH_2 at aa 251–254 [61]. Deisenhofer also found that SPA Fb binds to a second Fc site under the conditions used to form Fc/SPA Fb crystals. This binding site includes residues located in different BRs within CH_3, BR2 (aa 383–390) and BRHe (aa 413–421). This second Fc site includes 15 residues, of which 7 are in BR2, CH_3 (aa 383, 384, 386, 387, 388, 389, 390), 6 are in or adjacent to BRHe, CH_3 (aa 411, 412, 413, 416, 419, 421) and 2 are in a loop which contacts BRHe, CH_3 and is homologous to the CH_2/SPA Fb contact loop discussed above (aa 355, 362).

Cytophilia-Blocking IgG Decapeptide

The decapeptide described by Ciccimarra able to block IgG binding to monocytes is located in IgG, CH_3 at aa 407–416 [308]. The only four residues of this peptide that are exposed in the intact Fc fragment are aa 413–416, as shown in Figures 20 and 21, and are probably responsible for the peptide's cytophylia-blocking activity. These exposed residues are located in BRHe, CH_3 which includes aa 413–421.

Immunoreactive β-Endorphin

Julliard et al. recently isolated a high-molecular-weight protein from human placental extracts that had significant crossreactivity with antisera specific for β-endorphin [430]. The crossreactive determinant proved to be identical to a tryptic fragment of the human IgG H chain at aa 363–377 and surprisingly had 43% homology with the known antigenic determinant of the β-endorphin molecule. A synthetic peptide identical in sequence to IgG aa 363–379 was shown to competitively displace β-endorphin from its specific antisera, thus confirming the determinant's location. This fragment includes all of BR1 of IgG, CH_3 (aa 371–379).

While the biologic significance, of this peptide region is unknown, it is interesting to note that homology with another biologically active peptide, β-endorphin, occurs as in Ig BR.

Superoxide Dismutase

According to our theory all molecules having an Ig-fold domain structure, regardless of their biologic function, should use residues spatially equivalent to Ig HV regions to mediate specific biologic functions. This concept is supported by studies of the enzyme superoxide dismutase (SOD). SOD is an enzyme present in all prokaryocytes and eukaryocytes that live in an oxygen-rich environment. SOD catalyzes the conversion of the toxic superoxide anion, O_2^- to H_2O_2, which is subsequently converted by another enzyme, catalase, to H_2O and O_2 [431]. X-ray crystallographic studies of SOD show that its tertiary structure closely resembles Ig domains [432,433]. Although no obvious sequence homology exists between Igs and SOD, its Ig-fold structure suggests the possibility of an evolutionary relationship. This possibility is supported by the recent demonstration that SOD activity in mice is linked to the H-2 loci, whose gene product is evolutionarily related to Ig domains [144,148,434]. Each of the two 16,000-dalton SOD units have a single catalytic active site that contains two metal atoms, copper (Cu) and zinc (Zn) in eukaryocytes. Both atoms are held about 6 Å apart by two long amino acid loops. These loops occur at domain locations equivalent to the loops which form HV_2 and HV_3 in Ig V domains and are therefore termed BR2 and BR3. These loops are schematically illustrated in Figure 28.

Thymopoietin

Thymopoietin is a 49 amino acid protein first isolated from the thymus by Goldstein [435]. It induces differentiation of T lymphocyte stem cells and inhibits the differentiation of B lymphocytes *in vitro* [436]. Thymopoietin is thought to be a member of a family of thymus hormones that regulate the differentiation of lymphoid stem cells in the thymus and in lymphopoietic tissues throughout the body [437]. Recently a pentapeptide (TP5) corresponding to aa 32–36 of thymopoietin was shown to possess the immunologic activity of the parent molecule and is thought to represent an active site of the molecule [438]. We have recently demonstrated that thymopoietin is

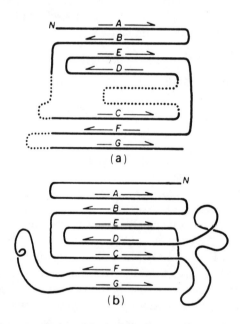

Fig. 28. Schamatic representation of the Ig-fold structure of (a) an immunoglobulin variable domain and (b) of bovine copper, zinc superoxide dismutase. Each horizontal line, labeled A–G, represents a β-strand. The dotted sections in (a) represent the complementary-determining hypervariable regions of variable domains. The enzyme's copper and zinc-containing catalytic active site is located among residues in the two long loops, which occur in superoxide dismutase at regions equivalent to HV_2 and HV_3 in the immunoglobulin variable domain. We therefore designate these enzyme loops BR2 and BR3. (Reproduced with permission from Richardson et al. [432].)

homologous to Igs and related cellular recognition molecules, including histocompatibility antigens (HLA-B7), β_2-microglobulin and the Thy-1 antigen [151]. Figure 29 displays the TP5 region of thymopoietin aligned with amino acid sequences in the region of BRHe in rabbit IgG, CH_3 (aa 413–421), human IgE, CH_4 (aa 502–510), human β_2-microglobulin (aa 71–77), the carboxy-terminal domain of HLA-B7 (aa 248–256), and rat brain Thy-1 antigen (aa 73–81). The overlapping boundaries of the five BRHe, underlined in Figure 29, can be seen to form an He "envelope," designated by a dashed box, which entirely contains the TP5 active site of thymopoietin. Of special interest is the homology between the BRHe sequence in rabbit IgG: Gln-Arg-Gly-Asp-Val-Phe and the sequence in thymopoietin: Gln-Arg-Lys-Asp-Val-Tyr, which includes TP5; Arg-Lys-Asp-Val-Tyr.

When an average of 1.3 gaps per molecule were inserted in each sequence to maximize the number of residues identical to thymopoietin, the degree of homology with the other molecules was found to markedly increase over the entire 49 residues of thymopoietin. Computer-generated alignments of each molecule with thymopoietin are shown in Figure 30. When all 49 residues of thymopoietin were compared to the sequences of the other molecules in Figure 29, statistically significant homology was found between β_2-microg-

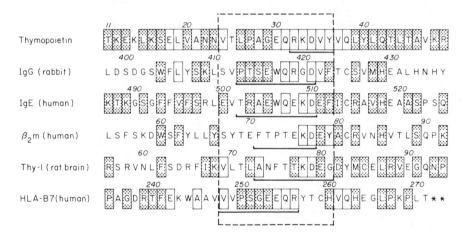

Fig. 29. Comparison of the TP5 active site region of thymopoietin with the BRHe regions of IgG CH_3, IgE CH_4, β_2-microglobulin, Thy-1 antigen, and the HLA-B7 carboxy-terminal domain. Residues identical to thymopoietin are boxed. Single-base mutations that would convert a thymopoietin residue to a residue in any of the other five molecules are indicated by shaded boxes. The TP5 active site of thymopoietin and the BRHe in each of the other molecules are underlined. The dashed line encloses the BRHe envelope. Residues in HLA-B7 beyond 271 are indicated by asterisks. One-letter symbols for amino acid residues are listed in the legend of Figure 1. (Reproduced from Hahn and Hamburger [151] with permission.)

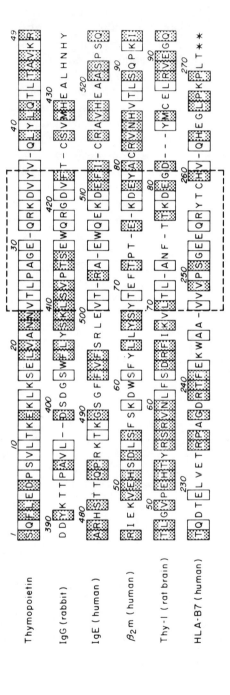

Fig. 30. Comparison of the entire thymopoietin molecule with approximately one-half of IgG CH₃, IgE CH₄, β₂-microglobulin, Thy-1 antigen, and the carboxy-terminal domain of HLA-B7. Gaps were inserted to maximize residues identical to those in thymopoietin. To minimize the possibility that gaps might spuriously increase identities, gaps were inserted only when they resulted in two or more new identities. Most identities can be seen to occur in the BRHe envelope within the dashed lines. Functionally conserved amino acids are those designated by Dayhoff [144] from chemical similarity and accepted point mutation data and consist of (A,P,G), (N,Q), (D,E), (S,T), (C), (V,I,M,L), (K,R,H) and (F,Y,W). See legend of Figure 1 for one-letter symbols for amino acids. (Reproduced from Hahn and Hamburger [151] with permission.)

lobulin and thymopoietin (22% identities, $P = 0.03$). Our statistical analysis revealed a comparable degree of similarity between β_2-microglobulin and CH_3 of human IgG (24% identities, $P = 0.007$) and between CH_1 and CH_2 of human IgG (26% identities, $P = 0.003$). We concluded that thymopoietin may be derived from approximately one half of the ancestral 100 residue domain common to immunoglobulins and related cellular recognition molecules.

Genetic Events Involving Binding Regions

Analysis of amino acid and nucleotide sequences within or adjacent to BRs reveals unusual distributions that suggest recombinational events. Tucker et al. recently reported the complete nucleotide sequence of the constant region of the murine IgG_{2b} H chain messenger RNA and observed three nearly identical 17 nucleotide homology regions in the CH_1 and CH_2 domains [439]. Two of these homology regions are located in the CH_1 domain and correspond to aa 183–188 and aa 199–204. The third region spans CH_2, aa 308–314. The regions beginning at aa 183 and 308 occur at exactly corresponding positions in CH_1 and CH_2 when invariant cysteine residues are aligned. These three homology regions delineate the upper and lower boundaries of BRHe, CH_1 (aa 189–199) and the lower boundary of BRHe, CH_2 (aa 307–317). Moreover, it is at or near the lower boundary of BRHe in CH_2 that IgG_{2b}/IgG_{2a} crossover event occurred in variant MPC 11 myeloma antibody isolated by Birshtein et al. The resulting mutant IgG has a IgG_{2b}/IgG_{2a} hybrid H chain [440].

A Gm antigen whose determinant derives from a deleted residue also occurs near the beginning of BRHe, CH_2 at aa 309 of human IgG_4. The deletion of Leu 309 from the sequence Val-Leu-His forms the G4m (b) determinant, the G4m (a) determinant consisting of the intact sequence [44].

Shinoda et al. recently reported that the human $C\delta3$ domain contains two homologous 8 residue segments with an unusual concentration of proline residues at aa 446–453 and aa 467–474 [155] (Fig. 2). The latter segment includes all but one residue of BRHe, CH_3 (aa 467–475) (Fig. 2). Shinoda suggested that the observed homology strongly implies that the sequences arose by partial duplication during evolution of the $C\delta3$ domain. The biological significance of these unusual segments is unclear; however, the occurrence of one of them in BRHe suggests that this domain region may be subject to unique genetic processing. The high degree of homology of the two segments (75%) suggests that their nucleotide sequences are very similar and thus resemble the three repeated nucleotide sequences which flank BRHe in murine IgG_{2b}. Tucker suggested that repeated homologous nucleotide sequences might function as sites for recombination between two domains and might be important for domain evolution [439]. Such recombinational events surrounding a BR may have produced the "half-domain" fragment that is thymopoietin. A "free" BR active site, not having the regulatory influences imposed by a domain's "framework" residues, might be constantly active, and could thus serve a hormonal function in immune regulation.

THERAPEUTIC IMPLICATIONS OF IMMUNOGLOBULIN "ACTIVE SITE" PEPTIDES

An understanding of the molecular mechanisms of how antibodies activate and regulate immune defense systems may lead to the development of new therapeutic modalities.

For therapeutic purposes, peptides identical to immunoglobulin active sites would have a considerable advantage over the passively administered parent Ig for several reasons: 1) Active sites of Igs become functional in only limited *in vivo* circumstances; 2) there are only limited supplies of pure human Igs, whereas small peptides can be synthesized cheaply and in large amounts; and 3) a small peptide (under ten amino acids long) is unlikely to induce an allergic response which large proteins frequently elicit.

Peptides able to block IgE binding to mast cell and basophil receptors could prevent IgE-mediated allergies since binding must occur in order for antigen to induce degranulation. C_1q-blocking peptides could prevent the tissue damage caused by the inappropriate complement activation which accompanies autoantibody-associated autoimmune diseases such as sytemic lupus erythematosus and rheumatoid arthritis. Peptides with phagocytosis or ADCC-blocking activity might prevent the cytolysis that occurs when non-destructive viral antigens are expressed on host cells which are subsequently killed. Diseases in which such a pathogenesis has been implicated include chronic active hepatitis, hemolytic anemias and demyelinating neurologic disease such as multiple sclerosis [441].

Peptides having immunostimulatory activity could be very useful in treating infections or neoplastic disease. Already, one Ig-derived peptide, tuftsin, has proved to be efficacious in treating neoplasms in animals. Such peptides might also be used as adjuvants to enhance the immune response to injected antigens [241]. The possibilities, as evidenced by this brief list, are almost limitless.

ACKNOWLEDGMENTS

I thank Dr. Richard O'Connor and Dr. Robert Hamburger for critically reviewing the manuscript, Dr. Alex Lucas for helpful discussions, Richard Rogo for artwork, and Steve Dempsey for expert advice and assistance in the use of the UCSD Molecular Modeling System. The UCSD Research Resource Computer Facility is funded by PHS Grant RR00757. GSH is partially funded by National Institutes of Health Immunology Training Grant 5T32 CA 09174 and by a grant from Immunetech, Inc.

REFERENCES

1. Natvig JB, Kunkel HG: Immunoglobulins: Classes, subclasses, genetic variants, and idiotypes, Adv Immunol 16:1, 1973.
2. Cunningham BA, Gottlieb PD, Pelumm MN, Edelman GM: Immunoglobulin structure: Diversity, gene duplication and domains. In Amos B (ed): "Progress in Immunology." New York: Academic Press, 1971, pp 3–24.
3. Putnam FW, Titani K, Wikler M, Shinoda T: Structure and evolution of kappa and lambda light chains. Cold Spring Harbor Symp Quant Biol 32:9–29, 1967.
4. Milstein C: Interchain disulphide bridge in Bence-Jones proteins and in gamma-globulin beta chains. Nature (London) 205:1171, 1965.
5. Porter RR: Immunoglobulin structure, defense and recognition. In Porter RR (ed): "Biochemistry Series One." Vol. 10, London: Butterworths, 1973, pp 159–197.
6. Mole JE, Bhoun AS, Bennett JC: Primary structure of human J chain: Alignment of peptides from chemical and enzymatic hydrolyses. Biochemistry 16:3507, 1977.
7. Metzger H: Structure and function of gamma-M macroglobulins. Adv Immunol 12:57, 1970.
8. Heremans J: The IgA system in connection with local and systemic immunity. In Mestecky J, Lawton A (eds): "The Immunoglobulin A System." Adv Exp Med Biol Vol. 45, New York: Plenum, 1974, pp 3–12.
9. Rogers J, Early P, Carter C, Calame K, Bond L, Hood L, Wall L: Two mRNAs with different 3' ends encode membrane-bound and secreted forms of immunoglobulin mu chain. Cell 20:303, 1980.
10. Neuberger M, Rajewsky K: Switch from hapten-specific immunoglobulin M to Immunoglobulin D secretion in a hybrid mouse cell line. Proc Natl Acad Sci USA 78:1138, 1981.
11. Tyler BM, Cownan AF, Adams JM, Harris AW: Generation of long mRNA for membrane immunoglobulin gamma 2a chains by differential splicing. Nature (London) 293:406, 1981.
12. Edelman GM: The covalent structure of a human γ G-immunoglobulin. XI. Functional implications. Biochemistry 9:3197, 1970.
13. Hill RL, Delaney R, Fellows RE Jr, Lebovitz HE: The evolutionary origins of immunoglobulins. Biochemistry 56:1762, 1966.
14. Singer SJ, Doolittle RF: Antibody active sites and immunoglobulin molecules. Science 153:13, 1966.
15. Appella E, Perham RN: The structure of immunoglobulin light chains. Cold Spring Harbor Symp Quant Biol 32:37–44, 1967.
16. Beale D, Feinstein A: Structure and function of the constant regions of immunoglobulins. Q Rev Biophys 9:150, 1976.
17. Lin LC, Putnam FW: Structural studies of human IgD: Isolation by a two-step purification procedure and characterization by chemical and enzymatic fragmentation. Proc Natl Acad Sci USA 76:6572, 1979.
18. Jerry LM, Kunkel HG, Grey HM: Absence of disulfide bonds linking the heavy and light chains: A property of a genetic variant of αA2 globulins. Proc Natl Acad Sci USA 65:557, 1970.
19. Hahn GS: Unpublished observations.
20. Cohen FE, Sternberg JE, Taylor WR: Analysis and prediction of beta-sheet structures by a combinatorial approach. Nature (London) 285:378, 1980.
21. Hilschmann N, Craig LC: Amino acid sequence studies with Bence-Jones proteins. Proc Natl Acad Sci USA 53:1403, 1965.
22. Titani K, Putnam FW: Immunoglobulin structure: Amino and carboxyl-terminal peptides of Type I Bence-Jones proteins. Science 147:1304, 1965.

23. Wu TT, Kabat EA: An analysis of the sequences of the variable regions of Bence-Jones proteins and myeloma light chains and their implications for antibody complementarity. J Exp Med 132:211, 1970.
24. Kabat EA, Wu TT: Attempts to locate complementarity determining residues in the variable positions of light and heavy chains. Ann NY Acad Sci 190:382, 1971.
25. Capra JD, Kehoe MJ: Variable region sequences of five human immunoglobulin heavy chains of the V_HIII subgroup: Definitive identification of four heavy chain hypervariable regions. Proc Natl Acad Sci USA 71:845, 1974.
26. Hamovich J, Eisen HN, Hurwitz E, Givol D: Localization of affinity labeled residues on the heavy and light chain of two myeloma proteins with anti-hapten activity. Biochemistry 11:2389, 1972.
27. Amzel LM, Poljak RJ, Saul F, Varga JM, Richards FF: The three-dimensional structure of a combining region—ligand complex of immunoglobulin New at 3.5-Å resolution. Proc Natl Acad Sci USA 71:1427, 1974.
28. Segal DM, Padlan EA, Cohen GH, Rudikoff S, Potter M, Davies DR: The three-dimensional structure of a phosphorylcholine-binding mouse immunoglobulin Fab and the nature of the antigen binding site. Proc Natl Acad Sci USA 71:4298, 1974.
29. Padlan, EA: Structural basis for the specificity of antibody-antigen reactions and structural mechanisms for the diversification of antigen-binding specifications. Q Rev Biophys 10:35, 1977.
30. Epp O, Lattman EE, Schiffer M, Huber R, Palm W: The molecular structure of a dimer composed of the variable portions of the Bence-Jones protein REI refined at 2.0-Å resolution. Biochemistry 14:4943, 1975.
31. Epp O, Colman P, Fehlhammer H, Bode W, Schiffer M, Huber R, Palm W: Crystal and molecular structure of a dimer composed of the variable portions of the Bence-Jones protein REI. Eur J Biochem 45:513, 1974.
32. Porter RR: The hydrolysis of rabbit γ-globulin and antibodies with crystalline papain. Biochem J 73:119, 1959.
33. Isenman DE, Ellerson JR, Painter RH, Dorrington KJ: Correlation between the exposure of aromatic chromophores at the surface of the F_c domains of immunoglobulin G and their ability to bind complement. Biochemistry 16:233, 1977.
34. Ellerson JR, Yasmeen D, Painter, RH, Dorrington KJ: Structure and function of immunoglobulin domains III. Isolation and characterization of a fragment corresponding to the Cγ2 homology region of human immunoglobulin G. J Immunol 116:510, 1976.
35. Connell GE, Porter RR: A new enzymatic fragment (Facb) of rabbit immunoglobulin G. Biochem J 124:53, 1971.
36. Nisonoff A, Markus G, Wissler FC: Separation of univalent fragments of rabbit antibody by reduction of a single labile disulphide bond. Nature (London) 189:293, 1961.
37. Ishizaka K, Ishizaka T: Immune mechanisms of reversed type reaginic hypersensitivity. J Immunol 103:588, 1969.
38. Solomon A: Bence-Jones proteins and light chains of immunoglobulins. N Engl J Med 294:91, 1976.
39. Franklin EC, Frangione B: Structural variants of human and murine immunoglobulins. In Inman FP, Mandy WJ (eds): "Contemporary Topics in Molecular Immunology." Vol. 4, New York: Plenum, 1975, pp 89–126.
40. Franklin EC, Prelli F, Frangione B: Human heavy chain disease protein WIS: Implications for the organization of immunoglobulin genes. Proc Natl Acad Sci USA 76:452, 1978.
41. Biewenga J, Frangione B, Franklin EC, Van Loghem E: A γ1 heavy-chain disease protein (EST) lacking the entire V_H and CH$_1$ domains. Scand J Immunol 11:601, 1980.
42. Glenner GG, Terry W, Harada M, Isersky C, Page DL: Amyloid fibril proteins: Proof of homology with immunoglobulin light chains. Science 172:1150, 1971.
43. Glenner GG, Page DL: Amyloid, amyloidosis and amyloidogenesis. Int Rev Exp Pathol

15:1, 1976.

44. Kabat EA, Wu TT, Bilofsky H: Sequences of immunoglobulin chains. US Dept of HEW Publication 80–2008:141, 1979.

45. Putnam FW, Takahashi N, Tetaert D, Debuire B, Lin LC: Amino acid sequence of the first constant region domain and the hinge region of the δ heavy chain of human IgD. Proc Natl Acad Sci USA 78:6168, 1981.

46. Putnam FW, Liu YV, Low TLK: Primary sturcture of a human IgA1 immunoglobulin IV. Streptococcal IgA1 protease digestion, Fab and Fc fragments, and the complete amino acid sequence of the α-1 heavy chain. J Biol Chem 254:2865, 1979.

47. Yguerabide J, Epstein HF, Stryer L: Segmental flexibility in an antibody molecule. J Mol Biol 51:573, 1970.

48. Valentine RC, Green NM: Electron microscopy of an antibody—hapten complex. J Mol Biol 27:615, 1967.

49. Schlessinger IZ, Steinberg IZ, Givol D, Hochman J, Pecht I: Antigen-induced conformational changes in antibodies and their Fab fragment studied by circular polarization of fluorescence. Proc Natl Acad Sci USA 72:2775, 1975.

50. Poljak RJ: Three-dimensional structure, function and genetic control of immunoglobulins. Nature (London) 256:373, 1975.

51. Davies DR, Padlan EA: Three-dimensional structure of immunoglobulins. Ann Rev Biochem 44:639, 1975.

52. Silverton EW, Navia MA, Davies DR: Three-dimensional structure of an intact human immunoglobulin. Proc Natl Acad Sci USA 74:5140, 1977.

53. Poljak RJ: Correlations between three-dimensional structure and function of immunoglobulins. CRC Crit Rev Biochem 5:45, 1978.

54. Padlan EA, Davies DR: Variability of three-dimensional structure in immunoglobulins. Proc Natl Acad Sci USA 72:819, 1975.

55. Padlan EA: Structural implications of sequence variability in immunoglobulins. Proc Natl Acad Sci USA 74:2551, 1977.

56. Poljak RJ, Amzel LM, Chen BL, Phizackerley RP, Saul F: The three-dimensional structure of the Fab fragment of a human myeloma immunoglobulin at 2.0-Å resolution. Proc Natl Acad Sci USA 71:3440, 1974.

57. Schechter B, Schechter I, Sela M: Antibody combining sites to a series of peptide determinants of increasing size and defined structure. J Biol Chem 245:1438, 1970.

58. Marquart M, Deisenhofer J, Huber R: Crystallographic refinement and atomic models of the intact immunoglobulin molecule Kol and its antigen-binding fragment at 3.0-Å and 1.0-Å resolution. J Mol Biol 141:369, 1980.

59. Steiner LA, Lopes AD: The crystallizable human myeloma protein Dob has a hinge-region deletion. Biochemistry 18:4054, 1979.

60. Toraño A, Tsuzukida Y, Liu YV, Putnam FW: Location and structural significance of the oligosaccharides in human IgA1 and IgA2 immunoglobulins. Proc Natl Acad Sci USA 74:2301, 1977.

61. Deisenhofer J: Crystallographic refinement and atomic models of a human Fc fragment and its complex with fragment B of protein A from staphylococcus at 2.9 and 2.8-Å resolution. Biochemistry 20:2361, 1981.

62. Schenkein I, Uhr J: Immunoglobulin synthesis and secretion. I. Biosynthetic studies of the addition of the carbohydrate moieties. J Cell Biol 46:42, 1970.

63. Takayasu T, Takahashi N, Shinoda T: Amino acid sequence and location of the three glycopeptides in the Fc region of human immunoglobulin D. Biochem Biophys Res Commun 97:635, 1980.

64. Wu TT, Kabat EA, Bilofsky H: Some sequence similarities among cloned mouse DNA segments that code for λ and κ light chains of immunoglobulins. Proc Natl Acad Sci USA 76:4617, 1979.

65. Solomon A: Bence-Jones proteins and light chains of immunoglobulins. N Engl J Med 294:17, 1976.
66. Mackenzie MR, Warner NL, Linscott WD, Fudenberg HH: Differentiation of human IgM subclasses by the ability to interact with a factor resembling the first component of complement. J Immunol 103:607, 1969.
67. Yount WJ, Dorner MM, Kunkel HG, Kabat EA: Studies on human antibodies. VI. Selective variations in subgroup composition and genetic markers. J Exp Med 127:633, 1968.
68. Oudin J: The genetic control of immunoglobulin synthesis. Proc R Soc Lond [Biol] 166B:207, 1966.
69. Capra JD, Kehoe MJ: Structure of antibodies with shared idiotypy: The complete sequence of the heavy chain variable regions of two IgM anti-gamma globulins. Proc Natl Acad Sci USA 71:4032, 1974.
70. Eichmann K: Expression and function of idiotypes on lymphocytes. Adv. Immunol 26:195, 1978.
71. Oudin J, Cazenave PA: Similar idiotypic specificities in immunoglobulin fractions with different antibody functions or even without detectable antibody function. Proc Natl Acad Sci USA 68:2616, 1971.
72. Dryer WJ, Bennett JC: The molecular basis of antibody formation: A paradox. Proc Natl Acad Sci USA 54:864, 1965.
73. Jearne NK: The somatic generation of immune recognition. Eur J Immunol 1:1–9, 1971.
74. Cohn M: The take-home lesson. Ann NY Acad Sci 190:529, 1971.
75. Kabat EA: Origins of antibody complementarity and specificity—Hypervariable regions and the minigene hypothesis. J Immunol 125:961, 1980.
76. Kabat EA, Wu TT, Bilofsky H. Evidence supporting somatic assembly of the DNA segments (minigenes), coding for the framework, and complementary-determining segments of immunoglobulin variable regions. J Exp Med 149:1299, 1979.
77. Hood L, Campbell J, Elgin S: The organization, expression and evolution of antibody genes and other multigene families. Ann Rev Genet 9:305, 1975.
78. McKean DJ, Bell M, Potter M: Mechanisms of antibody diversity: Multiple genes encode for structurally related mouse κ variable regions. Proc Natl Acad Sci USA 75:3913, 1978.
79. Blomberg B, Traunecker A, Eisen H, Tonegawa S: Organization of four mouse λ light chain immunoglobulin genes. Proc Natl Acad Sci USA 78:3765, 1981.
80. Marx JL: Antibodies: Getting their genes together. Science 212:1015, 1981.
81. Valbuena O, Marcu KB, Weigart M, Perry RP: Multiplicity of germline genes specifying a group of related mouse κ chains with implications for the generation of immunoglobulin diversity. Nature (London) 276:780, 1978.
82. Max EE, Seidman JG, Leder P: Sequences of five potential recombination sites encoded close to an immunoglobulin κ constant region gene. Proc Natl Acad Sci USA 76:3450, 1979.
83. Rudikoff S, Rao DN, Glaudemans CPJ, Potter M: κ chain joining segments and structural diversity of antibody combining sites. Proc Natl Acad Sci USA 77:4270, 1980.
84. Sakano H, Rogers JH, Hüppi K, Brack C, Traunecker A, Maki R, Wall R, Tonegawa S: Domains and the hinge region of an immunoglobulin heavy chain are encoded in separate DNA segments. Nature (London) 277:627, 1979.
85. Bentley DL, Rabbitts TH: Human V_κ immunoglobulin gene number: Implications for the origin of antibody diversity. Cell 24:613, 1981.
86. Burnet M: "Cellular Immunology." London: Melbourne University Press, Cambridge University Press, 1969, p 14.

87. Brack C, Hirama M, Lenhard-Schuller R, Tonegawa S: A complete immunoglobulin gene is created by somatic recombination. Cell 15:1, 1978.
88. Early P, Huang H, Davis M, Calame K, Hood L: An immunoglobulin heavy chain variable region gene is generated from three segments of DNA: V_H, D and J_H. Cell 19:981, 1980.
89. Sakano H, Kurosawa Y, Weigert M, Tonegawa S: Identification and nucleotide sequence of a diversity DNA segment (D) of immunoglobulin heavy chain genes. Nature 290:562, 1981.
90. Gough NM, Bernard O: Sequences of the joining region genes for immunoglobulin heavy chains and their role in generation of antibody diversity. Proc Natl Acad Sci USA 78:509, 1981.
91. Davis MM, Calame K, Early PW, Livant DL, Joho R, Weisman IL, Hood L: An immunoglobulin heavy-chain gene is formed by at least two recombinational events. Nature (London) 283:733, 1980.
92. Sakano H, Maki R, Kurosawa Y, Roeder W, Tonegawa S: Two types of somatic recombination are necessary for the generation of complete immunoglobulin heavy-chain genes. Nature (London) 286:676, 1980.
93. Molgard HV: Assembly of immunoglobulin heavy chain genes. Nature (London) 286:657, 1980.
94. Hengartner H, Meo T, Müller E: Assignment of genes for immunoglobulin κ and heavy chains to chromosomes 6 and 12 in mouse. Proc Natl Acad Sci USA 75:4494, 1978.
95. Honjo T, Kataoka T: Organization of immunoglobulin heavy chain genes and an allelic deletion model. Proc Natl Acad Sci USA 75:2140, 1978.
96. Nishida Y, Kitaoka T, Ishida N, Nakai S, Kishimoto T, Böttcher I, Honjo T: Cloning of mouse immunoglobulin ε gene and its location within the heavy chain gene cluster. Proc Natl Acad Sci USA 78:1581, 1981.
97. Liu CP, Tucker PW, Mushinski JF, Blattner FR: Mapping of heavy chain genes for mouse immunoglobulins M and D. Science 209:1348, 1980.
98. Max EE, Seidman JG, Miller H, Leder P: Variation in the crossover point of kappa immunoglobulin gene V-J recombination: Evidence for a cryptic gene. Cell 21:793, 1980.
99. Pech M, Höchtl J, Schnell H, Zachau HG: Differences between germ-line and rearranged immunoglobulin V_κ coding sequences suggest a localized mutation mechanism. Nature (London) 291:668, 1981.
100. Bothwell ALM, Paskind M, Reth M, Imanishi-Kari T, Rajewsky K, Baltimore D: Heavy chain variable region contribution to the NP^b family of antibodies: Somatic mutation evident in a γ2a variable region. Cell 24:625, 1981.
101. Wuilmart C, Urbain J, Givol D: On the locations of palindromes in immunoglobulin genes. Proc Natl Acad Sci USA 74:2526, 1977.
102. Ben-Sasson S: Immunoglobulin differentiation is dictated by repeated recombination sequences within the V region prototype gene: A hypothesis. Proc Natl Acad Sci USA 76:4598, 1979.
103. Pernis B, Forni L, Luzzati AL: Synthesis of multiple immunoglobulin classes by single lymphocytes. Cold Spring Harbor Symp Quant Biol 41:175, 1976.
104. Goding JW, Scott DW, Layton JE: Genetics, cellular expression and function of IgD and IgM receptors. Immunol Rev 37:152, 1977.
105. Davis MM, Kim SK, Hood L: DNA sequences mediating class switching in α-immunoglobulins. Science 209:1360, 1980.
106. Early P, Hood L: Allelic exclusion and nonproductive immunoglobulin gene rearrangements. Cell 24:1, 1981.

107. Harris H: "The Principles of Human Biochemical Genetics." 2nd ed, New York: American Elsevier, 1975.
108. Hieter PA, Korsmeyer SJ, Waldman TA, Leder P: Human immunoglobulin κ light-chain genes are deleted or rearranged in λ producing B-cells. Nature 290:368, 1981.
109. Bouvet JP, Feingold J, Oriol R, Liacopoulos P: Statistical study of double paraproteinemias. Evidence for a common cellular origin of both myeloma globulins. Biomedicine 22:517, 1975.
110. Bachmann R: Simultaneous occurrence of two immunologically different M-components in serum. Acta Med Scand 177:593, 1965.
111. Penn GM, Kunkel HG, Grey HM: Sharing of individual antigenic determinants between a γG and a γM protein in the myeloma serum. Proc Soc Exp Biol Med 135:660, 1970.
112. Rudders RA, Yakulis V, Heller P: Double myeloma: Production of both IgG type lambda and IgA type lambda myeloma proteins by a single plasma cell line. Am J Med 55:215, 1973.
113. Oriol R, Huerta J, Bouvet JP, Liacopoulos P: Two myeloma globulins, IgG1κ and IgG1λ, from a single patient (Im). Immunology 27:1081, 1974.
114. Kuan TK, Tung E, Wang IY, Wang AC: Three monoclonal immunoglobulins, an IgG2(κ), and an IgM(κ) and an IgM/A hybrid, in one patient. II. Sharing of common variable regions. Immunology 44:265, 1981.
115. Morse HC III, Pumphrey JG, Potter M, Asofsky R: Murine plasma cells secreting more than one class of immunoglobulin heavy chain. I. Frequency of two or more M-components in ascitic fluids from 788 primary plasmacytomas. J Immunol 117:541, 1976.
116. Morse HC III, Neiders ME, Lieberman R, Lawton AR III, Asofsky R: Murine plasma cells secreting more than one class of immunoglobulin heavy chain. II. SAMM 388— A plasmacytoma secreting IgG2b_κ and IgA_κ. Immunoglobulins which do not share idiotypic determinants. J Immunol 118:1682, 1977.
117. McKeever PE, Neiders ME, Nero GB, Asofsky R: Murine plasma cells secreting more than one class of immunoglobulin. VII. Analysis of the IgG2_b and IgA precursors within the cytoplasm of spontaneous myeloma SAMM 368 in culture shows segregation of heavy chains. J Immunol 124:541, 1980.
118. Klein M, Haeffner-Cavaillon N, Isenman DE, Rivat C, Navia MA, Davies DR, Dorrington KJ: Expression of biological effector functions by immunoglobulin G molecules lacking the hinge region. Proc Natl Acad Sci USA 78:524, 1981.
119. Michaelsen TE, Frangione B, Franklin EC: Primary structure of the "hinge" region of the human IgG3: Probable quadruplication of a 15-amino acid residue basic unit. J Biol Chem 252:883, 1977.
120. Stryer L. "Biochemistry." 2nd ed, San Francisco: WH Freeman, 1981, p 559.
121. Francus T, Dharmgrongartama B, Campbell R, Scharff D, Birshtein BK: IgG2a-producing variants of an IgG2b-producing mouse myeloma cell line. J Exp Med 147:1535, 1978.
122. Natvig JB, Kunkel HG: A hybrid IgG4—IgG2 immunoglobulin. J Immunol 112:1277, 1974.
123. Miyata T, Yasunaga T, Yamawaki-Kataoka Y, Obata M, Honjo T: Nucleotide sequence divergence of mouse immunoglobulin γ1 and γ2b chain genes and the hypothesis of intervening sequence-mediated domain transfer. Proc Natl Acad Sci USA 77:2143, 1980.
124. Marchalonis JJ: Phylogenetic origins of antibody structure. Transplant Proc 2:318, 1970.
125. Marchalonis JJ, Edelman GM: Phylogenetic origins of antibody structure. III. Antibodies in the primary immune response of the sea lamprey, Petromyzon Marinus. J Exp Med 127:891, 1968.
126. Linthicum DS, Hildemann WH: Immunologic responses of pacific hagfish. III. Serum antibodies to cellular antigens. J Immunol 105:912, 1970.

127. De Ioannes AE, Hildemann WH: Preliminary structural characterization of pacific hagfish immunoglobulin. Adv Exp Med Biol 64:151, 1975.
128. Marchalonis JJ, Cone RE: The phylogenetic emergence of vertebrate immunity. Aust J Exp Biol Med Sci 51:461, 1973.
129. Shulkind ML, Robbins JB, Clem LW: Reactivities of shark 19S and 7S IgM antibodies to Salmonella typhimurium. Nature (New Biol) 230:182, 1971.
130. McCumber LJ, Clem LW: A comparative study of J chain: Structure and stoichiometry in human and nurse shark IgM. Immunochem 13:479, 1976.
131. Sledge C, Clem LW, Hood L: Antibody structure: Amino terminal sequences of nurse shark light and heavy chains. J Immunol 112:941, 1974.
132. Marchalonis JJ: Isolation and characterization of immunoglobulin-like proteins of the Australian lungfish (Neoceratodus forsteri). Aust J Exp Biol Med Sci 47:405, 1969.
133. Steiner LA, Mikoryak CA, Lopes AD, Green C: Immunoglobulins in ranid frogs and tadpoles. Adv Exp Med Biol 64:173, 1975.
134. Marchalonis JJ, Cohen N: Isolation and partial characterization of immunoglobulin from a urodele amphibian (Necturus masculosus). Immunology 24:395, 1973.
135. Leslie GA, Clem LW: Phylogeny of immunoglobulin structure and function. VI. 17S, 7.5S and 5.7S anti-DNP of the turtle, Pseudamys scripta. J Immunol 108:1656, 1972.
136. Mehta PD, Reichlin M, Tomasi TB Jr: Comparative studies of vertebrate immunoglobulins. J Immunol 109:1272, 1972.
137. Bienenstock J, Perey DYE, Gauldie J, Underdown BJ: Chicken immunoglobulin resembling γA. J Immunol 109:403, 1972.
138. Neoh SH, Jahoda DM, Rowe DS: Immunoglobulin classes in mammalian species identified by cross-reactivity with antisera to human immunoglobulin. Immunochem 10:805, 1973.
139. Guttman RM, Tebo T, Edwards J, Barboriak JJ, Fink JN: The immune response of the pigeon (Columba Livia). J Immunol 106:392, 1971.
140. Halliwell REW, Schwartzman RM, Rockey JH: Antigenic relationship between human IgE and canine IgE. Clin Exp Immunol 10:399, 1972.
141. Liakopoulou A, Perelmutter L: Antigenic relationship between human IgE immunoglobulin and rat homocytotropic antibody. J Immunol 107:131, 1971.
142. Doolittle RF: Similar amino acid sequences: Chance or common ancestry? Science, 214:149, 1981.
143. Fitch WM: Aspects of molecular evolution. Ann Rev Genet 7:343, 1973.
144. Barker WC, Dayhoff MO: Detecting distant relationships: Computer methods and results. In "Atlas of Protein Sequence and Structure." Vol 5, Washington, D.C.: National Biomedical Research Foundation, 1972, pp 101–110.
145. Hill RL, Delaney R, Fellows RE Jr, Lebovitz HE: The evolutionary origins of immunoglobulins. Biochemistry 56:1762, 1966.
146. Singer SJ, Doolittle RF: Antibody active sites and immunoglobulin molecules. Science 153:13, 1966.
147. Strominger JL, Engelhard VH, Guild BC, Kostyk TG, Lancet D, Lopez de Castro JA, Orr IIT, Parham P, Ploegh HL, Pober JS: Complete primary structure of human histocompatibility antigen HLA-B7: Evolutionary and functional implications. Curr Top Dev Biol 14:97, 1980.
148. Peterson PA, Cunningham BA, Berggard I, Edelman GM: β_2-microglobulin—A free immunoglobulin domain. Proc Natl Acad Sci USA 69:1697, 1972.
149. Cohen FE, Novotny J, Sternberg MJE, Campbell DG, Williams AF: Analysis and structural similarities between brain Thy-1 antigen and immunoglobulin domains. Biochem J 195:31, 1981.

150. Osmond AP, Gewurz H, Friedenson B: Partial amino acid sequences of human and rabbit C-reactive proteins: Homology with immunoglobulin domains and histocompatibility antigens. Proc Natl Acad Sci USA 74:1214, 1977.
151. Hahn GS, Hamburger RN: Evolutionary relationship of thymopoietin to immunoglobulins and cellular recognition molecules. J Immunol 126:459, 1981.
152. Soloski MJ, Uhr JW, Flaherty L, Vitetta ES: Qa-2, H-2K and H-2D alloantigens evolved from a common ancestral gene. J Exp Med 153:1080, 1981.
153. Urbain J: Evolution of immunoglobulins and ferredoxins and the occurrence of pseudosymmetrical sequences. Biochem Genet 3:249, 1969.
154. Wuilmart C, Wijns L, Urbain J: Linear and inverted repetitions in protein sequences. J Mol Evol 5:259, 1975.
155. Shinoda T, Takahashi N, Takayasu T, Okuyama T, Shimizu A: Complete amino acid sequence of the Fc region of a human δ chain. Proc Natl Acad Sci USA 78:785, 1981.
156. Barker WC, Ketcham LK, Dayhoff MO: Origins of immunoglobulin heavy chain domains. J Mol Evol 15:113, 1980.
157. Lin LC, Putnam FW: Primary structure of the Fc region of human immunoglobulin D: Implications for evolutionary origin and biological function. Proc Natl Acad Sci USA 78:504, 1981.
158. Putnam FW, Florent G, Paul C, Shinoda T, Shimizu A: Complete amino acid sequence of the Mu heavy chain of a human IgM immunoglobulin. Science 182:287, 1973.
159. Tucker PW, Marcu KB, Newell N, Richards J, Blattner FR: Sequence of the cloned gene for the constant region of murine γ2b immunoglobulin heavy chain. Science 206:1303, 1979.
160. Yamawaki-Kataoka Y, Miyata T, Honjo T: The complete nucleotide sequence of mouse immunoglobulin γ2a gene and evolution of heavy chain genes: Further evidence for intervening sequence-mediated domain transfer. Nucleic Acids Res 9:1365, 1981.
161. Buckley RH, Dees SC, O'Fallon WM: Serum immunoglobulins: I. Levels in normal children and in uncomplicated childhood allergy. Pediatrics 41:600, 1968.
162. Josephs SH, Buckley RH: Serum IgD concentrations in normal infants, children, and in adults and in patients with elevated IgE. J Pediatrics 96:417, 1980.
163. Kjellman NIM, Johansson SGO, Roth A: Serum IgE levels in healthy children quantified by a sandwich technique (PRIST). Clin Allergy 6:51, 1976.
164. Nye L, Merrett TG, Landon J, White RJ: A detailed investigation of circulating IgE levels in a normal population. Clin Allergy 1:13, 1975.
165. Morell A, Skvaril F, Barandun S: Serum concentrations of IgG subclasses. In Back F, Good R (eds): "Clinical Immunobiology." New York: Academic Press, 1976, pp 37–56.
166. Wells JV: Immunoglobulins: biosynthesis and metabolism. In Fudenberg H, Stites D, Caldwell J, Wells J (eds): "Basic and Clinical Immunology." 3rd ed, Los Altos: Lange Medical Publications, 1980, pp 64–78.
167. Virella G, Parkhouse RME: Papain sensitivity of heavy chain subclasses in normal human IgG and localization of antigenic determinants for the subclasses. Immunochem 8:243, 1971.
168. Molgaard HV, Weir L, Kenten J, Cramer F, Klukas CK, Gould H, Birch JR: Isolation of immunoglobulin messenger ribonucleic acid from human lymphoblastoid cell lines. Biochemistry 20:4467, 1981.
169. Fukumoto T, Brandon MR: The site of IgG$_{2a}$ catabolism in the rat. Mol Immunol 18:741, 1981.
170. Virella G, Nunes AS, Tamagnini G: Placental transfer of human IgG subclasses. Clin Exp Immunol 10:476, 1972.

171. Van Furth R, Schuit HRE, Hijmans W: The immunological development of the human fetus. J Exp Med 122:1173, 1965.
172. Brambell FWR: "Frontiers of Biology." Vol. 18, Amsterdam: North Holland, 1970.
173. Kohler PF, Farr RS. Elevation of cord over maternal IgG immunoglobulin: Evidence for an active placental IgG transport. Nature (London) 210:1070, 1966.
174. Gitlin D: Development and metabolism of the immune globulins. In Kagan B, Stiehm R (eds): "Immunologic Incompetence." Chicago: Year Book Medical Publishers, 1971, pp 1–16.
175. Van Der Muelen JA, McNabb TC, Haeffner-Cavaillon N, Klein M, Dorrington KJ: The Fc gamma receptor on human placental plasma membrane. I. Studies on the binding of homologous and heterologous immunoglobulin G. J Immunol 124:500, 1980.
176. Hyvarinen M, Zeltzer P, Oh W, Stiehm ER: Influence of gestational age on serum levels of alpha-1-fetoprotein, IgG globulin and albumin in newborn infants. J Pediatr 82:430, 1973.
177. Bandilla KK, McDuffie FC, Gleich GJ: Immunoglobulin classes of antibodies produced in the primary and secondary responses in man. Clin Exp Immunol 5:627, 1969.
178. Woodland RT, Cantor H: Idiotype specific T helper cells are required to induce idiotype-positive B memory cells to secrete antibody. Eur J Immunol 8:600, 1978.
179. Sullivan JL, Ochs HD, Schiffman G, Hammerschlag MR, Miser J, Vichinsky E, Wedgwood RJ: Immune response after splenectomy. Lancet 1:178, 1978.
180. Likhite VV: Immunological impairment and susceptibility to infection after splenectomy. J Am Med Assoc 236:1376, 1976.
181. Terry WD, Fahey JL: Subclasses of human gamma-2-globulin based on differences in the heavy polypeptide chains. Science. 146:400, 1964.
182. Wang AC, Tung E, Fudenberg HH: The primary structure of a human IgG$_2$ heavy chain: Genetic, evolutionary and functional implications. J Immunol 125:1048, 1980.
183. Connell GE, Parr DM, Hofmann T: The amino acid sequences of the three heavy chain constant region domains of a human IgG$_2$ myeloma protein. Can J Biochem 57:758, 1979.
184. Spiegelberg HL: Biological activities of immunoglobulins of different classes and subclasses. Adv Immunol 19:259, 1974.
185. Isenman DE, Dorrington KJ, Painter RH: The structure and function of immunoglobulin domains. II. The importance of interchain disulfide bonds and the possible role of molecular flexibility in the interaction between immunoglobulin G and complement. J Immunol 114:1726, 1975.
186. McNabb T, Koh TY, Dorrington KJ, Painter RH: Structure and function of immunoglobulin domains. V. Binding of immunoglobulin G and fragments to placental membrane preparations. J Immunol 117:882, 1976.
187. Spiegelberg HL, Fishkin BG, Grey HM: Catabolism of human γG-immunoglobulins of different heavy chain subclasses. I. Catabolism of γG-myeloma proteins in man. J Clin Invest 47:2323, 1968.
188. Augener W, Grey HM: Studies on the mechanism of heat aggregation of human γG. J Immunol 105:1024, 1970.
189. Seegan GW, Smith CA, Schumaker VN: Changes in quaternary structure of IgG upon reduction of the interheavy-chain disulfide bond. Proc Natl Acad Sci USA 76:907, 1979.
190. Capra JD, Kunkel HG: Aggregation of γG proteins. Relevance to the hyperviscosity syndrome. J Clin Invest 49:610, 1970.
191. Simmons JG, Fuller CR, Buchanan PD, Yount WJ: Distribution of surface, cytoplasmic and secreted IgG subclasses in human lymphoblastoid cell lines and normal peripheral blood lymphocytes. Scand J Immunol 14:1, 1981.

192. Nisonoff A, Hopper JE, Spring SB: "The Antibody Molecule." New York: Academic Press, 1975, p 303.

193. Austrian R: Pneumococci. In Davis B, Dulbecco R, Eisen H, Ginsberg H, (eds): "Microbiology." 3rd ed, San Francisco: Harper and Row, 1980, p 604.

194. Frame M, Mollison PL, Terry WD: Gamma G4-Globulin antibody causing inhibition of clotting factor VIII. Nature 217:174, 1968.

195. Frame M, Mollison PL, Terry WD: Anti-Rh activity of human gamma G4 proteins. Nature (London) 225:641, 1970.

196. Johnson PM, Faulk WP: Rheumatoid factor: Its nature, specificity and production in rheumatoid arthritis. Clin Immunol Immunopathol 6:414, 1976.

197. Schur PH, Bianco NE, Panush RS: Antigammaglobulins in normal individuals and in patients with adult and juvenile rheumatoid arthritis and osteoarthritis. Rheumatology 6:155, 1975.

198. Dresser DW: Most IgM-producing cells in the mouse secrete autoantibodies (rheumatoid factor). Nature (London). 274:480, 1978.

199. Elkon KB, Caeiro F, Gharavi AE, Patel BM, Ferjencik PP, Hughes GRV: Radioimmunoassay profile of antiglobulins in connective tissue diseases: Elevated level of IgA antiglobulin in systemic sicca syndrome. Clin Exp Immunol 46:547, 1981.

200. Dunne JV, Carson DA, Spiegelberg HL, Alspaugh MA, Vaughan JH: IgA rheumatoid factor in the sera and saliva of patients with rheumatoid arthritis and Sjögren's syndrome. Ann Rheum Dis 38:161, 1979.

201. Gaarder PI, Natvig JB: The reaction of rheumatoid anti-Gm antibodies with native and aggregated Gm-negative IgG. Scand J Immunol 3:559, 1974.

202. Natvig JB, Gaarder PI, Turner MW: IgG antigens of the Cγ2 and Cγ3 homology regions interacting with rheumatoid factors. Clin Exp Immunol 12:177, 1972.

203. Deisenhofer J, Jones TA, Huber R: Crystallization, crystal structure analysis and atomic model of the complex formed by a human Fc fragment and fragment B of protein A from Staphylococcus aureus. Hoppe-Seyler's Z. Physiol Chem 359:975, 1978.

204. Ishizaka K, Ishizaka T, Hornbrook MM: Physicochemical properties of human reaginic antibody. IV. Presence of a unique immunoglobulin as a carrier of reaginic activity. J Immunol 97:75, 1966.

205. Kepron MR, Conrad DH, Froese A: The cross-reactivity of rat IgE and IgG with solubilized receptors of rat basophilic leukemia cells. International Symposium on the Structure and Function of Fc Receptors, Winnipeg, Abstract 23, June 1–3, 1981.

206. Prausnitz C, Küstner H. Studies on Super Sensitivity. Translated In: Gell PGH, Coombs RRA (eds): "Clinical Aspects of Immunology." 2nd ed, Philadelphia: F.A. Davis Co., 1968, p 1298.

207. Ishizaka K, Ishizaka T, Arbesman CE: Induction of passive cutaneous anaphylaxis in monkeys by human γ E antibody. J Allergy 39:254, 1967.

208. Stanworth DR, Smith AK: Inhibition of reagin-mediated PCA reactions in baboons by the human IgG₄ subclass. Clin Allergy 3:37, 1973.

209. Nakagawa T, Stadler BM, Heiner DC, Skvaril F, De Weck AL: Flowcytometric analysis of human basophil degranulation. II. Degranulation induced by anti-IgE, anti-IgG₄ and the calcium ionophore A23187. Clin Allergy 11:21, 1981.

210. Vijay HM, Perlmutter L: Inhibition of reagin-mediated PCA reactions in monkeys and histamine release from human leukocytes by human IgG₄ subclass. Int Archs Allergy Appl Immunol 53:78, 1977.

211. Ishizaka T, Debernardo R, Tomioka H, Lichtenstein LM, Ishizaka K: Identification of basophil granulocytes as a site of allergic histamine release. J Immunol 108:1000, 1972.

212. Bryant DH, Burns MW, Lazarus L: Identification of IgG antibody as a carrier of reagenic activity in asthmatic patients. J Allergy Clin Immunol 56:417, 1975.

213. Ovary Z, Caiazza SS, Kojima: PCA reactions with mouse antibodies in mice and rats. Int Archs Allergy Appl Immunol 48:16, 1975.

214. Almosawi T, Gwynn C, Stanworth DR: Immunological studies on anaphylactic antibodies of the IgG class. In Abstracts of the Proceedings of the Fourth Charles Blackley Symposium on The Clinical Aspects of Allergic Disease, Nottingham, England, July 1981.

215. Kimura I, Tanizaki U, Sato S, Takahashi K: Differences in response to anti-IgE and to anti-IgG in basophils from patients with bronchial asthma. Clin Allergy 11:31, 1981.

216. Porter RR: The Croonian Lecture, 1980: The complex proteases of the complement system. Proc R Soc Lond [Biol] 210B:477, 1980.

217. Knobel HR, Villeger W, Isliker H: Chemical analysis and electron microscopy studies of human Clq prepared by different methods. Eur J Immunol 5:78, 1975.

218. Hughes-Jones NC, Gardner B: Reaction between the isolated globular sub-units of the complement component Clq and IgG complexes. Mol Immunol 16:697, 1979.

219. Yasmeen D, Ellerson JR, Dorrington KJ, Painter RH: The structure and function of immunoglobulin domains. IV. The distribution of some effector functions among the Cγ2 and Cγ3 homology regions of human IgG. J Immunol 116:518, 1976.

220. Kehoe JM, Bourgois A, Capra JD, Fougereau M: Amino acid sequence of a murine immunoglobulin fragment that possesses complement fixing activity. Biochemistry 13:2499, 1974.

221. Johnson BJ, Thames KE: Investigations of the complement fixing sites of immunoglobulins. J Immunol 117:1491, 1976.

222. Boackle RJ, Johnson BJ, Caughman GB: An IgG primary sequence exposure theory for complement activation using synthetic peptides. Nature 282:742, 1979.

223. Lukas TJ, Muñoz H, Erickson BW: Inhibition of C1-mediated immune hemolysis by monomeric and dimeric peptides from the second constant domain of human immunoglobulin G J Immunol 127:2555, 1981.

224. Cohen S, Becker EL: The effect of benzylation or sequential amidination and benzylation on the ability of rabbit γG-antibody to fix complement. J Immunol 100:403, 1968.

225. Vivanco-Martínez F, Bragado R, Albar JP, Juarez C, Ortíz-Masllorens F: Chemical modification of carboxyl groups in human Fc gamma fragment: Structural role and effect on the complement fixation. Mol Immunol 17:327, 1980.

226. Allan R, Isliker H: Studies on the complement-binding site of rabbit immunoglobulin G. I. Modification of tryptophan residues and their role in anticomplementary activity of rabbit IgG. Immunochem 11:175, 1974.

227. Cohen S: The requirement for the association of two adjacent rabbit γG-antibody molecules in the fixation of complement by immune complexes. J Immunol 100:407, 1968.

228. Scribner DJ, Fahrney D: Neutrophil receptors for IgG and complement: Their roles in the attachment and ingestion phase of phagocytosis. J Immunol 116:892, 1976.

229. Wood WB, Davis BD: Host-parasite relations in bacterial infections. In Davis B, Dulbecco R, Eisen H, Ginsberg H, (eds): "Microbiology." 3rd ed, San Francisco: Harper and Row, 1980, pp 551–571.

230. Messner RP, Jelinek J: Receptors for human γG globulin on human neutrophils. J Clin Invest 49:2165, 1970.

231. Henson PM, Johnson HB, Spiegelberg HL: The release of granule enzymes from human neutrophils stimulated by aggregated immunoglobulins of different classes and subclasses. J Immunol 109:1182, 1972.

232. Schanfield MS, Schoeppner SL: Additional studies on differences in the ability to promote phagocytosis by human IgG$_1$ and IgG$_3$ allo and autoantibodies. International Symposium on the Structure and Function of Fc receptors. Winnipeg, Abstract 5, June 1–3, 1981.

233. Schanfield MS: Genetic markers of immunoglobulins. In Fudenberg H, Stites D, Caldwell J, Wells J (eds): "Basic and Clinical Immunology." Los Altos: Lange Medical Publications, 1978, p 64.

234. MacLennan ICM, Connell GE, Gotch FM: Effector activating determinants on IgG. II. Differentiation of the combining sites for Clq from those for cytotoxic K cells and neutrophils by plasmin digestion of rabbit IgG. Immunology 26:303, 1974.

235. Barnett-Foster DE, Dorrington KJ, Painter RH: Structure and function of immunoglobulin domains. VII. Studies on the structural requirements of human immunoglobulin G for granulocyte binding. J Immunol. 120:1952, 1978.

236. Dossett JH, Kronvall G, Williams RC Jr, Quie PG: Antiphagocytic effects of staphylococcal protein A. J Immunol 103:1405, 1969.

237. Kronvall G, Frommel D: Definition of staphylococcal protein A reactivity for human immunoglobulin G fragments. Immunochem 7:124, 1970.

238. Najjar VA, Nishioka K: Tuftsin: A natural phagocytosis stimulating peptide. Nature 228:672, 1970.

239. Nishioka K, Constantopoulos A, Satoh PS, Najjar VA: The characteristics, isolation and synthesis of the phagocytosis stimulating peptide Tuftsin. Biochem Biophys Res Commun 47:172, 1972.

240. Florentin I, Schultz J, Bruley-Rosset M, Kiger N, Martinez J, Mathé G: In vivo immunomodulating properties of two synthetic agents: Azimexon and Tuftsin. Recent Results Cancer Res 75:153, 1980.

241. Nishioka K, Amoscato AA, Babcock GF: Tuftsin: A hormone-like tetrapeptide with antimicrobial and antitumor activities. Life Sci 28:1081, 1981.

242. Phillips JH, Babcock GF, Nichioka K: Tuftsin: A naturally occurring immunopotentiating factor. I. In vitro enhancement of murine natural cell mediated cytotoxicity. J Immunol 126:915, 1981.

243. Tzehoval E, Segal S, Stabinsky Y, Fridkin M, Spirer Z, Feldman M: Tuftsin (an Ig-associated tetrapeptide) triggers the immunogenic function of macrophages: Implications for activation of programmed cells. Proc Natl Acad Sci USA 75:3400, 1978.

244. Stabinsky Y, Gottlieb P, Zakuth V, Spirer Z, Fridkin M: Specific binding sites for the phagocytosis stimulating peptide Tuftsin on human polymorphonuclear leukocytes and monocytes. Biochem Biophys Res Commun 83:599, 1978.

245. Nair RMG, Ponce B, Fudenberg HH: Interactions of radiolabeled Tuftsin with human neutrophils. Immunochem 15:901, 1978.

246. Bar-Shavit Z, Stabinsky Y, Fridkin M, Goldman R: Tuftsin-macrophage interaction: Specific binding and augmentation of phagocytosis. J Cell Physiol 100:55, 1979.

247. Unkeless JC, Eisen HN: Binding of monomeric immunoglobulins to Fc receptors of mouse macrophages. J Exp Med 142:1520, 1975.

248. Veretennikova NI, Chipens GI, Nikiforovich GV, Betinsh YR: Rigin, another phagocytosis-stimulating tetrapeptide isolated from human IgG. Int J Pep Protein Res 17:430, 1981.

249. Huber R, Deisenhofer J, Colman PM, Matsushima M, Palm W: Crystallographic structural studies of an IgG molecule and an Fc fragment. Nature (London) 264:415, 1976.

250. Barnett-Foster DE, Sjoquist J, Painter RH: The effect of fragment B of staphylococcal protein A on the binding of rabbit IgG to human granulocytes and monocytes. Mol Immunol 19:407, 1982.

251. Shen L, Lydyard PM, Penfold P, Roitt IM: Evidence for antibody-dependent cell-mediated cytotoxicity by T cells bearing receptors for IgG. Clin Exp Immunol 35:276, 1979.

252. Gale RP, Zighelboim J: Polymorphonuclear leukocytes in antibody-dependent cellular cytotoxicity. J Immunol 114:1047, 1975.

253. Kohl S, Starr SE, Oleske JM, Shore SL, Ashman RB, Nahmias AJ: Human monocyte-macrophage-mediated antibody-dependent cytotoxicity to herpes simplex virus-infected cells. J Immunol 118:729, 1977.

254. Capron M, Rousseaux J, Mazingue C, Bazin H, Capron A: Rat mast cell-eosinophil interaction in antibody-dependent eosinophil cytotoxicity to shistosoma mansoni schistosomula. J Immunol 121:2518, 1978.

255. Rager-Zisman B, Allison AC: Mechanism of immunologic resistance to herpes simplex virus 1 (HSV-1) infection. J Immunol 116:35, 1976.

256. Ziegler HK, Henney CS: Antibody-dependent cytolytically active human leukocytes: An analysis of inactivation following in vitro interaction with antibody-coated target cells. J Immunol 115:1500, 1975.

257. Ferrarini M, Moretta L, Abrile L, Durante M: Receptors for IgG molecules on human lymphocytes forming spontaneous rosettes with sheep red cells. Eur J Immunol 5:70, 1975.

258. Wisloff F, Michaelsen TE, Froland SS: Inhibition of antibody-dependent human lymphocyte-mediated cytotoxicity by immunoglobulin classes, IgG subclasses and IgG fragments. Scan J Immunol 3:29, 1974.

259. MacLennan ICM, Connell GE, Gotch FM: Effector activating determinants on IgG. II. Differentiation of the combining sites for Clq from those for cytotoxic K cells and neutrophils by plasmin digestion of rabbit IgG. Immunology 26:303, 1974.

260. Austin RM, Daniels CA: Inhibition by rheumatoid factor, anti-Fc and staphylococcal protein A of antibody-dependent cell-mediated cytolysis against herpes simplex virus-infected cells. J Immunol 117:602, 1976.

261. Baker RF, Loosli CG: The ultrastructure of encapsulated Diplococcus pneumoniae type 1 before and after exposure to type-specific antibody. Lab Invest 15:716, 1966.

262. Hoover RG, Lynch RG: Lymphocyte surface membrane immunoglobulin in myeloma: II. T cells with IgA-Fc receptors are markedly increased in mice with IgA plasmacytomas. J Immunol 125:1280, 1980.

263. Hoover RG, Hickman S, Gebel HM, Rebbe N, Lynch RG: Expansion of Fc receptor-bearing T cells in patients with IgG and IgA myeloma. J Clin Invest 67:308, 1981.

264. Hoover RG, Gebel HM, Dieckgraefe BK, Hickman S, Rebbe NF, Hirayama N, Ovary Z, Lynch RG: Occurrence and potential significance of increased numbers of T cells with Fc receptors in myeloma. Immunol Rev 56:115, 1981.

265. Mckenzie IFC, Potter T: Murine lymphocyte surface antigens. Adv Immunol 27:181, 1979.

266. Moretta L, Ferrarini M, Cooper MD: Characterization of human T cell subpopulations as defined by specific receptors for immunoglobulin. Contemp Top Immunobiol 8:19, 1978.

267. Hayashi H: The intracellular neutral SH-dependent protease associated with inflammatory responses. Int Rev Cytol 40:101, 1975.

268. Yamamoto S, Nishiura M, Hayashi H: The natural mediator for PMN emigration in inflammation. V. The site of structural change in the chemotactic generation of immunoglobulin G by inflammatory SH-dependent protease. Immunology 24:791, 1973.

269. Higuchi Y, Ishida M, Hayashi H: A lymphocyte chemotactic peptide released from immunoglobulin G by neutrophil neutral thiol protease. Cell Immunol 46:297, 1979.

270. Ishida M, Honda M, Hayashi H: In vitro macrophage chemotactic generation from serum immunoglobulin G by neutrophil neutral seryl protease. Immunology 35:167, 1978.

271. Fridman WH, Rabourdin-Combe C, Neauport-Sautes C, Gisler RH: Characterization and function of T cell Fc$_\gamma$ receptor. Immunol Rev 56:51, 1981.

272. Joskowicz M, Rabourdin-Combe C, Neauport-Sautes C, Fridman WH: Characterization of suppressive immunoglobulin-binding factor (IBF). J Immunol 121:777, 1978.

273. Berman MA, Spiegelberg HL, Weigle WO: Lymphocyte stimulation with Fc fragments. I. Class, subclass, and domain of active fragments. J Immunol 122:89, 1979.

274. Morgan EL, Thoman ML, Weigle WO: Enhancement of T lymphocyte functions by Fc fragments of immunoglobulins. I. Augmentation of allogeneic mixed lymphocyte culture reactions requires I-A or I-B-subregion differences between effector and stimulator cell populations. J Exp Med 153:1161, 1981.

275. Thoman ML, Morgan EL, Weigle WO: Fc fragment activation of T lymphocytes. I. Fc fragments trigger Lyt 1 + 23 − T lymphocytes to release a helper T cell replacing activity. J Immunol 126:632, 1981.

276. Miller F: The carbohydrate moieties of mouse immunoglobulins: Composition and evidence against a role in transplacental transport. J Immunol 107:1161, 1971.

277. Johanson RA, Shaw AR, Schlamowitz M: The CH_2 domain of rabbit IgG is the site of the receptor recognition unit for maternofetal transport. Fed Proc 39:481, 1980.

278. Arend WP, Webster DE: Catabolism and biologic properties of two species of rat IgG$_{2a}$ Fc fragments. J Immunol 118:395, 1977.

279. Weitzman S, Palmer L, Grennon M: Serum decay and placental transport of a mutant mouse myeloma immunoglobulin with defective polypeptide and oligosaccharide structure. J Immunol 122:12, 1979.

280. Kronvall G, Seal US, Finstad J, Williams RC Jr: Phylogenetic insight into evolution of mammalian Fc fragment of γG globulin using staphylococcal protein A. J Immunol 104:140, 1970.

281. Johnsson S, Kronvall G: The use of protein A-containing S. aureus as a solid phase anti-IgG reagent in radioimmunoassays as exemplified in the quantitation of alpha-fetoprotein in normal human adult serum. Eur J Immunol 4:29, 1974.

282. Brunda MJ, Minden P, Grey H: Heterogeneity of binding of human IgA subclasses to protein A. J Immunol 123:1457, 1979.

283. Lind I, Harboe M, Fölling I: Protein A reactivity of two distinct groups of human monoclonal IgM. Scand J Immunol 4:483, 1975.

284. Johansson SGO, Inganäs M: Interaction of polyclonal human IgE with protein A from Staphylococcus aureus. Immunol Rev 41:248, 1978.

285. Endresen C: The binding to protein A of immunoglobulin G and of Fab and Fc fragments. Acta Pathol Microbiol Scand [C] 87:185, 1979.

286. Sjödahl J: Repetitive sequences in protein A from Staphylococcus aureus: Arrangement of five regions within the protein, four being highly homologous and Fc binding. Eur J Immunol 73:343, 1977.

287. Recht B, Frangione B, Franklin E, van Loghem E: Structural studies of a human γ3 myeloma protein (Goe) that binds staph protein A. J Immunol 127:917, 1981.

288. Deisenhofer J, Colman PM, Epp O, Huber R: Crystallographic structural studies of a human Fc fragment. II. Complete model based on a fourier map at 3.5-Å resolution. Hoppe-Seyler's Z. Physiol Chem 357:1421, 1976.

289. Biguzzi S: Interaction of anti-staphylococcal protein A antisera with Fc receptor-bearing human normal lymphocytes. Eur J Immunol 9:52, 1979.

290. Pfueller SL, Lüscher EF: The effects of aggregated immunoglobulins on human blood platelets in relation to their complement-fixing abilities. I. Studies of immunoglobulins of different types. J Immunol 109:517, 1972.

291. Henson PM, Spiegelberg HL: Release of serotonin from human platelets induced by aggregated immunoglobulins of different classes and subclasses. J Clin Invest 52:1282, 1973.

292. Cheng CM, Hawiger J: Affinity isolation and characterization of immunoglobulin G Fc fragment-binding glycoprotein from human blood platelets. J Biol Chem 254:2165, 1979.

293. LuBuglio AF, Cotran RS, Jandl JH: Red cells coated with immunoglobulin G: Binding and sphering by mononuclear cells in man. Science 158:1582, 1967.

294. Lawrence DA, Weigle WO, Spiegelberg HL: Immunoglobulins cytophilic for human lymphocytes, monocytes, and neutrophils. J Clin Invest 55:368, 1975.

295. Anwar ARE, Kay AB: Membrane receptors for IgG and complement (C_4, C_{3b} and C_{3d}) on human eosinophils and neutrophils and their relation to eosinophilia. J Immunol 119:976, 1977.

296. Butterworth AE, Remold HG, Houba V, David JR, Franks D, David PH, Sturrock RF: Antibody-dependent eosinophil-mediated damage to ^{51}Cr-labeled schistosomula of Schistosoma mansoni. III. Mediation by IgG and inhibition by antigen-antibody complexes. J Immunol 118:2230, 1977.

297. Kay AB: The eosinophil in infectious diseases. J Infect Dis 129:606, 1974.

298. Metcalfe DD, Gadek JE, Raphael GD, Frank MM, Kaplan AP, Kaliner M: Human eosinophil adherence to serum-treated sepharose: Granule-associated enzyme release and requirement for activation of the alternative complement pathway. J Immunol 119:1744, 1977.

299. Minta JO, Painter RH: A reexamination of the ability of pFc' and Fc' to participate in passive cutaneous anaphylaxis. Immunochem 9:1041, 1972.

300. Ovary Z, Saluk PH, Quijada L, Lamm ME: Biologic activities of rabbit immunoglobulin G in relation to domains of the Fc region. J Immunol 116:1265, 1976.

301. Klein M, Neauport-Sautes C, Ellerson JR, Fridman WF: Binding site of human IgG subclasses and their domains for Fc receptors of activated murine T cells. J Immunol 119:1077, 1977.

302. Froland SS, Natvig JB: Surface-bound immunoglobulin on lymphocytes from normal and immunodeficient humans. Scand J Immunol 1:1, 1972.

303. Oi VT, Bryan VM, Herzenberg LA, Herzenberg LA: Lymphocyte membrane IgG and secreted IgG, are structurally and allotypically distinct. J Exp Med 151:1260, 1980.

304. Huber H, Douglas SD, Nusbacher J, Kochwa S, Rosenfield RE: IgG subclass specificity of human monocyte receptor sites. Nature 229:419, 1970.

305. Hay FC, Torrigiani G, Roitt IM: The binding of human IgG subclasses to human monocytes. Eur J Immunol 2:257, 1972.

306. Alexander MD, Andrews JA, Leslie RGQ, Wood NG: The binding of human and guinea-pig IgG subclasses to homologous macrophage and monocyte Fc receptors. Immunol 35:115, 1978.

307. Okafor GO, Turner MW, Hay FC: Localization of monocyte binding site of human immunoglobulin G. Nature (London) 248:228, 1974.

308. Ciccimarra F, Rosen FS, Merler E: Localization of the IgG effector site for monocyte receptors. Proc Natl Acad Sci USA 72:2081, 1975.

309. Dorrington KJ: Properties of the FC receptor on macrophages and monocytes. Immunol Commun 5:263, 1976.

310. Guyre PM, Crabtree GR, Bodwell JE, Munck A: MLC-conditioned media stimulate an increase in Fc receptors on human macrophages. J Immunol 126:666, 1981.

311. Crabtree GE: Fc receptors of a human promyelocytic cell line: Evidence for two types of receptors defined by binding of the staphylococcal protein—A-IgG, complex. J Immunol 125:448, 1980.

312. Anderson CL, Grey HM: Physicochemical separation of two distinct Fc receptors on murine macrophage-like cell lines. J Immunol 121:648, 1978.

313. Walker WS: Mediation of macrophage cytolytic and phagocytic activities by antibodies of different classes and subclass—specific Fc receptors. J Immunol 119:367, 1977.

314. Haeffner-Cavaillon N, Dorrington KJ, Klein M: Studies on the $Fc\gamma$ receptor of the murine macrophage-like cell line P388D$_1$. II. Binding of human IgG subclass proteins and their proteolytic fragments. J Immunol 123:1914, 1979.

315. Diamond B, Birshtein BK, Scharff MD: Site of binding of mouse IgG$_{2b}$ to the Fc receptor on mouse macrophages. J Exp Med 150:721, 1979.

316. Yasmeen D, Ellerson JR, Dorrington KJ, Painter RH: Evidence for the domain hypothesis: Location of the site of cytophilic activity toward guinea-pig macrophages in the C_H3 homology region of human immunoglobulin G. J Immunol 110:1706, 1973.

317. Dissanayake S, Hay FC: Investigation of the binding site of mouse IgG subclasses to homologous peritoneal macrophages. Immunology 29:1111, 1975.

318. Tomasi TB, McNabb PC: The secretory immune system. In Fudenberg H, Stites D, Caldwell J, Wells J (eds): "Basic and Clinical Immunology." 3rd ed, Los Altos: Lange Medical Publications, 1980, pp 240–250.

319. Tomasi TB: The concept of local immunity and the secretory system. In Dayton D Jr, Small P Jr, Chanuck R, Kaufman H, Tomasi T (eds): "The Secretory Immune System." DHEW publication, Wash., D.C.: US Govt Printing Office, 1971, p 3.

320. Tomasi TB, Larson L, Challacombe S, McNabb P: Mucosal immunity: The origin and migration pattern of cells in the secretory immune system. J Allergy Clin Immunol 65:12, 1980.

321. Husband AJ, Gowans JL: The origin and antigen-dependent distribution of IgA-containing cells in the intestine. J Exp Med 148:1146, 1978.

322. Kaartinen M, Imir M, Klockars T, Sandholen M, Mäkelä O. IgA in blood and thoracic duct lymph: Concentration and degree of polymerization. Scand J Immunol 7:299, 1978.

323. Turesson I: Distribution of immunoglobulin-containing cells in human bone marrow and lymphoid tissues. Acta Med Scand 199:293, 1976.

324. Heremans JF: Immunoglobulin A. In Sela M (ed): "The Antigens." Vol. II, London: Academic Press, 1974, pp 365–522.

325. Keren DF, Kern SE, Bauer PJ, Porter S, Porter P: Direct demonstration in intestinal secretions of an IgA memory response to orally administered Shigella Flexneri antigens. J Immunol 128:475, 1982.

326. Toraño A, Putnam FW: Complete amino acid sequence of the $\alpha 2$ heavy chain of a human IgA2 immunoglobulin of the A2m (2) allotype. Proc Natl Acad Sci USA 75:966, 1978.

327. Pardo AG, Lamm ME, Plaut AG, Frangione B: Secretory component is covalently bound to a single subunit in human secretory IgA. Mol Immunol 16:477, 1979.

328. Nagura H, Brandtzaeg P, Nakane PK, Brown WR: Ultrastructural localization of J chain in human intestinal mucosa. J Immunol 123:1044, 1979.

329. Parkhouse RME, Della Corte E: Assembly and secretion of immunoglobulin A. In Mestecky J, Lawton A (eds): "The Immunoglobulin A System." Adv Exp Med Biol Vol. 45, New York: Plenum, 1974, p 139.

330. Brandtzaeg P: Presence of J chain in human immunocytes containing various immunoglobulin classes. Nature (London) 252:418, 1974.

331. Tomasi TB, Hauptman S: Modulation of the assembly of immunoglobulin subunits by J chain. In Mestecky J, Lawton A (eds): "The Immunoglobulin A System." Adv Exp Med Biol Vol. 45, New York: Plenum, 1974, pp 111.

332. Kühn LC, Kraehenbuhl JP: The membrane receptor for polymeric immunoglobulin is structurally related to secretory component. J Biol Chem 256:12490, 1981.

333. Strober W, Krakauer R, Klaeveman HL, Reynolds HY, Nelson DL: Secretory component deficiency. A disorder of the IgA immune system. N Engl J Med 294:351, 1976.

334. Orlans E, Peppard J, Reynolds J, Hall J: Rapid active transport of immunoglobulin A from blood to bile. J Exp Med 147:588, 1978.

335. Plaut AG, Wistar R Jr, Capra JD: Differential susceptibility of human IgA immunoglobulins to streptococcal IgA protease. J Clin Invest 54:1295, 1974.

336. Hanson LA, Ahlstedt S, Carlsson B, Kaijser B, Larsson P, Mattsby Baltzer I, Sohl Akerlund A, Svanborg Edén C, Svennerholm A-M: Secretory IgA antibodies to enterobacterial virulence antigens, their induction and possible relevance. In McGhee J, Mestecky J, Babb JL (eds): "Secretory Immunity and Infection." Adv Exp Med Biol, New York: Plenum, 107:165, 1978.

337. Svanborg Edén C, Hanson LA, Jodal U, Lindberg U, Sohl Akerlund A: Variable adherence to normal human urinary tract epithelial cells of Escherichia coli strains associated with various forms of urinary tract infection. Lancet 2:490, 1976.

338. Dayton DH, Small PA, Chanock RM, Kaufman HE, Tomasi TB (eds): "The Secretory Immunologic System." DHEW publication, Wash., D.C.: U.S. Govt. Printing Office, 1971.

339. Buckley RH: Clinical and immunologic features of selective IgA deficiency. In Bergsma D, Good R, Finstad J, Paul N (eds): "Immunodeficiency in Man and Animals, Birth Defects Original Article Series." Vol. XI, No. 1, Sunderland, Mass: Sinauer Associates, 1975, pp 134–142.

340. Stokes CR, Soothill JF, Turner MW: Immune exclusion is a function of IgA. Nature (London) 255:745, 1975.

341. Buckley RH, Dees SC: Correlation of milk precipitins with IgA deficiency. N Engl J Med 281:465, 1969.

342. Ammann AJ, Hong R: Selective IgA deficiency and autoimmunity. Clin Exp Immunol 7:833, 1970.

343. Vyas GN, Perkins HA, Fudenberg HH: Anaphylactoid transfusions associated with anti-IgA. Lancet 2:312, 1968.

344. Iida K, Fujita T, Inai S, Sasaki M, Kato T, Kobayashi K: Complement fixing abilities of IgA myeloma proteins and their fragments: The activation of complement through the classical pathway. Immunochem 13:747, 1976.

345. Burritt MF, Calvanico NJ, Mehta S, Tomasi TB Jr: Activation of the classical complement pathway by Fc fragment of human IgA. J Immunol 118:723, 1977.

346. Shen L, Fanger MW: Secretory IgA antibodies synergize with IgG in promoting ADCC by human polymorphonuclear cells, monocytes and lymphocytes. Cell Immunol 59:75, 1981.

347. Grov A: Human colostral IgA interacting with staphylococcal protein A. Acta Pathol Microbiol Scand [C] 84(1):71, 1976.

348. Patrick CC, Virella G, Koistman J, Fudenberg HH: Differential binding of IgA proteins of different subclasses and allotypes to staphylococcal protein A. Z Immunitaetsforsch 153:466, 1977.

349. Fanger MW, Shen L, Pugh J, Bernier GM: Subpopulations of human peripheral granulocytes and monocytes express receptors for IgA. Proc Natl Acad Sci USA 77:3640, 1980.

350. Lum LG, Keren MD, Koski JD, Kiski I, Strober W, Blaese RM: A receptor for IgA on human T lymphocytes. J Immunol 122:65, 1979.

351. Lum LG, Muchmore AV, O'Connor N, Strober W, Blaese RM: Fc receptors for IgA on human B and human non-B non-T lymphocytes. J Immunol 123:714, 1979.

352. Fanger MW, Pugh J, Bernier GM: The specificity of receptors for IgA on human peripheral polymorphonuclear cells and monocytes. Cell Immunol 60:324, 1981.

353. Gupta S, Pahwa R, O'Reilly RO, Good RA, Siegal FP: Ontogeny of lymphocyte subpopulations in human fetal liver. Proc Natl Acad Sci USA 73:919, 1976.

354. Cathou RE: Solutional conformation and segmental flexibility of immunoglobulins. In Litman G, Good R (eds): "Immunoglobulins." New York: Plenum, 1978, pp 37–83.

355. Vassalli P, Tedghi R, Lisowska-Bernstein B, Tartakoff A, Jaton JC: Evidence for hydrophobic region within heavy chains of mouse B lymphocyte membrane-bound IgM. Proc Natl Acad Sci USA 76:5515, 1979.

356. Feinstein A: Conclusions: An IgM model. In Brent L, Holborow J (eds): "Progress in Immunology II." Vol. 1, New York: American Elsevier Publishing Company, 1974, p 115.

357. Bush ST, Swedlund HA, Gleich GJ: Low molecular weight IgM in human sera. J Lab Clin Med 73:194, 1969.

358. Kehry M, Sibley C, Fuhrman J, Schilling J, Hood LE: Amino acid sequence of a mouse immunoglobulin μ chain. Proc Natl Acad Sci USA 76:2932, 1979.

359. McCumber LJ, Capra JD: The complete amino-acid sequence of a canine μ chain. Mol Immunol 16:565, 1970.

360. Kim YD, Karush F: Equine anti-hapten antibody. VII. Anti-lactoside antibody induced by a bacterial vaccine. Immunochem 10:365, 1971.

361. Romans DG, Tilley CA, Crookston MC, Falk RE, Dorrington KJ: Conversion of incomplete antibodies to direct agglutinins by mild reduction. Evidence for segmental flexibility within the Fc fragment of immunoglobulin G. Proc Natl Acad Sci USA 74:2531, 1977.

362. Feinstein A, Munn EA, Richardson NE: The three-dimensional conformation of γM and γA globulin molecules. Ann NY Acad Sci 190:104, 1971.

363. Ishizaka T, Tada T, Ishizaka K: Fixation of C' and C'la by rabbit γG and γM antibodies with particulate and soluble antigens. J Immunol 100:1145, 1968.

364. Faulk WP, Kiyasu WS, Cooper MD, Fudenberg HH: Deficiency of IgM. Pediatrics 47:399, 1971.

365. Grov A: Antigenicity of human IgM in relation to interaction with staphylococcal protein A. Acta Pathol Microbiol Scand [C] 83:325, 1975.

366. Hurst MM, Volanakis JE, Hester RB, Stroud RM, Bennett JC: The structural basis for binding of complement by immunoglobulin M. J Exp Med 140:1117, 1974.

367. Hurst MM, Volanakis JE, Stroud RM, Bennett JC: C_1 fixation and classical complement pathway activation by a fragment of the $C\mu4$ domain of IgM. J Exp Med 142:1322, 1975.

368. Shen L, Lydyard PM, Roitt IM, Fanger MW: Synergy between IgG and monoclonal IgM antibodies in antibody-dependent cell cytotoxicity. J Immunol 127:73, 1981.

369. Lamon EW, Shaw MW, Lidin B, Walia AS, Fuson EW: Antibody-dependent cell-mediated cytotoxicity in the moloney sarcoma virus system: Differential activity of IgG and IgM with different subpopulations of lymphocytes. J Exp Med 145:302, 1977.

370. Fuson EW, Whitten HD, Ayers RD, Lamon EW: Antibody-dependent cell mediated cytotoxicity by human lymphocytes. I. Comparison of IgM and IgG-induced cytotoxicity. J Immunol 120:1726, 1978.

371. Aoki T, Shimizu A, Yamamura Y: Leucocyte chemotactic factor generated by tryptic digestion of human IgM. Immunochem 13:461, 1976.
372. Preud'homme JL, Gonnot M, Tsapis A, Brouet JC, Mihaesco C: Human T lymphocyte receptors for IgM: Reactivity with monomeric 8S subunit. J Immunol 119:2206, 1977.
373. Burns GF, Cawley JC, Barker CR: Characterization of the receptor for IgM present on human B lymphocytes. Immunology 36:569, 1979.
374. Reynolds HY, Atkinson JP, Newball HH, Frank MM: Receptors for immunoglobulin and complement on human alveolar macrophages. J Immunol 114:1813, 1975.
375. Boltz-Nitulescu G, Bazin H, Spiegelberg H: Specificity of Fc receptors for IgG_{2a}, IgG_1/IgG_{2b} and IgE on rat macrophages. J Exp Med 154:374, 1981.
376. Moretta L, Webb SR, Grossi CE, Lydard PM, Cooper MD: Functional analysis of two human T-cell subpopulations: Help and suppression of B-cell responses by T cells bearing receptors for IgM or IgG. J Exp Med 146:184, 1977.
377. Pichler WJ, Broder S: In vitro functions of human T cells expressing Fc-IgG or Fc-IgM receptors. Immunol Rev 56:163, 1981.
378. Conradie JD, Bubb MO: $C\mu4$ domain of IgM has cytophilic activity for human lymphocytes. Nature (London) 265:160, 1977.
379. Rowe DS, Fahey JL: A new class of human immunoglobulins. I. A unique myeloma protein. J Exp Med 121:171, 1965.
380. Van Boxel JA, Paul WE, Terry WD, Green I: IgD-bearing human lymphocytes. J Immunol 109:648, 1972.
381. Rowe DS, Hug K, Forni L, Pernis B: Immunoglobulin D as a lymphocyte receptor. J Exp Med 138:965, 1973.
382. Dunnette SL, Gleich GJ, Miller RD, Kyle RA: Measurement of IgD by a double antibody radioimmunoassay: Demonstration of an apparent trimodal distribution of IgD levels in normal human sera. J Immunol 119:1727, 1977.
383. Jancelewicz Z: IgD multiple myeloma. Arch Int Med 135:87, 1975.
384. Eidels L: IgD is present on the cell surface of murine lymphocytes in two forms: δ_2L_2 and δL. J Immunol 123:896, 1979.
385. Pollock R, Mescher MF: Murine cell surface immunoglobulin: Two native IgD structures. J Immunol 124:1668, 1980.
386. Pollock RR, Dorf ME, Mescher MF: Genetic control of murine IgD structural heterogeneity. J Immunol 77:4256, 1980.
387. Tucker PW, Liu CP, Mushinski JF, Blattner FR: Mouse immunoglobulin D: Messenger RNA and genomic DNA sequences. Science 209:1353, 1980.
388. Vitetta ES, Uhr JW: Immunoglobulin receptors revisited: A model for the differentiation of bone marrow-derived lymphocytes is described. Science 189:964, 1975.
389. Kettman JR, Cambier JC, Uhr JW, Ligler F, Vitetta ES: The role of receptor IgM and IgD in determining triggering and induction of tolerance in murine B cells. Immunol Rev 43:69, 1979.
390. Bazin H, Platteau B, Beckers A, Pauwels R: Differential effect of neonatal injections of anti-μ or anti-δ antibodies on the synthesis of IgM, IgD, IgE, IgA, IgG_1, IgG_{2a}, IgG_{2b} and IgG_{2c} immunoglobulin classes. J Immunol 121:2083, 1978.
391. Henney CS, Welscher HD, Terry WD, Rowe DS: The lack of skin-sensitizing and complement fixing activities of IgD. Immunochemistry 6:445, 1969.
392. Spiegelberg HL: The structure and biology of human IgD. Immunol Rev 37:3, 1977.
393. Forsgren A, Grubb AO: Many bacterial species bind human IgD. J Immunol 122:1468, 1979.
394. Sjöberg O: Presence of receptors for IgD on human T and non-T lymphocytes. Scand J Immunol 11:377, 1980.

395. Waldmann TA, Iio A, Ogawa M, McIntyre OR, Strober W. The metabolism of IgE: Studies in normal individuals and in a patient with IgE myeloma. J Immunol 117:1139, 1976.
396. Tada T, Ishizaka K: Distribution of γ E-forming cells in lymphoid tissues of the human and monkey. J Immunol 104:377, 1970.
397. Chiorazzi N, Fox DA, Katz DH: Hapten-specific IgE antibody responses in mice. VI. Selective enhancement of IgE antibody production by low doses of X-irradiation and by cyclophosphamide. J Immunol 117:1629, 1976.
398. Chiorazzi N, Fox DA, Katz DH: Hapten-specific IgE antibody responses in mice. VII. Conversion of IgE "non-responder" strains to IgE "responders" by elimination of suppressor T cell activity. J Immunol 118:48, 1977.
399. Stiehm ER, Fulginiti VA: "Immunologic Disorders in Infants and Children." 2nd ed, Philadelphia: W.B. Saunders Company, 1980.
400. Radermecker M, Bekhti A, Poncelet E, Salmon J: Serum IgE levels in protozoal and helminthic infections. Int Arch Allergy 47:285, 1974.
401. Hamburger RN, Orgel HA, Bazaral M: Genetics of human serum IgE levels. In Goodfriend L, Sehon A (eds): "Mechanisms in Allergy, Reagin-Mediated Hypersensitivity." New York: Marcel Decker, 1973, pp 131–139.
402. Marsh DG, Bias WB, Ishizaka K: Genetic control of basal serum immunoglobulin E level and its effect on specific reagin sensitivity. Proc Natl Acad Sci USA 71:3588, 1974.
403. Willcox HNA, Marsh DG: Genetic regulation of antibody heterogeneity: Its possible significance in human allergy. Immunogenetics 6:209, 1978.
404. Hamburger RN: Development of atopic allergy in children. In Johansson S (ed): "Diagnosis and Treatment of IgE-mediated diseases." Amsterdam: Exerpta Medica, 1981, p 30.
405. Bennich H, Bahr-Lindström H: Structure of Immunoglobulin E (IgE). In Brent L, Holborow J (eds): "Progress in Immunology II." Vol. I, New York: American Elsevier Publishing Company, 1974, p 49.
406. Nezlin RS, Zagyansky A, Käiväräinen I, Stefani DV: Properties of myeloma immunoglobulin E (Yu), chemical, fluorescence polarization and spin-labeled studies. Immunochem 10:681, 1973.
407. Bennich HH, Dorrington K: Structure and conformation of immunoglobulin E (IgE). In Ishizaka K, Dayton D (eds): "The Biological Role of the Immunoglobulin E System." HEW Publication, 1972, p 19.
408. Dorrington K, Bennich H: Thermally induced structural changes in immunoglobulin E. J Biol Chem 248:8378, 1973.
409. Takatsu K, Ishizaka T, Ishizaka K: Biologic significance of disulfide bonds in human IgE. J Immunol 114:1838, 1975.
410. Kulczycki A Jr, Vallina VL: Specific binding of nonglycosylated IgE to FCε receptor. Immunochem 18:723, 1981.
411. Ishizaka K, Ishizaka T: Mechanisms of reaginic hypersensitivity and the IgE antibody response. Immunol Rev 41:109, 1978.
412. Metzger H: The IgE—mast cell system as a paradigm for the study of antibody mechanisms. Immunol Rev 41:186, 1978.
413. Steinberg P, Ishizaka K, Norman PS: Possible role of IgE—mediated reaction in immunity. J Allergy Clin Immunol 54:359, 1974.
414. Jarrett EEE, Jarrett WFH, Urquhart GM: Quantitative studies in the kinetics of establishment and expulsion of intestinal nematode population in susceptible and immune hosts. Parasitology 59:625, 1968.

415. Haque A, Ouaissi A, Joseph M, Capron M, Capron A: IgE antibody of eosinophil and macrophage—mediated in vitro killing of Dipetalonema viteae microfilariae. J Immunol 127:716, 1981.
416. Gonzalez-Molina A, Spiegelberg H: A subpopulation of normal human peripheral B lymphocytes that bind IgE. J Clin Invest 59:616, 1977.
417. Spiegelberg HL, Melewicz M: Fc receptors specific for IgE on subpopulations of human lymphocytes and monocytes. Clin Immunol Immunopathol 15:424, 1980.
418. Anderson CL, Spiegelberg HL: Macrophage receptors for IgE: Binding of IgE to specific IgE Fc receptors on a human macrophage cell line U937. J Immunol 126:2470, 1981.
419. Spiegelberg HL: Lymphocytes bearing Fc receptors for IgE. Immunol Rev 56:199, 1981.
420. Suemura M, Shiho O, Deguchi H, Yamamura Y, Böttcher I, Kishimoto, T: Characterization and isolation of IgE class-specific suppressor factor (IgE-TsF) I. The presence of the binding site(s) for IgE and of the H-2 gene products in IgE-TsF. J Immunol 127:465, 1981.
421. Yodoi J, Harashima M, Ishizaka K: Lymphocytes bearing Fc receptors for IgE. VI Suppressive effect of glucocorticoids on the expression of Fcε receptors and glycosylation of IgE-binding factors. J Immunol 127:471, 1981.
422. Hamburger RN: Peptide inhibition of the Prausnitz-Küstner reaction. Science 189:389, 1975.
423. Bennich H, Ragnarsson V, Johansson SGO, Ishizaka K, Ishizaka T, Levy DA, Lichtenstein LM: Failure of the putative IgE pentapeptide to compete with IgE for receptors on basophils and mast cells. Int Archs Allergy Appl Immunol 53:459, 1977.
424. Vardinon N, Spirer Z, Fridkin M, Schwartz J, Ben-Efraim S: Influence of the synthetic pentapeptide L-Asp-Ser-Asp-Pro-Arg on the direct and indirect mast cell degranulation induced by reaginic antibodies. Acta Allergol 32:291, 1977.
425. Stanworth DR, Kings M, Roy PD, Moran DM: Investigation of the reputed inhibition of the Prausnitz-Küstner reaction by the pentapeptide Asp-Ser-Asp-Pro-Arg. Int Archs Allergy Appl Immunol 56:409, 1978.
426. Hamburger RN: Inhibition of IgE binding to tissue culture cells and leucocytes by pentapeptide. Immunology 38:781, 1979.
427. Stanworth DR, Kings M, Roy PD, Moran JM, Moran DM: Synthetic peptides comprising sequences of the human immunoglobulin E heavy chain capable of releasing histamine. Biochem J 180:665, 1979.
428. Hahn GS, Hamburger RN: A theory of receptor binding sites in immunoglobulins and cellular recognition molecules. Pediatr Res 14:546, 1980.
429. Hahn GS, Hamburger RN: Conservation of active sites in molecules with immunoglobulin fold domain structure. In Nakamura R, Dito W, Tucker E (eds): "Immunologic Analysis: Recent Progress in Diagnostic Laboratory Immunology." New York: Masson Publishing Company, 1982 (in press).
430. Julliard JH, Shibasaki T, Ling N, Guillemin R: High molecular weight immunoreactive β-endorphin in extracts of human placenta is a fragment of immunoglobulin G. Science 208:183, 1980.
431. Fridovich I: The biology of oxygen radicals. Science 201:875, 1978.
432. Richardson JS, Thomas KA, Rubin BH, Richardson DC: Crystal structure of bovine Cu, Zn superoxide dismutase at 3Å resolution: Chain tracing and metal ligands. Proc Natl Acad Sci USA 72:1349, 1975.
433. Richardson JS, Richardson DC, Thomas KA, Silverton EW, Davies DR: Similarity of three dimensional structure between the immunoglobulin domain and the copper, zinc superoxide dismutase subunit. J Mol Biol 102:221, 1976.

434. Novak R, Bosze Z, Matkovics B, Fachet J: Gene affecting superoxide dismutase activity linked to the histocompatibility complex in H-2 congenic mice. Science 207:86, 1979.
435. Schlesinger DH, Goldstein G: The amino acid sequence of thymopoietin II. Cell 5:361, 1975.
436. Scheid MP, Goldstein G, Boyse EA: The generation and regulation of lymphocyte populations. J Exp Med 147:1727, 1978.
437. Goldstein G, Scheid M, Boyse EA, Brand A, Gilmour DG: Thymopoietin and burso-poietin induction signals regulating early lymphocyte differentiation. Cold Spring Harbor Symp Quant Biol 41:5, 1977.
438. Goldstein G, Scheid MP, Boyse EA, Schlesinger DH, Wauwe JV: A synthetic penta-peptide with biological activity characteristic of the thymic hormone thymopoietin. Science 204:1309, 1979.
439. Tucker PW, Marcu KB, Slightom JL, Blattner FR: Structure of the constant and 3' untranslated regions of the murine γ_{2b} heavy chain messenger RNA. Science 206:1299, 1979.
440. Kenter AL, Birshtein BK: Genetic mechanism accounting for precise immunoglobulin domain deletion in a variant of MPC 11 myeloma cells. Science 206:1307, 1979.
441. Sampter M: "Immunological Diseases." Boston: Little Brown and Company, 1978.
442. Stiehm ER: The B lymphocyte system. In Stiehm E, Fulginiti V (eds): "Immunological Disorders in Infants and Children." Philadelphia: W.B. Saunders Company, 1980, p 73.
443. Velpo JA, Irjala K, Viljanen MK, Klemi P, Kouvonen I, Rönnem AA: δ-heavy chain disease: A study of a case. Clin Immunol Immunopathol 17:584, 1980.
444. Hieter PA, Hollis GF, Korsmeyer GJ, Waldmann TA, Leder P: Clustered arrangement of immunoglobulin λ constant region genes in man. Nature 294:536, 1981.

Physiology of Immunoglobulins: Diagnostic and
Clinical Aspects, pages 305–351
© 1982 Alan R. Liss, Inc., 150 Fifth Avenue, New York, NY 10011

10

Immunoglobulin E:
Diagnostic and Clinical Manifestations

Konrad J. Wicher, DM Sc, PhD

INTRODUCTION

γE immunoglobulin (IgE) is a carrier of reaginic activity. Behind this simple statement lie many years of studies and a colorful history. The term reagin has a historic connotation; it was applied to a serum factor in allergic individuals which, when injected into the skin of a nonallergic subject, reacts upon challenge with a proper allergen. This reaction was observed in the 1920s by two German scientists, Dr. Carl Prausnitz and Dr. Heinz Küstner. Doctor Küstner, a gynecologist, was allergic to cooked fish, but his serum did not react with an extract of cooked fish in any of the tests then known. However, when his serum was injected into the skin of Dr. Prausnitz's forearm and the same spot was challenged 24 hours later with the fish extract, a severe erythema and induration developed within minutes. This procedure, known as the Prausnitz-Küstner (P-K) test [118], was until 1967 the most used and most reliable test for skin-sensitizing (reaginic, homocytotropic) antibodies, which we now call IgE antibodies. The P-K test is very rarely used today, and because of the possibility of transmitting hepatitis virus it is banned in most states in the USA.

IgE is primarily (but not exclusively) associated with atopic allergy. The term allergy was introduced by an Austrian pediatrician, Dr. Clemens von Pirquet, in 1906 to describe an altered reactivity resulting from primary sensitization. Dr. Arthur F. Coca, an American allergoimmunologist (in the modern sense), introduced the term atopy to denote a type of hypersensitivity subject to hereditary influence.

This chapter is dedicated to Carl E. Arbesman, Buffalo General Hospital, Buffalo, NY, on the occasion of his 70th birthday.

For over 40 years investigators tried to identify the serum factor responsible for reaginic activity. Reports associating this activity first to known protein fractions and later to globulin classes were soon followed by publications refuting such findings.

In 1966 Kimishige and Teruko Ishizaka and their technical group working in Denver, Colorado, reported [63] the identification of a unique immuno-globulin (Ig) as the carrier of reaginic activity. The newly described Ig was designated as E. The Ishizaka studies are an example of foresight and me-ticulously executed experiments.

At almost the same time two researchers in Sweden, Gunnar Johansson and Hans Bennich, isolated from the serum of a patient (N.D.) a unique myeloma protein which was different from the IgG, IgM, IgA, and IgD classes [68]. These authors called the protein IgND. Radioimmunoassay with antiserum to IgND showed that normal sera contain small amounts of IgND. However, IgND concentrations were higher in some allergic patients. This observation and the physicochemical properties of the IgND, which were similar to the newly described IgE, led to the conclusion that IgND and IgE were of the same class of globulins. In February 1968, at a joint conference sponsored by the World Health Organization (WHO) in Lausanne, Switz-erland, the results obtained by the Ishizakas group and the Bennich-Johansson group were compared and analyzed. WHO then issued a report [17] that IgND is a myeloma protein of IgE and that IgE is the carrier of the biologic properties of reaginic antibody.

The first myeloma IgE (IgND) contributed significantly to knowledge of the physicochemical properties of IgE, which, because of the low yield of IgE from sera of allergic patients, had not been complete. In 1969 the second report of myeloma IgE was published [106]. The monoclonal IgE cases reported thus far are summarized in Table I.

The discovery of the new immunoglobulin class which carried the reaginic antibody activity responsible for allergic reactions encouraged the develop-ment of new diagnostic procedures in the field of allergy.

STRUCTURE AND PHYSICOCHEMICAL CHARACTERISTICS OF IgE

The IgE molecule is composed of two heavy (H) and two light (L) chains (Fig. 1, Table II). The H (ϵ) chain is estimated to weigh 75,000 daltons, the L chain 22,500, and the intact protein 200,000 daltons. The Fc portion of the molecule can be split off by papain digestion, and depending on the digestion conditions, a subfragment, Fc', can be obtained. The Fc portion has two non-cross-reacting groups of antigenic determinants, $D_{\epsilon 1}$ and $D_{\epsilon 2}$. $D_{\epsilon 1}$ is associated with the Fc' fragment, $D_{\epsilon 2}$ with the carboxyl-terminal end

TABLE I. Published Reports of IgE Monoclonal Gammopathy, 1967–1980

Group	Case no.	Year published	Reference no.	Country	Patient	Sex	Age (years)	Plasma cell leukemia	Skeletal lesions	Type L-chain	Bence Jones protein in urine	Serum IgE (g/dl)
Monoclonal IgE gammopathy	1	1967	68	Sweden	ND	M	50	+	−	λ	+	3.80
	2	1969	106	USA	PS	M	60	+	−	λ	+	7.50
	3	1972	43	USA	Hea	F	65	−	−[a]	κ	Trace	2.70
	4	1972	113[b]	USA	DB	F	55	−	+	κ	−	1.80
	5	1972	131	USSR	Yu	M	51	−	−	κ	−	0.18
	6	1976	100	UK	FK	M	59	−	−	κ	−	0.60
	7	1976	81	W. Germany	KM	F	48	−	+	κ	−	6.30
	8	1976	144	USA	HL	F	69	−	+	κ	−	2.10
	9	1976	140	USA	DH	M	57	−	−	κ	+	0.06
	10	1976	151	Japan	KG	M	54	+	+	κ	+	2.70
	11	1977	119	USA	?	M	69	−	+	κ	−	4.17
	12	1977	38	France	Gui	F	64	−	+	κ	−	2.42
	13	1978	153	Czechoslovakia	?	F	65	−	+	κ	−[c]	5.50
	14	1979	138	Belgium	Des	F	55	−	−	κ	Trace	4.55
	15	1980	39	Italy	GM	F	60	−	+	λ	+	3.80
	16	1981	42A	Japan	?	M	68	−	−	κ	+	3.10
Unusual monoclonal IgE gammopathy	U-1[d]	1976	11	W. Germany	?	F	70	−	−	κ	?	0.026
	U-2[e]	1977	28	USA	?	M	67	Lymphocytic lymphoma	?	κ	−	?
	U-3[f]	1978	128	Japan	?	F	76	−	−	λ	−	?
	U-4[g]	1980	91	Austria	?	F	−71	−	−	λ	−	0.535

[a]Osteosclerosis absent at onset of disease but present after six months of treatment.
[b]In the abstract two cases of IgE myeloma are described, Hea and DB.
[c]Peptides considered to be incomplete Fc fragments and IgE specific Fab fragments were identified in urine.
[d]Questionable IgE myeloma appeared after preceding IgA (κ) myeloma disappeared.
[e]Double paraproteinemia: IgM (κ) with 1.9 to 2.3 g/dl and IgE (κ). Since only one of a few antisera to IgE detected the presence of IgE and no serum IgE concentration was established, it is doubtful whether the case can be considered as IgM-IgE paraproteinemia.
[f]Waldenström's macroglobulinemia (6.7 g/dl) with IgE M component; IgE serum concentration was not determined.
[g]This patient seemed to have a benign monoclonal IgE gammapathy for at least 14 years without turning into rapid malignant proliferation.

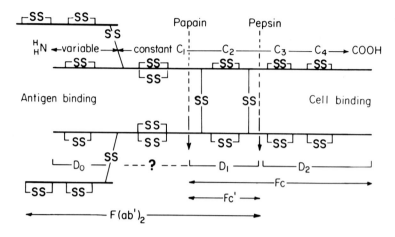

Fig. 1. Diagrammatic representation of IgE molecule. For a detailed description see the text. (From Ishizaka and Ishizaka [61] and Bennich and von Bahr-Lindström [20].)

TABLE II. Physicochemical Properties of IgE

Molecular weight	200,000 daltons
Molecular weight, H chain	75,000 daltons
Molecular weight, L chain	22,500 daltons
Sedimentation coefficient	8.0 S
Electrophoretic mobility	γ_1
Carbohydrate content	12.0%
Rate of synthesis (μg/kg body weight/day)	3.8
Half-life	2.7 days
Synthetic rate	Low
Catabolic rate	High

Some of the data may vary slightly depending on the protein and methods used.

of the H chain. Both determinants are characteristic for the IgE class, but rabbit antiserum to $D_{\epsilon 2}$ seems to have higher affinity for IgE. The $D_{\epsilon 0}$ region contains idiotypic antigenic determinants characteristic for the monoclonal protein. The H chain is composed of 550 amino acid residues, forming four constant and one variable region. Pepsin digestion of the molecule yields an F(ab')$_2$ fragment, which is composed of two L chains and a portion of the H chain that includes the Fd fragment. The H-chain portion of the F(ab')$_2$ fragment includes the $D_{\epsilon 0}$ and $D_{\epsilon 1}$ antigenic determinants. The IgE molecule contains 40 half-cystein residues, 30 in the two H chains and 10 in the L chains. The kinetics of the reduction by 2-mercaptoethanol (2-ME) indicate a rapid cleavage of the H-L-chain disulfide bonds, but the remaining disulfides are reduced at a much slower rate. Complete reduction with 0.1 mol/L 2-ME takes 20 hours, but with 10 mmol/L dithiothreitol the reduction is accomplished in 4 hours.

The sedimentation coefficient is 8.0S; the electrophoretic mobility is γ_1; the carbohydrate content is 12.0%. The rate of synthesis in normal individuals is 3.8 μg/kg body weight/day, and the half-life is 2.7 days. Thus IgE differs from the other Ig in having the lowest synthetic rate and the highest fractional catabolic rate. Total circulating IgE is 4.1 μg/kg body weight, and 41% of the IgE is in the intravascular space [142]. However, in patients with E myeloma the synthetic rate increases, while the functional catabolic rate decreases, resulting in serum IgE concentrations usually measured in mg/mL [142]. The physicochemical properties of IgE antibodies in experimental animals such as the monkey, rabbit, rat, mouse, or the rat IgE myeloma are similar to that described in man. (For more details on physicochemical properties of IgE see [15,16,18,20,41].)

BIOLOGIC PROPERTIES OF IgE

The IgE class is distinct among proteins because of its biologic properties (Table III) and the role it plays in atopic diseases. Its most important biologic properties are the ability to sensitize tissues of homologous species or closely related species (e.g., human IgE sensitizes monkey cells) but not tissues of heterologous species. The target cells to which IgE is bound are basophilic granulocytes and mast cells. The Fc fragment at the carboxyl terminal is responsible for binding, via receptors, with the target cells. The long time needed for passive sensitization of the target cells, i.e. the latent period, is another unique feature of IgE. The molecule requires 24 to 72 hours to combine firmly with the receptors of the target cells [57,59]. The reason for this long period is unclear. Also, the persistence of the IgE fixed to the cell is uniquely long; the average half-life of the passively attached IgE is 13 days [32].

IgE is heat-labile. Heating at 56°C causes irreversible conformational changes [19,66] in the Fc fragment, preventing the molecule from attaching to the target cells. The degree of change depends on the duration of exposure, but heating at 56°C for even 30 minutes causes disfiguration and prevents cellular sensitization. F(ab')$_2$ and Fc' are heat-stable, and heating does not affect the antigen-binding site. Thus heated IgE antibody cannot sensitize a target cell but will react with antigen *in vitro*.

IgE is also susceptible to reducing agents. The degree of molecular change depends on the concentration of the reducing agent and the duration of

TABLE III. Biologic Properties of Human IgE Antibody

Sensitizes cells of homologous species (basophils and mast)	+
Sensitizes cells of heterologous species[a]	−
Latent period	24–72 h
Half-life in passively sensitized skin	13 d
Labile to heat (56°C)	+
Labile to reducing agents	+
Fixes complement	−
Divalent	+
Placenta passing	−

[a]It does sensitize cells of higher monkeys.

exposure. Reduction of the disulfide bonds affects the Fc portion responsible for cell attachment. Circular dichroism studies [19] have shown that the changes caused by reduction are different from those induced by heating. Reduction changes are likely to involve more extensive regions of the molecule than those affected by heating. Molecules subjected to reduction and alkylation will, to various degrees, lose their antigen-binding capacity.

IgE antibody does not fix complement, although aggregated IgE binds complement through the alternative pathway. IgE antibody can agglutinate red blood cells coated with antigen, indicating that the antibodies are at least divalent. IgE is not transmitted across the intact placenta. (For more details see [18,57,72,155].)

GENETIC AND CELLULAR ASPECTS OF IgE PRODUCTION

The factors which determine atopy are not known. Genetic factors seem to play a role, but environmental factors are also important. Not all allergic individuals have elevated serum IgE, and not all nonallergic subjects have normal concentration of IgE [93]. Highly elevated IgE concentrations were found in nonatopic individuals with parasitic infestation [71] or bacterial [52] or fungal [74] infection and in patients with some primary immunodeficiency diseases [30].

Gerrard and associates [47], after examining serum IgE concentrations in 80 families, concluded that the IgE production in man may be under control by two dominant genes. A similar conclusion was reached by Levine and Vaz [86] and Levine [85] on the basis of experiments in mice. These authors found that two genes are involved in control of reaginic antibodies: one (unrelated to the H-2 major histocompatibility complex) controls the production and possibly the concentrations of IgE, while the other (linked to major histocompatibility complex) controls antigen-specific immune responsiveness per se. Marsh et al. [93] speculated, on the basis of their studies of 28 families, that inheritance of high serum IgE could be a Mendelian recessive trait and that there is no linkage between *HLA* haplotype and IgE concentration. From their observation on multiple- and single-allergen hypersensitivity the authors concluded that the gene regulating IgE production may mask the role played by the *Ir* genes linked to a *HLA* haplotype in controlling the expression of a specific IgE antibody response to different allergens and that a genetic factor capable of controlling total IgE production in man may correspond to a factor controlling IgE antibody production in mice.

Early studies of IgE production suggested that this Ig, like IgG and IgA, is T-cell-dependent, requiring the cooperation of T-helper cells. However, the high IgE serum concentrations in patients with absent or impaired T-cell function cast some doubt on the requirement of T-helper cell cooperation in IgE production. Tada and his group [108,134] reported that they could augment IgE antibody production in rats by treatment with antithymocyte serum or various chemical immunosuppressants, by whole-body irradiation, or by adult thymectomy and splenectomy before or immediately after immunization. These workers suggested that the augmentation results from depletion of T-dependent regulatory cells, possibly suppressor T cells, which under normal circumstances terminate the IgE antibody response. Maia et al. [92] and Takatsu and Ishizaka [135] also showed in mice that suppressor T cells are involved in regulation of IgE antibody production. An antigen-specific T-cell-suppressive factor with affinity for carrier determinants was found by Tada and Okumura [134] in rats and characterized as being of low molecular weight ($\leq 60,000$) and specific for IgE antibody response.

Further discussion of the immunoregulatory mechanism of IgE synthetis is beyond the scope of this review, since more explicit descriptions of very complex experiments would have to be described and many links for full understanding of regulation of IgE synthesis are still missing. As a general conclusion it may be stated that IgE synthesis requires T-helper cells for initiation and is under active T-cell-suppressor control. The association of increased IgE serum concentrations in immunodeficiency disorders with thymus-dependent function supports the involvement of the T-cell system in regulation of the IgE biosynthesis (for more details see [56,61,94]).

IgE SERUM CONCENTRATIONS IN HEALTHY PERSONS

The literature on serum IgE concentrations presents confusing data. Prior to the establishment of the WHO IgE standard, concentrations were reported in ng/mL. Difficulties in standardization of IgE were foreseen and discussed at the WHO International Reference Center for Immunoglobulins in Lausanne, Switzerland, in 1968. A research standard (68/341) was made available in 1970 [122] and was estimated by Johansson et al. [72] to contain approximately 10,000 ng/mL. Consequently, nanograms and units were used interchangeably. A few years later it was reported that 1 WHO unit contains 2.42 [13] or 2.35 [152] ng of IgE. It is now accepted that 1 Unit = 2.4 ng. In this review, to facilitate comparison, all values reported in ng have been recalculated and expressed in units (Tables IV–VII).

Another problem contributing to discrepancies on reported IgE concentrations is the diversity of methods used for detection. The practical methods are the radioimmunosorbent test (RIST), the paper radioimmunosorbent test (PRIST), and the double-antibody radioimmunoassay (DARIA). The RIST seems to measure some additional serum protein and therefore gives higher apparent IgE concentrations. The PRIST, because of its simplicity and reliability, is the most frequently used. For sera with very low IgE, the DARIA, being the most sensitive test, is more reliable; but the DARIA is not a simple test, requires many days of incubation, and is primarily a research tool. The varying serum concentrations in atopic patients are another cause of the discrepancies in the literature. IgE may increase for a certain period when the patient is exposed to allergen(s). Since exposure to various allergens is seasonal, the concentrations of IgE may vary seasonally, Patients with multiple allergies have higher IgE than patients sensitive to a single allergen.

An additional factor influencing the discrepancies in reported IgE concentrations is the selection of the groups of individuals examined. Various percentages of the "apparently healthy individuals" used for studies in various countries may be atopic or may have parasitic infections which prevent objective evaluation. Statistical approaches will also affect the interpretation of the reported results. The variations in the unselected populations may also be genetically influenced. Marsh et al. [93], reporting the bimodal distribution for 28 allergic families, had given the cutoff between allergic high-IgE phenotypes and nonallergic normal IgE phenotypes at 95 U/mL. Gerrard et al. [47], in a study of more than 80 unselected families, proposed a cutoff point between allergic and nonallergic individuals as 150 U/mL.

All of these factors help to explain the differences in the reported serum IgE concentrations (Table IV). Although the fetus has the capacity to produce IgE [99], the low values for cord serum indicate that it actually produces very little protein E. The cord serum-IgE results of Johansson [67a], who used the RIST, are higher than those of Bazaral et al. [14], Kjellman et al. [80], or Michel [97]. Although Bazaral and associates also used the RIST, they employed different reagents than Johansson. The values of IgE measured in cord sera by the PRIST are the lowest and most likely the most objective. The serum IgE of selected infants (6 weeks–6 months) in Sweden assayed

TABLE IV. IgE Concentrations in Sera of Cord Blood and Apparently Healthy Individuals

| Individuals | | Method of examination | Units/mL | | References |
Source/age	No.		Range	Mean	
Neonates (cord)	37	RIST	6.7–40.6	15.3	Johansson [67a]
	33	RIST	< 0.1–7.5	2.1	Bazaral et al. [14]
	24	PRIST	< 0.1–1.5	0.2	Kjellman et al. [80]
	136	PRIST	< 0.1–5.5	0.3	Michel et al. [97]
6 wk - infants	17	PRIST	< 0.1–2.8	0.7	Kjellman et al. [80]
6 wk - infants	23	RIST	< 0.1–31.6	5.5	Bazaral et al. [14]
6 mo - infants	17	RIST	2.1–229.0	57.6	Bazaral et al. [14]
6 mo - infants	15	PRIST	0.9–28.0	2.7	Kjellman et al. [80]
1 yr	12	PRIST	1.1–10.2	3.5	Kjellman et al. [80]
4 yr	7	PRIST	2.4–34.8	8.6	Kjellman et al. [80]
10 yr	17	PRIST	0.3–215.0	23.7	Kjellman et al. [80]
14 yr	19	PRIST	1.9–159.0	20.1	Kjellman et al. [80]
Ethiopian children 1–5 yr; negative for *A. lumbricoides*	19	RIST	50.0–2187.5	358.3	Johansson et al. [71]
Ethiopian children 1–5 yr; positive for *A. lumbricoides*	25	RIST	100.0–5958.3	1833.3	Johansson et al. [71]
Swedish children 1–5 yr	23	RIST	20.8–225.0	66.7	Johansson et al. [71]
Healthy adults	125	RIST	27.5–752.5	103.3	Johansson [67a]
	24	RIST	19.4–540.0	148.5	Bazaral et al. [14]
	96	DARIA	0.41–1125.0	74.6	Gleich et al. [49]
	183[a]	SRRD	< 10.0–3687.5	90.8	Arbesman et al. [4]

[a]Random samples from blood bank; atopic individuals not excluded.

TABLE V. Serum IgE Concentrations in Atopic Disease

Disease	Method of examination	No. of sera	Units/mL		Elevated IgE in samples (%)	Comments	References
			Range	Mean			
Seasonal allergic rhinitis/asthma	RIST	28	58–1164	358	54	Children 1–15 yr	Berg and Johansson [21]
	SRRD	74	17–1461	209	58	Six children, 68 adults	Arbesman et al. [4]
Extrinsic bronchial asthma	RIST	16	51–1680	662	63	Adults, mean age 35 yr	Johansson [67]
Atopic dermatitis	RIST	13	40–1667	509	77	Children, 5–12 yr	Berg and Johansson [21]
	SRRD	23	17–4948	1065	78	Three patients were under 12 yr	Arbesman et al. [4]
Bronchopulmonary aspergillosis	DARIA	14	2500–30,000	14,160	100		Patterson et al. [111]
	SRRD	21	620–10,000	4880	100		Arbesman et al. [6]
Penicillin allergy	RIST	45	50–2800	568	NA	Values within 30 days after allergic reaction	Kraft et al. [82]
Penicillin allergy	RIST	38	< 1–12,083	561	24		Assem and Vickers [8]
Penicillin with other drug allergy	RIST	7	106–4167	982	43	Other drugs: aspirin, tetracycline cephaloridine, and others	Assem and Vickers [8]
Single allergy to various drugs	RIST	7	10–972	570	42	Single allergy to aspirin, griseofulvin, iodinated radio-contrast	Assem and Vickers [8]
Antituberculous drugs allergy	RIST	6	50–1333	611	66	Streptomycin, rifampicin para-aminosalicyclic acid, Isoniazid and others	Assem and Vickers [8]

TABLE VI. Serum IgE Concentrations in Nonatopic Diseases

Disease	Method of examination	No. of sera	Units/mL Range	Units/mL Mean	Elevated IgE in samples (%)	Comments	References
Infections with various microorganisms	RIST SRRD	Elevated IgE was observed in infections with various microorganisms.					See [5,12,25,52,55, 71,73,74,95, 111,120,127]
Infectious mononucleosis	RIST	24	13–1063	218	33	The levels are of 7–10 days after onset	Nordbring et al. [104]
Bullous pemphigoid	SRRD	39	40–10,000	2114	84		Arbesman et al. [5]
Hodgkin's disease	SRRD	31	20–6500	488	53	8 patients with elevated levels had personal or family history of atopy	Arbesman et al. [5]
Interstitial nephritis	RIST	5	217–1167	678	100	Drug-induced nephritis	Ooi et al. [109]

TABLE VII. Serum IgE Concentrations in Immunologic Disorders

Disease	Method of examination	No. of sera	Units/mL Range	Units/mL Mean	Elevated IgE in samples (%)	Comments	References
Wiscott-Aldrich	RIST	4	304–2542	1057	75		Berglund et al. [23]
	DARIA	4	135–720	381	100		Buckley and Fiscus [30]
Extreme hyperimmunoglobulinemia E	DARIA	20	2150–50,200	20,275	100		Buckley and Becker [31]
Selective IgA deficiency	DARIA	74	3–51,200	124	NA		Buckley and Fiscus [30]
Severe combined immunodeficiency	DARIA	9	1–82	2		Significantly low	Buckley and Fiscus [30]
X-linked agammaglobulinemia	DARIA	10	1–5	2		Significantly low	Buckley and Fiscus [30]
Non-X-linked agammaglobulinemia	DARIA	15	1–10	3		Significantly low	Buckley and Fiscus [30]
X-linked immunodeficiency with hyper IgM	DARIA	3	1–2	1		Significantly low	Buckley and Fiscus [30]
Ataxia telangiectasia	DARIA	7	1–54	7		Significantly low	Buckley and Fiscus [30]
Transient hypogammaglobulinemia	DARIA	8	2–31	6		Significantly low	Buckley and Fiscus [30]

by the PRIST was lower in range and geometric mean than that of a comparable group of infants in the United States assayed by RIST [14]. This difference probably reflects the different sensitivities of the methods.

IgE concentrations increase with age, and 10-year-old children have IgE concentrations as high as those of adults or even higher [80]. Higher IgE serum concentrations in children and teenagers (6–15 years old) have often been reported [48,53,149]. IgE serum concentrations in Ethiopian children, even in the group where parasitic infection by *Ascaris lumbricoides* could be excluded, were much higher than in comparable groups of Swedish children [71]. The Ethiopian children free of *A. lumbricoides* might still have been infested with other parasites which may produce the elevated serum IgE. In an apparently healthy adult population the ranges and means also differed depending on the method used.

Grundbacher [53] used the RIST to examine sera from 172 blacks and 154 whites (USA) aged 5–69 years and observed higher mean IgE concentrations in blacks (539.1 U/mL) than whites (243.9 U/mL). Gerrard et al. [48] found differences between Canadian white and Metis populations. The authors examined by the RIST 819 whites from 1 to 70 years old and 275 Metis from 1 to 61 years old. The geometric means were: whites, 81.3 U/mL; Metis, 275.5 U/mL. Wittig et al. [149], using the PRIST, measured IgE serum concentrations in an apparently healthy population (USA) aged 1–40 years and found a geometric mean of 32 U/mL.

These ethnic, age, and technical differences make it quite difficult to establish normal serum IgE values. Wittig et al. [149] suggest that in the USA PRIST geometric means of 64 U/mL for infants, 150 U/mL for school children, and 120 U/mL for older age groups appear to be the most acceptable.

IgE IN SECRETIONS AND TISSUES

Protein E has been detected in bronchial and nasal washings, urine, and colostrum. An estimated 90% of the IgE in these fluids is locally produced. The absolute concentrations of IgE are, however, very low except in colostrum [72]. In bronchial and nasal washings of patients subjected to bronchoscopy the concentrations vary between 0.04 and 4.2 U/mL [72]. Ishizaka and Newcomb [62] using the less sensitive radioimmunodiffusion method were able to detect IgE in nasal washings and sputum in only 30–50% of asthmatic children. The concentrations (264.0–1296 U/mL) were, however, higher than those reported by Johansson [72]. Tse et al. [137], using the SRRD test, detected IgE antibodies in nasal washings but not in parotid saliva in only approximately 15% of adult patients allergic to ragweed. When nasal mucosa is stimulated locally by histamine in healthy individuals or by specific allergens in allergic patients, the concentrations of IgE and other immunoglobulins and albumin in the nasal washings increase, suggesting an increased passage of serum proteins [72].

The absolute concentration of intact IgE in urine of healthy individuals, as determined by the RIST, does not exceed 5 U/mL [132]. However, IgE-specific peptides were found in a patient with IgE myeloma [153]. Vladutiu et al. [140] described a case of low-level monoclonal IgE globinopathy with renal failure; 0.6 mg/mL IgE was detected in the serum as well as in the urine.

In colostrum, IgE concentrations are rather high [18]. During the first 24 hours of lactation a decrease of IgE similar to that of IgA may be observed. IgE isolated from colostrum [18] and respiratory fluid [102] has physico-chemical properties similar to those of serum IgE; hence no secretory piece could be demonstrated in colostrum IgE. Brown and Lee [27] found 40,000-dalton IgE fragments in intestinal fluid and concluded that trypsin and chymotrypsin may degrade IgE secreted into the intestinal lumen. The fragments were probably the $D_{\epsilon 1}$ antigenic determinants.

The distribution of IgE-producing cells has been examined in man and monkey [133,145]. Most are in the tonsils, gastrointestinal tract, and lymph nodes.

IgE CONCENTRATIONS IN VARIOUS DISEASES
Atopic Diseases

Elevated IgE (Table V) has been found in approximately 50% of patients suffering from allergic rhinitis with complicating asthma [21]. A higher incidence was found in patients with extrinsic bronchial asthma [67,72]. Patients with atopic dermatitis frequently have high serum IgE [75,107,150]. Patients with acute urticaria have significantly elevated serum IgE, but because the acute stage is so brief, a survey of these patients may not reveal a high incidence of elevated IgE. Patients with bronchopulmonary allergic aspergillosis—but not those with aspergilloma, hypersensitivity pneumonitis, or chronic bronchitis and/or bronchiectases—have significantly elevated IgE [6,111].

Patients with acute reactions to various drugs, especially penicillin, have elevated IgE. However, as in patients with acute urticaria, the elevated concentrations persist only a few weeks after the reaction [8,82]. Patients with eosinophilia and no evidence of allergies or parasitic infestations may also have highly elevated serum IgE [4]. In most instances IgE concentrations correlate with the severity of clinical symptoms, but individual variations are too great to allow for prediction of individual cases. A significant correlation was found between high IgE concentrations during the first year of life in children with or without allergy and the appearance of atopic allergy during childhood [79]. Therefore determination of serum IgE by a reliable test may predict future allergic manifestations, especially in children of atopic parents.

Nonatopic Diseases

Elevated serum IgE is also found in a variety of nonatopic diseases (Table VI). A number of parasites, such as *A. lumbricoides* [71], *Toxocara canis* [55], *Capillaris philippinensis* [120], and *Nippostrongylus brasiliensis* [73], cause increased IgE production. Other parasitic infestations associated with elevated serum IgE have also been reported [12]. The mechanism by which the parasites lead to increased IgE production is uncertain, nor is it known why the elevated IgE usually is not specific for the parasites. Elevated IgE has also been reported in infections with *Treponema pallidum, Neisseria gonorrhoeae* and *Trichomonas vaginalis* [52], *Staphylococcus aureus* [127], and *Candida albicans* [95] and in certain mycoses [25,74]. High serum IgE was reported [5] in leprosy, but since parasitic infestation could not be excluded, this information awaits confirmation. Serum IgE was high in some patients with chronic bacterial infections, but whether the elevated IgE was due to infection or vice versa is difficult to say. Buckley et al. [29,154] observed that patients with hyper-IgE syndrome experienced severe chronic infections of the skin and lower respiratory tract associated with *S. aureus, Hemophilus influenzae,* group A streptococci, and other microorganisms. In some viral infections IgE serum concentrations are below normal levels [114].

Some patients with infectious mononucleosis have elevated serum IgE [104], but since other serum immunoglobulins were also high and the concentrations decreased rapidly after the onset of the disease, the elevation of IgE must be interpreted as part of a general immune response. Patients with bullous pemphigoid—but not those with pemphigus—have high serum IgE [5,25]. In pemphigoid the basement membrane of the skin is implicated, whereas in the pemphigus, the intracellular substances of the epidermis are responsible. Whether the disease affects mast cells, causing release of IgE, is not known.

Elevated serum IgE has been found in Hodgkin's disease [5,84,123,136,141], but as Landaas et al. [84] demonstrated, the serum IgE contains both κ- and λ-L chains, and patients with elevated IgE also have increased concentrations of other immunoglobulin classes. The authors conclude that increased serum IgE in Hodgkin's disease, where an atopic stage can be excluded, may reflect at least in some patients a more general defect in the regulatory T-cell function. This is supported by the correlation between serum IgE concentration and impaired cell-mediated immunity observed in Hodgkin's disease [123].

Elevated serum IgE was also observed in nephritis [109], probably drug-induced; in patients with chronic acral dermatitis without personal or family history of atopy [148]; and in some other diseases. (For review see [31,69,72,155].)

Immunodeficiency Diseases

Studies during the 1970s provided information on the augmentation of IgE biosynthesis in a number of immunodeficiency diseases (Table VII), where the IgE serum concentrations were associated with the T-cell system [46]. Elevated IgE was found in patients with Wiskott-Aldrich syndrome [23], thymic alymphoplasia (Nezelof syndrome) [78], and selective IgA deficiency [30]. In contrast, IgE serum concentrations were significantly lower in patients with a generalized defect of Ig synthesis [117]. (For review see [31,116,154].)

SIGNIFICANCE OF SERUM IgE ANTIBODIES

Present-day knowledge allows us to consider the IgE antibody as unique in function and purpose, both cell-bound and present in body fluids, and primarily involved in atopic diseases. IgE antibody can be detected by a variety of sensitive tests, whether fixed to target cells or in circulation. These tests help to establish the clinical diagnosis of allergic disease, define the allergen(s) responsible for the clinical symptoms, and measure the antibody concentrations produced in response to allergen(s) in the environment or to specific immunotherapy.

IgE antibody to inhalant allergens can rarely be detected in serum from nonatopic individuals [22,44]. Patients manifesting symptoms of immediate hypersensitivity to such allergens as grasses, weeds, trees, foods, molds, house dusts, drugs, or stinging insects have various concentrations of IgE antibodies in sera and occasionally in secretions. The concentrations fluctuate considerably depending on the exposure. Higher IgE antibody concentrations may be observed during season than out of season, and antibody concentrations during immunotherapy may increase in some individuals while decreasing in others. Similar situations may occur in nasal secretions [137,152]. IgE antibodies to various microorganisms have been reported [12,24,25,55,73,95,111,120,127], but the role of the antibodies in the infection process remains to be clarified.

Measurement of IgE-specific antibodies is used widely in the diagnosis of allergic diseases. Although its usefulness varies, it is sometimes invaluable—for example, to diagnose respiratory allergies in adults and children, to identify the causative allergen among a large number of potential offenders,

to monitor individuals allergic to venom or other substances of the hymenoptera for drug hypersensitivity, and to evaluate the results of immunotherapy. Measurement of IgE and IgG antibodies can provide important
information on an individual's state of protection to avoid an anaphylactic
response to an allergen.

METHODS OF IgE ANTIBODY DETECTION
Detection of Cell-Bound Antibodies

Long before it was known that immediate hypersensitivity is due to IgE
antibody and that an allergic reaction is based on cell-bound antibody-allergen
interaction, a state of allergy could be determined by various biologic methods.

Skin tests
Intradermal test. Injection of a properly diluted allergenic extract into the
forearm of a sensitive individual will cause, within minutes, erythema and
induration (Fig. 2). The same extract injected into nonallergic individuals
should not elicit any reaction. The principle of the skin test is that the reaction
between the injected allergenic extract and the mast cell-bound IgE antibody
releases histamine (and possibly other mediators), causing erythema alone
(mild reaction) or with induration.

The test is done by injecting intradermally in the volar surface of the
lower or upper arm 0.02 to 0.05 mL of a properly diluted allergenic extract.
The reaction is examined within 15 minutes. The mean diameters of the
erythema and induration are expressed in mm and, for convenience, graded
as ± to 4+. A change in sensitivity can be established by using an endpoint dilution of an allergen to which the patient is sensitive. The highest
dilution of an allergen giving a 1+ to 2+ reaction is considered the endpoint. It is important not to use high concentrations of extracts because
systemic reaction may occur. (For more details see [105,125].)

Prick test. The principle of the prick test is the same as that of the intradermal test, but the technique is slightly different. A single drop of properly
diluted allergenic solution is placed on the skin, and a 26-gauge needle is
passed through the drop and inserted into the skin, which is slightly lifted.
The remaining solution is gently wiped off. The diameters of reaction are
measured in mm, but the grading is slightly different from the intradermal
test, since the erythema and induration are less pronounced. Higher concentrations of the allergenic extracts are used for the prick tests. (For more
details see [105].)

Skin window. An allergic reaction can also be determined by gently abrad-
ing a small area of skin on the arm and applying the allergenic extract to it.

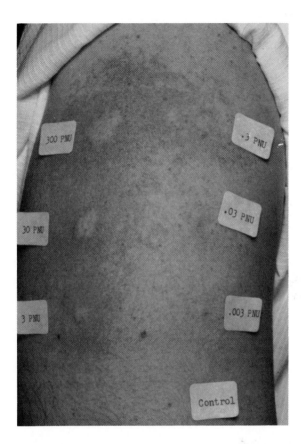

Fig. 2   Skin test. Various dilutions of an extract (here ragweed extract) injected intradermally into a patient's arm will produce induration and erythema. The reaction is graded from ± (5–10 mm of erythema and induration) to 4 + (≥ 15 mm of induration and ≥ 40 mm erythema). The lowest concentration of an allergen required for 1 + to 2 + reaction is considered the endpoint.

The test site is covered with a glass or plastic coverslip which is taped for 12–24 hours. The coverslip is then removed and stained for cells. With an allergic reaction many eosinophils are found on the slide. Skin-window results correlate with those of other *in vivo* methods measuring immediate hypersensitivity. It may also be used to study cell migration in a variety of allergic-type reactions. The technique is a research tool, with no applicability in daily diagnostic practice [42].

Inhalation and challenge methods. The inability of skin-testing to provide clear-cut results, especially for individuals with borderline susceptibility, has led to the use of allergenic-extract aerosols as inhalants. Inhalation challenge is a much more reliable index of clinically significant allergies than any other test, but it is more cumbersome and requires equipment to measure pulmonary function (forced expiratory volume). It is usually performed by specialized allergologists on patients with asthma. Nasal and conjunctival challenge were in the past done quite frequently. In particular, conjunctival testing was very popular many years ago, prior to the widespread use of skin testing. These days, even for research purposes, these tests are used infrequently. (For more details see [34,105].)

Leukocyte histamine release. An *in vitro* test to assess immediate hypersensitivity is performed by measuring histamine release (HR) from peripheral blood or other tissues [90]. The principle of the HR test is that the interaction of an allergenic extract with IgE antibodies bound to basophils in peripheral blood releases histamine from the cells. This release can be measured by bioassay with a contracting smooth muscle, such as guinea pig uterus or ileum [126], by spectrofluorometry [90], or by a radioenzyme method [88]. Results are expressed as the percent of total HR. The results of HR tests on peripheral blood leukocytes from patients with ragweed or grass allergy correlate well with the results of the prick test and the radioallergosorbent (RAST) test (described below). The correlation is less satisfactory for patients with borderline allergies, who may be positive in skin tests but negative in HR and RAST. (For more details see [50].)

Detection of Circulating Antibodies

Biologic methods

Passive transfer test with human skin. The P-K test [118], once the only available method for detection of serum reagenic antibodies, is nowadays rarely used for diagnostic purposes because of the hazard of transmission of hepatitis virus. The principle of this test is that the interaction of the mast cell, passively sensitized by the IgE antibody, and the injected allergen releases histamine (and possibly other mediators) from the mast cells. This increases vascular permeability and causes localized edema.

The passive transfer test is done by injecting a nonatopic recipient intradermally with 0.05–0.1 mL of sterile, hepatitis-virus-free fresh patient's serum. (The serum is usually diluted threefold or higher to reach the endpoint reaction). The sites of injection must be well marked so that antigen in a proper concentration and volume (0.02–0.05 mL) can be injected in the same place 24–48 hours later. The wheal and erythema reaction (similar to that seen in Fig. 2) may be observed within 15–20 minutes; it is measured and interpreted as in the skin test. The minimum concentration of IgE antibodies required for a positive P-K reaction is on the order of 4×10^{-5} µg/N/mL [64]. The reproducibility of the P-K test depends on the IgE antibody concentration, the activity of the allergen used for challenge, and—most important—on the recipient's susceptibility, which varies greatly.

Passive transfer test with monkey skin. The human IgE antibody sensitizes skin mast cells, not only in man, but also in nonhuman primates. The passive cutaneous anaphylaxis (PCA) test is based on the same principles as the P-K test, but the technique is slightly different. The monkey is injected intradermally with 0.05-mL portions of the patient's serum at various dilutions. After 24 hours (latent period) a properly diluted allergenic extract mixed with a dye (most frequently 0.5–1% Evans blue) is injected intravenously into the monkey. Approximately 1 mL of the antigen-dye mixture/kg body weight is used. Within 15–20 minutes of antigen injection the sensitized skin shows a blue spot marking the zone of the reaction (Fig. 3). Its diameter is measured. The degree of reaction varies, depending on the concentrations of IgE antibody and allergen. The blue discoloration disappears, usually within a few days. All the higher primates (*Macaca mulatta,* African green monkey, cynomologous monkey) demonstrate skin sensitization, but the primitive-primate-like insectivore known as tree shrew fails to accept human IgE antibody.

The PCA is less sensitive than the P-K test. The minimum concentration of IgE antibody needed for a positive PCA test is 10^{-3} µg/N/mL (64). In addition, not all monkeys accept human reagenic antibodies to the same degree, and a very small percentage of human IgE antibodies cannot fix to monkey skin. The reason for this inability is not clear. The PCA test was once popular, but today it has very little if any application because of its low sensitivity and the high cost of monkeys. However, it remains a very good research tool and can be used successfully to measure reagenic antibodies in various laboratory animals by using homologous recipients' skin for passive sensitization.

An outmoded test with no present diagnostic applicability is the Schultz-Dale (S-D) test which is based on interaction of actively or passively sensitized smooth muscle (uterus, ileum or others) with reagenic antibody. Challenge with a proper allergen releases histamine, causing contraction of the smooth muscle, which is measured with a polygraph (For details see [3].)

Radioimmunoassays. Almost simultaneously with the detection of IgE as the carrier of reagenic antibody (1966) and the first myeloma IgE (1967), Wide et al. [147] reported the development of a test based on principles of the classic antiglobulin method. They called the new technique the radioallergosorbent test (RAST).

The principle of the RAST (Fig. 4) is a reaction between the allergenic extract covalently coupled to a solid phase [10], such as Sepharose or a filter-

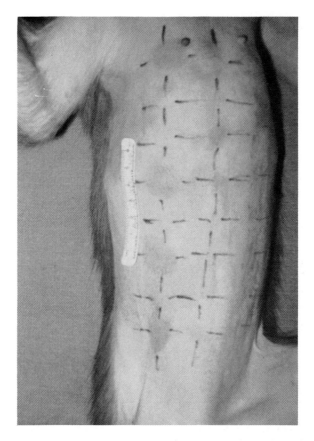

Fig. 3. Passive cutaneous anaphylaxis (PCA) test in monkey skin. In the marked area of the skin various dilutions of patient serum are injected intradermally, and 24 hours later a proper allergenic extract mixed with Evans blue is injected intravenously. Blue spots, appearing 20–30 minutes after injection, indicate a positive reaction. The reaginic antibody titer is expressed as the reciprocal of the last serum dilution giving an intense blue at least 5 mm in diameter.

paper disc, and IgE antibody in the test serum. The amount of IgE antibody bound is detected by reacting radiolabeled anti-human-IgE antiserum with the allergen-bound IgE antibody and measuring the radioactivity in a γ-counter. The more radioactivity is bound, the higher the IgE antibody concentration in the sample. The count-rate of the sample is compared directly with the count-rate of a reference material, which should have an estimated IgE antibody level. The result is expressed as a percent of binding compared to the reference sample or in arbitrary units or scores. Detailed technical information is given in each commercial kit.

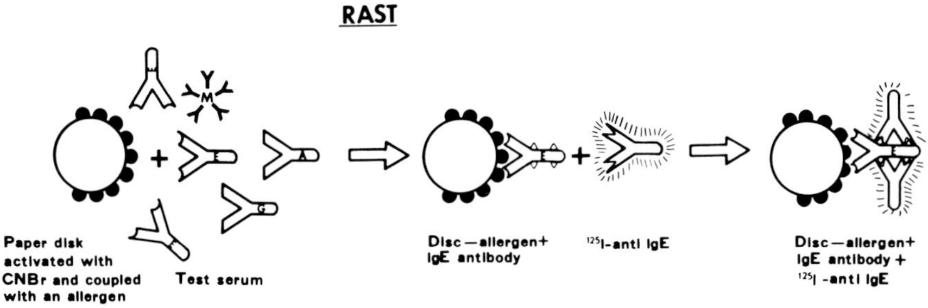

RAST

Fig. 4. Principle of the radioallergosorbent test (RAST). Covalently coupled allergen (●) on the surface of the cellulose carrier reacts with IgE antibody (E). Molecules labeled G, A, and M indicate serum immunoglobulins. The allergen-reacting IgE antibody is detected by radiolabeled anti-IgE.

Since a serum may also contain antibodies of other immunoglobulin classes reacting with the allergen on the carrier, will such antibodies react with the surface bound antigen and interfere in the IgE antibody-antigen interaction? IgG antibodies, if present in high concentration, may do so to some degree [139]. This IgG blocking effect may be lessened in the RAST by using a filter-paper disc rather than Sepharose [45]. Preferential interaction of serum IgE antibodies with the cellulose-bound allergen may also be explained by the fact that approximately 20% of the IgE has specific antibody activity, compared to approximately 5% in the IgG class.

The RAST has been widely used to detect serum IgE antibodies to such allergens as pollens, grasses, trees, weeds, various animal danders, house dust, mites, molds, foods, venom of stinging insects, and some drugs.

In the last decade the RAST has been the most challenged test in laboratory diagnosis of allergic diseases. In comparative studies with *in vivo* and *in vitro* tests the results varied, depending on the allergens and on whether the same quality of allergen was used in both the RAST and the challenging tests. Generally the RAST compared favorably with the P-K test and the leukocyte HR test. However, it was less sensitive than skin test or bronchial challenge.

The RAST offers some definite advantages over the remaining available tests, especially the skin test: 1) It is preferable in certain groups, such as infants, patients with widespread dermatosis, and patients with dermographism; 2) there is no risk to the patient, especially in drug allergy; 3) the results are not influenced by drugs a patient may be taking; 4) The changes in the antibody concentrations can be better monitored when expressed quantitatively; and 5) One serum sample can be tested for a variety of allergens and quantitated for IgE antibody to specific allergen or allergens in multiple allergy.

There are also some disadvantages: 1) The results are not available as fast as with the skin test; 2) in some instances the RAST may give erroneous results; and 3) because it requires expensive equipment and the know-how to handle radioactive reagents, the test is limited to certain institutions. (For reviews see [1,2].)

A successful modification, the mini-RAST, has been reported by Gleich and associates [51], who achieved greater sensitivity by reducing the solid-phase support for allergen and anti-IgE. The near future will most likely see practical application of another modification, replacing the radioactive reagent with an enzymatic marker [143].

The RAST, in addition to measuring serum IgE antibodies, can be utilized to measure the potency of allergy extracts. At present no adequate method is available to standardize the potency of the large number of extracts used for treatment and tests. Current standardization of allergens expresses the protein nitrogen content or the weight/volume ratio but not the biologic potency of the extract.

METHODS OF MEASURING TOTAL IgE

The very low concentration of IgE in normal serum renders it difficult to detect by the single radial diffusion (RID) method widely applied to other Igs. Modifications of the RID have been developed to measure ng of serum IgE. Rowe's [121] two-antibody technique can detect approximately 100 U (40 ng) of IgE/mL, and Arbesman et al.'s [4] simplified one-step radial radioimmunodiffusion test can detect approximately 50 U (20 ng) of IgE/mL.

Radioimmunosorbent Test

Johansson et al. [70] applied the radioimmunosorbent technique of Wide and Porath [146] to develop the RIST. Its principle (Fig. 5) is competitive binding of unlabeled and labeled IgE to a class-specific antibody to human IgE, covalently bound to Sephadex particles. The IgE concentration in the sample is determined by its capacity to inhibit the binding of labeled IgE, added to the sample at a constant concentration, to the insolubilized anti-IgE. This inhibition is compared with the inhibition produced by IgE standards in serial concentrations. During the incubation labeled IgE and the IgE in the standard or sample compete for the anti-IgE binding sites on the immunosorbent. The bound IgE is separated from the unbound by centrifugation. The sedimented particles are washed, and the radioactive IgE bound to the anti-IgE is examined in a γ-counter. A standard curve is prepared with dilutions of the reference serum, and the sample IgE concentration is determined by extrapolation. When a very small amount of unlabeled IgE is present

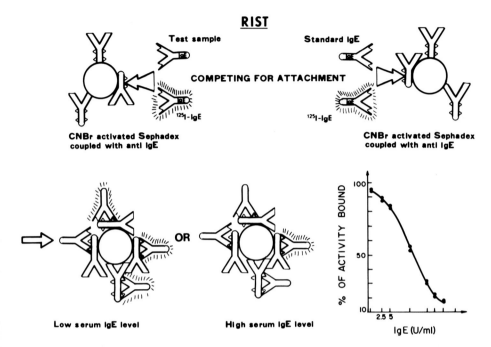

Fig. 5. Principle of the radioimmunosorbent test (RIST). Monospecific antibodies to IgE bound to the cellulose carrier react with IgE in the test or standard serum and/or with radiolabeled IgE added in a constant amount. Both labeled and unlabeled IgE compete for the anti-IgE. When the test or standard serum contains a low concentration of IgE, more labeled IgE will react with the cellulose-bound anti-IgE, and vice versa.

in the sample, a high percentage of the labeled IgE will be bound, and vice versa.

This procedure can determine IgE levels from 10 to 4000 U/mL.

Paper Disc Radioimmunosorbent Test

The RIST has been replaced [33] by a noncompetitive binding radioimmunoassay, the PRIST (Fig. 6). Monospecific antibody to human IgE is coupled to paper discs previously activated with cyanogen bromide. The serum to be tested and various dilutions of a reference serum are incubated with the discs. After exhaustive washings the discs are incubated with ^{125}I-labeled monospecific antiserum to IgE. The discs are washed again and examined in a γ-counter; the radioactive counts increase with the amount of IgE on the disc. The concentration in the sample is interpreted from a standard curve, which covers a wide range (1.0–10.000 U/mL). The PRIST is simpler

PRIST

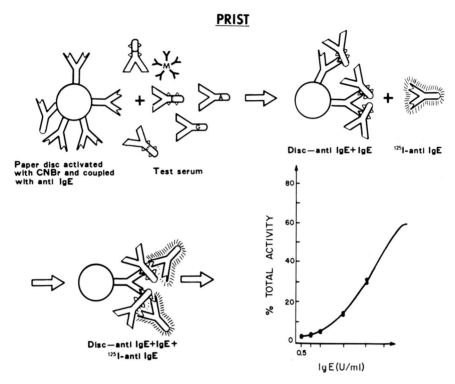

Paper disc activated
with CNBr and coupled
with anti IgE

Test serum

Disc—anti IgE+IgE

^{125}I-anti IgE

Disc—anti IgE+IgE+
^{125}I-anti IgE

% TOTAL ACTIVITY

IgE (U/ml)

Fig. 6. Principle of the paper disc radioimmunosorbent test (PRIST). Monospecific antibodies to IgE bound to the paper disc react with the serum IgE (E). Molecules labeled G, A, and M indicate serum immunoglobulins. The presence of IgE is detected by radiolabeled anti-IgE. The higher the IgE concentration in the standard or test sample, the more radioactive anti-IgE molecules are bound, and the higher the radioactive count.

to perform and more sensitive than the RIST. It is available commercially and is currently the most popular test.

Double-Antibody Radioimmunoassay

Although the RIST and PRIST satisfy the laboratory diagnostic need for determination of IgE in most sera, the DARIA of Morgan and Lazarow [101], applied by Gleich et al. [49] for IgE, is the most sensitive tool for detecting very low concentrations. Its principle (Fig. 7) is as follows: At the first step the test serum or IgE standard is mixed with highly diluted (1:50,000) rabbit anti-IgE, and a predetermined concentration of radiolabeled IgE is added. This mixture is incubated for 1 to 4 days. During that time the labeled and unlabeled IgE compete for the rabbit anti-IgE. At the second step goat

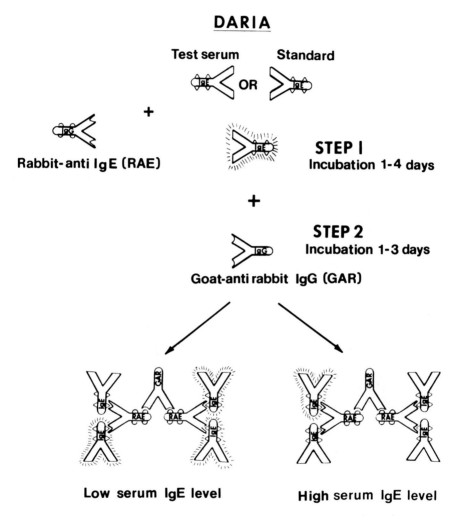

Fig. 7. Principle of the double-antibody radioimmunoassay (DARIA). During the first incubation period, IgE in the test sample or standard competes with a constant amount of radiolabeled IgE for rabbit antibody (IgG fraction) to IgE. In the second incubation period goat antibody (IgG fraction) to rabbit IgG reacts with the rabbit anti-IgE carrying labeled or unlabeled IgE. The radioactive count will be higher in sera with low IgE levels, and vice versa.

anti-rabbit γ globulin is reacted for 1 to 3 days with the rabbit anti-IgE carrying the human IgE. After washing down and centrifugation of the precipitate, the latter is measured for radioactivity in a γ-counter. The amount of the labeled IgE bound is inversely proportional to the concentration of IgE in the test serum. A standard curve is prepared for each test, and sample IgE concentrations are determined from it. The test as described can detect 0.4 U of IgE/mL. If the rabbit antiserum to human IgE is diluted further, e.g. 1:500,000 instead of 1:50,000, and the incubation time properly extended, the sensitivity can be increased. Buckley and Becker [31] were able to detect 50 pg of IgE/mL.

Other tests measuring IgE have also been developed [54,124]. The enzyme immunoassay for IgE [54] was neglected for almost a decade, but in an improved form is commercially available for measuring IgE and/or specific IgE antibodies. The sensitivity of the nonradioimmunoassay is similar to that which applies to radiolabelled reagents.

Monoclonal antibodies opened a new avenue in laboratory medicine. The antibodies can be accurately characterized, allowing selection of antibodies to the most specific part of an antigen molecule. A commercial RIA kit utilizing monoclonal antibodies for detection of IgE is available (interested readers may find details of product and commercial companies producing the kits in most professional journal advertisements).

MECHANISM OF ANAPHYLACTIC REACTION

One major property of IgE is to fix to target cells, the mast cell (Fig. 8) and the basophilic granulocyte (Fig. 9). Both cells possess receptors for IgE and contain granules which store pharmacologically active mediators, but the cells differ in distribution. In humans mast cells are found in subcutaneous and submucous tissues, while basophilic granulocytes are found in the blood (approximately 0.5%). In man the basophils also contain larger granules than the mast cells. The target cells in various species may contain different pharmacologically active mediators. Human mast cells and basophils contain histamine but no serotonin, whereas rat mast cells contain large amount of serotonin and less histamine.

The biologic function of the target cells, relevant to allergic reaction, is to release pharmacologically active mediators. Human target cells can synthesize and release histamine, slow reactive substance of anaphylaxis (SRS-A), eosinophilic chemotactic factor of anaphylaxis (ECF-A), platelet-activating factor (PAF), and basophilic kallikrein of anaphylaxis (BK-A), which generates kininlike peptides from serum kininogen [9,56,60,115].

The surfaces of both basophils and mast cells of a nonallergic individual contain receptors for IgE, plus IgE with no identified antibody specificity;

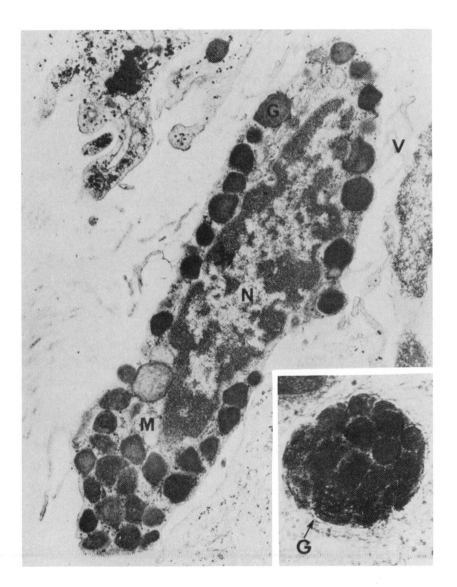

Fig. 8.   Electronmicrograph of human skin mast cell showing mitochondrion (M), nucleus (N), granules (G) and villi (V). *Insert:* Enlargement of a granule from a human bronchiolar mast cell. (From Orr [110b].)

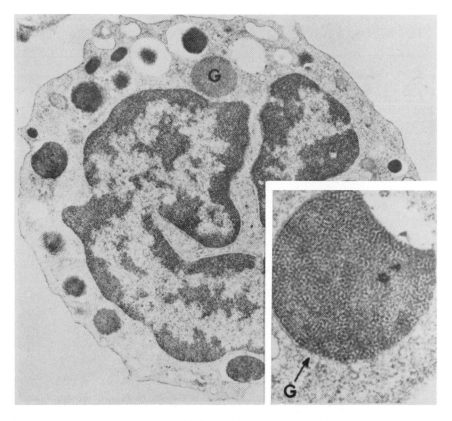

Fig. 9. Electronmicrograph of basophil from peripheral human blood showing granules (G). *Insert:* Enlargement of a granule showing inner ultrastructure. (From Parwaresch [110c].)

while the cells of an allergic individual will in addition have IgE antibodies with specificity for certain allergen(s) (Fig. 10). The receptors are present in approximately the same number on cells of allergic or nonallergic individuals. Human basophils are estimated to have from 4×10^4 to 9×10^4 receptors [65]. The IgE in allergic as well as in nonallergic individuals' target cells are bound by means of IgE receptors. The number of IgE molecules on human basophils was estimated to average between 1×10^4 to 4×10^4, indicating that not all receptors are occupied by IgE molecules [65]. Binding of IgE by cell receptors is reversible, and the number of cell-bound IgE does not parallel the concentration of serum IgE [65]. Rat basophilic leukemia cells contain 10^6 IgE-receptors/cell [83], and normal rat peritoneal mast cells contain 3×10^5 receptors/cell [35]; but since the rat mast cell surface is two

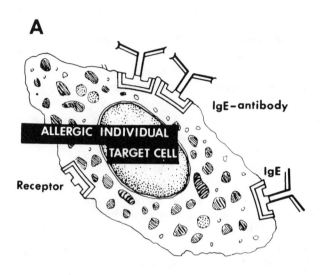

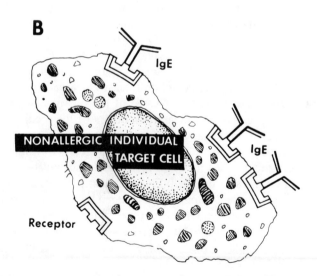

Fig. 10.   Diagrammatic representation of mast cell surface from allergic (A) and nonallergic (B) individuals. The mast cells of an allergic individual contain IgE antibody with specificity to certain (known) allergen(s), IgE without known antigen specificity, and unoccupied receptors. The mast cells of a nonallergic individual are similar except that they do not contain IgE antibody to certain (known) allergen(s).

to three times larger than that of the human basophil, the density of receptors per unit area may be the same in both rat mast cells and human basophilic granulocytes.

Investigators disagree about the molecular size of the target-cell receptors. Depending on the method employed the molecular-weight estimates vary from 62,000 to 260,000 [36,96]. It has been suggested [103] that the receptor molecule is composed of subunits of 45,000 daltons each, that only a small portion of a receptor molecule is exposed on the cell surface, and that a single IgE molecule can completely cover the receptor area. Tentative information indicates that the IgE receptor is a glycoprotein, but further studies and more detailed characterization of the receptors are needed.

Experimental evidence obtained thus far suggests that in biological conditions interaction between an allergen and the cell-bound IgE antibody triggers a complex event known as the allergic or immediate hypersensitivity reaction. The bridging hypothesis postulated by Ishizaka and Ishizaka [60] and Ishizaka et al. [58] explains to some degree the mechanism of an anaphylactic reaction. The IgE antibody is anchored to the target-cell receptor by the Fc fragment, leaving the antigen-combining sites free. To initiate a reaction a divalent antigen must bridge the cell-bound IgE antibodies (Fig. 11B). Univalent allergens are incapable of eliciting a reaction (Fig. 11A). Complexes of three cell-bound antibodies with two antigen molecules are the most effective in releasing pharmacologically active mediators. Since direct bridging of receptors by antibodies to receptors (Fig. 11C) will cause histamine release [58], it can be assumed that the IgE antibody-antigen interaction involves participation of the receptors through the bound antibodies. The antibody-antigen interaction releases a cascade of not well documented biochemical reactions until some of the pharmacologic mediators stored in the cell granules are released or others of the mediators are synthesized and released immediately.

Target-cell mediator release can also be triggered by numerous other stimuli, including antibodies to IgE (Fig. 11D); concanavalin A, which interacts with carbohydrates on the IgE molecules; polymerized IgG, which binds to different receptors; calcium flux induced by an ionophore (A23187); aspirin, morphine, polymyxin B, and other drugs; physical stress, as in exercise-induced asthma; anaphylatoxin (C_3a and C_5a); and antiserum against peritoneal rat mast cells in the presence of complement, but not without complement. (For review see [89,115].)

The biochemical events occurring during HR are rather complex. In general terms HR is modulated by cyclic adenosine monophosphate (cAMP); thus, any agent or reaction which raises the intracellular concentration of cAMP inhibits HR. Histamine release proceeds through two-stage reaction and only the first stage is affected by cAMP. The secretion in the second

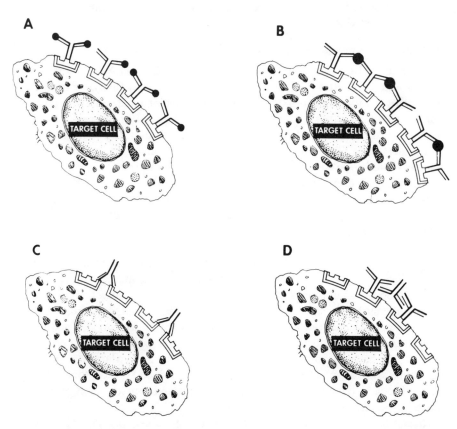

Fig. 11. Conditions for histamine release: (A) Interaction of bound IgE antibodies with monovalent antigen; no HR. (B) Interaction of bound IgE antibodies with divalent antigen; HR. (C) Antibodies to IgE receptors reacting with IgE receptors; HR. (D) Antibodies to IgE reacting with cell-bound IgE; HR.

stage is dependent upon Ca^{2+} and is affected by the microtubular system. Excess of released histamine can feed back and block HR by acting on receptors stimulating adenylcyclase, which influences the production of cAMP. More studies are needed to learn what happens in the cells after the antigen-antibody interaction.

Histamine, which is the most important mediator known thus far to be released in an anaphylactic reaction, induces smooth muscle contraction, manifested by bronchoconstriction; separation of endothelial cells, manifested by edema; increased mucous secretion, manifested by rhinitis and/or bronchial obstruction; and vasomotor collapse, which in the extreme is manifested by anaphylactic shock.

Mediators of Immediate Hypersensitivity

Histamine. Histamine [5-(2-aminoethyl) imidazole, $C_5H_9N_3$] is by far the most prominent mediator of the allergic response. It is synthesized from L-histidine by histidine decarboxylase, which is present in mast cells, basophilic granulocytes, and other cells. Histamine is synthesized in the cell plasma; the mechanism of transportation from plasma to granules and storage is not well understood. Once histamine is inside the granules, it appears to be retained there, possibly for many weeks, through firm ionic bulkage to carboxyl groups on granule proteins. Release of histamine from the granules is probably a physicochemical event, but it can be induced by variety of stimuli. Once released, it is converted in minutes to inactive derivatives, such as N-methylhistamine or N-methylamidazol.

The physiologic effects of histamine include contraction of smooth muscles, dilation of blood vessels, and stimulation of secretion from exocrine glands. These effects are mediated by interaction of histamine with specific receptors on the membranes of cells in various target tissues. The receptor on smooth muscle is said to contain a histidyl radical as part of its active center. Two different types of histamine receptors are known, H_1 and H_2. Some of the effects of histamine on H_1 receptors on smooth muscles, bronchi, and gut can be antagonized by such antihistamines as pyrilamine, diphenhydramine and others. These antagonists do not work on H_2 receptors, which can be blocked by newly developed histamine antagonists, such as burimamide, metiamide, or cimetidine.

Histamine can be assayed *in vitro* by using guinea pig ileum, which contracts in the presence of histamine, or by a fluorometric method or RIA. (For review see [77,87,110,115].)

Slow-reacting substance of anaphylaxis. In contrast to histamine, which acts within seconds, SRS-A requires several minutes to produce a maximum response. This substance does not exist preformed in the cells; rather it is synthesized as a consequence of an anaphylactic reaction and is secreted into the blood. SRS-A is formed in and released from lung leukocytes and other tissues during IgE antibody-antigen mediated reactions as well as in response to a variety of nonimmunologic stimuli, e.g., a calcium ionophore A-23187, (such substance is termed SRS). SRS-A presumably acts, like histamine, via specific receptors. An experimental drug, FLP 55712, appears to be a SRS-A antagonist, but the drug also blocks histamine and inhibits the release of other mediators.

SRS-A or SRS have only recently been characterized. The substance generated by lipoxygenase pathway of arachidonate metabolism is hydroxylated derivative of arachidonic acid with tripeptide substituents. The molecule has characteristic ultraviolet absorbance (280 nm), due to the conjugated triene, and has been named leukotriene (derived from leukocytes). As of now, leukotriene C, C_1, and D have been identified. The SRS may be one of the leukotrienes or a mixture of two, e.g., leukotriene C and D.

Human small airway muscle is very sensitive to SRS-A, causing airway constriction in bronchial asthma. *In vitro,* the SRS-A causes prolonged contraction of guinea pig ileum, rabbit jejunum, and duodenum; and vascular permeability of monkey skin. It has no effect on the gerbil colon, which is very sensitive to prostaglandin, or on the rat uterus, which is sensitive to serotonin and bradykinin. Histamine and SRS-A probably act synergistically on smooth muscle and blood vessels, and each of the agents may cause a secondary release of prostaglandin. SRS-A can be detected or quantitated *in vitro* by measuring prolonged contraction of guinea pig ileum, which is compared to the effect of a standard concentration of SRS-A. (For review see [26,88a,101a,110a,115].)

Eosinophilic chemotatic factor of anaphylaxis. ECF-A, a factor released from human lung tissue after challenge with an allergen [76], is defined by its ability to cause specific eosinophil chemotaxis in a Boyden chamber. It is a small-molecular-weight (400 daltons) peptide derived from the mast cell or basophil. It appears to exist in a preformed state in mast cells, but in basophils it is synthesized rapidly after cell stimulation. Release of ECF-A, like that of histamine and SRS-A, is controlled by cyclic nucleotide levels. While it is not a mediator in the pharmacologic sense, its presence explains one aspect of the allergic response *in vivo,* namely, the abundance of eosinophils in the area of allergic reaction. However, histamine, kallikrein, and C_5a also have eosinophilic chemotactic activity and may act synergistically with ECF-A. Elevated blood concentrations of ECF-A have been detected in humans in experimental cold urticaria and anaphylaxis. (For review see [115,130].)

Additional substances, such as neutrophil chemotactic factor, PAF, and BK-A, may be released from the target cells as consequence of an antigen-antibody interaction, but their roles in anaphylactic reaction have not yet been established.

THERAPY OF ALLERGIC DISEASES

Allergic diseases must be treated by both pharmacologic and immunologic approaches. The former uses a variety of pharmacologically active drugs. The latter uses selective allergenic extract(s) for immunotherapy; it is also referred to as desensitization (or more popularly as "shots").

Pharmacologic Therapeutics

Since most of the known allergic reactions are consequences of IgE antibody-allergen interaction, the pharmacologic therapeutics are designed to prevent such a reaction, to inhibit the release of biogenic amines, or to act selectively on adrenoceptors involved in contraction or relaxation of various tissues.

Allergic reactions are numerous, but the most common are due to airborne allergens which cause airway obstruction (asthma). Apart from allergies to drugs and stinging insects, these are the most life-threatening reactions. Drug treatment of asthma is primarily based on β-stimulant bronchodilators, cromolyn sodium (sodium chromoglycate), and glucocorticoid steroids. Among the adrenergic drugs for treatment of airway obstruction epinephrine and isoproteranol will serve as examples. Both are β-adrenoreceptor stimulants used in bronchodilators. Epinephrine is less frequently used by inhalation but is usually administered by subcutaneous or intramuscular injection to relieve bronchospasm in asthmatic attack. Epinephrine activates both α- and β-receptors. Its therapeutic uses depend on its inhibitory effect on respiratory smooth muscle and its action on the cardiovascular system. Isoproterenol is a more active stimulant of all β-adrenoceptors but less active on α-receptors than epinephrine. Isoproterenol is used primarily as a bronchodilator; taken by inhalation it causes intense bronchodilation within seconds. Other analogs being used effectively include metaproterenol and albuterol, which are more selective β-2 than β-1 stimulators.

Theophylline and its derivatives, although long recognized for treatment of asthma, have only in the last decade been widely studied. Theophylline is presently most likely the primary drug for treatment of asthma. Another drug used for treatment of asthma is cromolyn sodium, which can prevent the development of bronchospasm when administered by inhalation prior to antigen challenge. Cromolyn is not effective when the bronchospasms have started. A number of other drugs with similar activity have recently been introduced for treatment of asthma, allergic rhinitis, allergic conjunctivitis, and other allergic conditions.

Steroids can suppress the symptoms of asthma, hay fever, and urticaria, but they are not effective in systemic anaphylactic reaction. The mechanism of action of steroids is not well known.

Allergic diseases are also treated successfully with antihistamines, which act on both types of histamine receptor, H_1 and H_2. Diphenhydramine and pyrilamine are examples of H_1 receptor inhibitors; burimamide, metiamide, and cimetidine are H_2 receptor inhibitors. The H_1 and H_2 receptor blockers differ in their pharmacologic properties and clinical use. The antihistamine drugs are used for a number of clinical indications, but are not effective for treatment of asthma. The H_2 antagonists are not effective in the treatment of allergic diseases. (For more details see [98].)

Immunotherapy

Immunotherapy stems from the very early work on microbial immunology. The first use of immunotherapy (in 1911) was based on the observation that pollen were the cause of seasonal rhinitis and that active or passive immunization against rabies, tetanus, and diptheria was successful in experimental animals. Immunotherapy employs subcutaneous injections of subclinical doses of allergenic extract(s) to which the patient is sensitive. The injection dose is increased as the patient becomes less sensitive to the allergen(s). This general pattern is varied with great flexibility by individual allergologists.

It is very difficult to conclude whether desensitization is useful for treatment of all allergic diseases. Only in recent years have methods been developed to standardize the patterns of allergenic extracts used for immunotherapy. Current studies of the immunochemical properties of allergenic extracts suggest possible improvements in a basic element of immunotherapy, quality control of the allergenic extracts. In well-controlled studies the effectiveness of immunotherapy has been demonstrated in certain allergic diseases, including allergic rhinitis due to ragweed, grass, and mountain cedar, as well as allergies to insects.

The mechanism of the beneficial effect of immunotherapy is not well understood. In a very simplistic, general view it is assumed that the subclinical doses of allergenic extract(s) cause the production of IgG antibodies at titers high enough for them to combine with the challenging allergen, blocking the reaction with IgE antibodies.

Extensive and prolonged immunotherapy causes a decrease of serum IgE. However, it is not certain whether the reduction is a response of individual patients, is genetically influenced, or is dependent on the allergen(s).

Even less is known about how mast cells or basophils behave during immunotherapy. Are they less susceptible to vasoamine release? Are they sensitized best with more or fewer antibodies? One new approach in research is to measure immune responses during or after immunotherapy for the number of T suppressor or helper cells, which are important in IgE production. This approach awaits further development.

Parallel with studies to reveal the mechanism of immunotherapy, efforts are being made to improve the methods. Research is directed toward 1) purification of allergenic extracts and isolation of the most effective fractions; 2) modifying allergens by polymerization; 3) retarding the absorption of the allergen from the injection site; 4) modifying the allergenic extract by eliminating or reducing its allergenicity, analogous to detoxification of toxins in production of toxoids; and 5) producing compounds known as allergoids, which will retain immunogenic properties. All efforts to find more suitable substances and methods of administration are directed to reducing or eliminating the IgE antibody production responsible for the allergic reaction. Whether this will be achieved on the T-cell or B-cell level, time will show.

At present, however, there is no real cure for allergy. The disappearance or significant reduction of symptoms observed in some allergic individuals is a poorly understood phenomenon. (For review see [112].)

LATE-PHASE IgE-MEDIATED REACTIONS

The IgE-mediated, type I [37] hypersensitivity reaction in human skin develops within minutes, reaches a peak usually in 15–30 minutes, and subsides within a few hours. Although late reactions in allergic individuals were observed long before the discovery of IgE antibody, Dolovich and associates' [40] careful observation of skin reaction was the first to link the late response to IgE antibody. This observation was confirmed and the involvement of IgE firmly documented by Solley et al. [129], who provided a macroscopic description of the reaction.

In late-phase responders the immediate reaction of pruritic wheal and flare reaches a peak between 15 and 30 minutes, subsides into the flare zone within 60–90 minutes, and remains quiescent for 4–5 hours. Exacerbation of inflammation peaks at 6–12 hours after antigen challenge. At this late-response peak the lesion is characterized by erythema, edema, pruritis, and tenderness more extensive than in the immediate response. The lesions usually subside within 24 hours after antigen challenge; in some cases they persist for 48 hours. Histologic examination of the skin during the late-phase response shows mixed cellular infiltration, predominantly by lymphocytes but also by eosinophils, neutrophils, and basophils.

That the dual immediate and late-phase reaction is IgE-dependent has been proven by producing this reaction in nonallergic individuals to whom the IgE antibody specific for certain antigens was passively transferred (P-K test). The serum factor responsible is heat-sensitive, can be removed by anti-IgE, is completely inhibited by dilution in IgE myeloma protein, and has a long duration in the skin.

The late-phase response was initially considered a unique reaction to very selective allergens injected at high concentrations. Solley et al. [129] observed the dual response in most ragweed-sensitive patients, but other allergens can also elicit the reaction. A stronger late-phase reaction is achieved by challenge with a higher concentration of the allergen but a mild late-phase reaction can be produced by a routine test dose.

The mechanism of the late-phase reaction is not clear. As a working hypothesis it is assumed that the challenge allergen reacts with the cell-bound IgE antibody, causing initially a local anaphylactic reaction. What causes the accumulation of the cells is not known. It is feasible that mast cells release chemotactic factors that attract the various leukocytes, including basophils, to which surface IgE antibodies react with the available allergen. In consequence a cascade of local reactions may take place, attracting more cells and inflammatory fluids and causing thickening and reactions of the skin. At this point it must be accepted that the late-phase, IgE-mediated reaction can cause a cascade of events which are separate from the Arthus reaction (type III, IgG-mediated) and from T-cell-mediated, delayed hypersensitivity, tuberculin type (type IV). Its clinical implications are under study.

The late-phase IgE-mediated response in man is similar to the cutaneous basophil hypersensitivity (CBH) produced in animals. The latter is quite complex and is beyond the scope of this chapter, but some general comments must be made in view of the confusion with the earlier described Jones-Mote reaction (JMR). Both CBH and JMR are late reactions; both can be T-cell- or antibody-mediated; and both are induced by Freund's incomplete adjuvant. The main difference is that in the JMR fewer basophils are accumulated than in the CBH. Ashkenase considers JMR a subcategory of CBH [7]. More time and work are needed to draw clear distinctions within the whole group of late hypersensitivity reactions—all of which are different from the immediate (IgE antibody), delay (T-cell-dependent, tuberculin type), or Arthus (IgG antibody) reactions.

OVERVIEW AND EXPECTATIONS

The list of etiologic events that have been implicated in anaphylactic reactions is very long. It includes pollen, grasses, molds, foods, products of various animals, venoms, drugs, antibiotics, chemicals, blood products, anesthetics, and hormones, and it is still incomplete. Our knowledge of allergic diseases involving some of these agents is very sketchy. Only a few groups of allergens have served as models for experimental approach; these include ragweed and tree pollen, venoms of hymenoptera, animal dandruff, and penicillin. Discussing the field of allergology we have in mind the more classical, widely investigated allergens. In the near future we may see also progress in such gray areas as allergies to various foods or drugs, where the involvement of IgE antibody has not been well documented.

Progress in allergology has occurred in phases and will doubtless continue to do so. From 1921, when Carl Prausnitz and Heinz Küstner demonstrated the reagenic factor responsible for anaphylactic reaction, until 1966 allergology did not make great progress. Then Kimishige and Teruko Ishizaka's discovery of IgE antibodies to ragweed initiated the *immunologic phase* and simultaneously opened the door to in-depth studies of the molecular and biological aspects of the mechanism of immediate hypersensitivity. The target cells—mast and basophils—were shown to have surface-bound IgE. Receptors to which the IgE molecules are bound have been identified, isolated, and to some degree characterized. It has also been shown that lymphocytes bear Fc receptors for IgE but its function is unknown. Great progress has been made in revealing the mechanism of HR. Other biogenic amines have been recognized and some isolated. These and other contributions have influenced significantly the pharmacotherapy of allergic diseases, enabling the industry to explore and introduce new and more effective drugs. A new generation of *in vitro* tests, measuring IgE concentrations and specific IgE antibodies in body fluids, were introduced. These tests are important in monitoring the kinetics of IgE antibody activity in various conditions.

Allergology also took advantage, during the last decade, of progress in cellular immunology and immunogenetics. There is suggestive evidence that atopy—and, in consequence, allergic diseases—are under genetic control. More studies in this area will follow. The role of T cells in an allergic state and the cooperation between subsets of T cells are under study. The results may reveal a new mechanism of activation or receding of symptoms in allergic individuals and may open the way to bioengineering.

The continuing *immunologic phase* and the ensuing *pharmacologic phase* were followed by the present trend, the *immunotherapy phase*. This approach is geared more toward bioengineering. Although immunotherapy has been practiced for many decades, research has recently been initiated on chemical conversion of allergenic substances into nonimmunogenic polymers or tolerogenic substances, which can be used to modulate T cells in IgE production. It is surely feasible to manipulate the cell systems, but will such engineering of biologic structure and organization be without deleterious consequences? Disturbing a biologic balance, though it may be imperfect, is not without serious risk. The next decade may show whether allergology will move toward bioengineering or toward pharmacologic control of the IgE-allergen interaction.

We may expect in the next decade that some allergic diseases will become public health problems. Allergic reactions to air pollutants or particulate allergens, chemical or biological, in air conditioners may one day be an issue. An outbreak of allergic reactions in a huge administrative building or plant may bring government action and involvement of public health officials. There may also be attempts to reduce or eliminate the sources of some natural allergens, such as ragweed. It may not be surprising to see in the next decade some practical devices to isolate an allergic individual from a polluted environment. Man's ingenuity in this regard is almost unlimited, and technology is much more advanced than medicine.

SUMMARY

IgE is a distinct class among proteins because of its biologic properties and the role it plays in atopic diseases. Through the Fc part of the molecule it can bind with homologous species' target cells, such as mast cells and basophils. Heating at 56 °C or treatment with 2-ME abolishes the cell binding property but does not interfere with antigen binding by the Fab portion. The mechanism of anaphylactic reaction is not known for certain, but in view of the available knowledge it is assumed that an allergen (which must be at least divalent) reacts with the cell-bound IgE antibodies, causing bridging of the antibodies, which in turn affects the IgE receptors. The antigen-antibody interaction releases a cascade of biochemical reactions, in consequence of which pharmacologically active amines (mediators) stored in the mast cells or basophilic granules are released. The major mediator is histamine, which upon release is modulated by cAMP. Histamine in an anaphylactic reaction in man induces smooth muscle contraction, separation of endothelial cells, increased mucous secretion, and vasomotor collapse. Histamine acts on the various tissues through histamine receptors, H_1 and H_2. An allergic reaction can be prevented or inhibited by various drugs or by immunotherapy.

IgE can be detected on the surface of the mast cells or basophils or in serum. However the concentrations in serum are rather low, and radioimmunoassays, detecting nanograms of the protein, must be employed. The most popular test is the PRIST. In IgE myeloma (thus far 18 cases have been reported) the concentrations are usually high (g/dL) and can be detected by RID or tests of similar sensitivity. IgE serum concentrations in healthy or allergic individuals vary widely, depending on the person's age, the geographic location, and the methods used for measuring. In the United States, with PRIST as the method of detection, the geometric means are 64 U/mL for infants, 150 U/mL for schoolchildren, and 120 U/mL for older age groups.

In some allergic diseases, including extrinsic or complicating bronchial asthma, acute urticaria, and bronchopulmonary aspergillosis, serum IgE concentrations are elevated. Elevated serum IgE may also be found in nonatopic individuals, e.g. in parasitic infestations, in some bacterial infections, or in immunologic disorders involving the T-cell system, such as Wiskott-Aldrich syndrome and Nezelof syndrome. In contrast, serum IgE is significantly lower in patients with a generalized defect of Ig synthesis.

Serum IgE antibodies with defined specificity to certain allergens are of basic importance in allergic diseases. Since the degree of allergic response can be modulated by immunotherapy, monitoring of serum IgE or cell-bound

IgE has a practical application. A variety of biologic and nonbiologic methods are available. The most popular are the RAST for measuring serum IgE antibodies and the leukocyte HR test for measuring actively or passively cell-bound IgE antibodies. (The P-K test is prohibited in many states because of the possibility of transferring hepatitis B virus.) Generally the RAST compares favorably with the P-K and leukocyte HR tests, but it is less sensitive than the skin test.

ACKNOWLEDGMENTS

I thank Robert Reisman, of Buffalo General Hospital, Buffalo, NY, for allowing me to use material for Figure 2, for review of the chapter, and for helpful comments.

REFERENCES

1. Adkinson NF: The radioallergosorbent test: Uses and abuses. J Allergy Clin Immunol 65:1, 1980.
2. Arbesman CE: Evaluation of the RAST in allergy. Proceedings of IX International Congress of Allergology, Buenos Aires, Argentina, 1976. Excerpta Medica International Congress series no. 414, p 392.
3. Arbesman CE, Girard P, Rose NR: Demonstration of human reagin in the monkey. II. *In vitro* passive sensitization of monkey ileum with the sera of untreated atopic patients. J Allergy 35:535, 1964.
4. Arbesman CE, Ito K, Wypych JI, Wicher K: Measurement of serum IgE by a one-step single radial radiodiffusion method. J Allergy Clin Immunol 49:72, 1972.
5. Arbesman CE, Wypych JI, Reisman RE: Serum IgE in human diseases. In Goodfriend L, Sehon A, Orange R (eds): "Mechanism in Allergy." New York: Marcel-Dekker, Inc., 1973.
6. Arbesman CE, Wicher K, Wypych JI, Reisman RE, Dickie H, Reed CE: IgE antibodies in sera of patients with allergic bronchopulmonary aspergillosis. Clin Allergy 4:349, 1974.
7. Askenase PW: Effector cells in late and delayed hypersensitivity reactions that are dependent on antibodies or T cells. In Fougereau M, Dausset J (eds): "Progress in Immunology IV." New York: Academic Press, 1980.
8. Assem, ESK, Vickers MR: Serum IgE and other *in vitro* tests in drug allergy. Clin Allergy 2:325, 1972.
9. Austen KF, Wasserman SI, Goetzl EJ: Mast cell-derived mediator: Structural and functional diversity and regulation of expression. In Johansson SGO, Strandberg K, Uvnas B (eds): "Molecular and Biological Aspects of the Acute Allergic Reaction." New York: Plenum Press, 1976.
10. Axén R, Porath J: Chemical coupling of enzymes to cross-linked dextran (Sephadex). Nature 210:367, 1966.
11. Baenkler HW: Monoclonal gammopathy of IgA and IgE type in a case of chronic lymphatic leukaemia. Acta Haematol (Basel) 56:189, 1976.
12. Ball, PAJ, Voller A, Tafts LF: Hypersensitivity to some nematode antigens. Br Med J 1:210, 1971.
13. Bazaral M, Hamburger RN: Standardization and stability of immunoglobulin E (IgE). J Allergy Clin Immunol 49:189, 1972.
14. Bazaral M, Orgel HA, Hamburger RN: IgE levels in normal infants and mothers and an inheritance hypothesis. J Immunol 107:794, 1971.

15. Bazin H, Beckers A, Querinjean P: Three classes and four subclasses of rat immunoglobulins: IgM, IgA, IgE, and IgG1, IgG2A, IgG2B, and IgG2C. Eur J Immunol 4:44, 1974.
16. Bennich H, Johansson SGO: Studies on a new class of human immunoglobulins. II. Chemical and physical properties. In Killander J (ed): "Gamma Globulin Structure and Control of Biosynthesis." Stockholm: Almquist & Wiksell, Interscience Publishers, A Division of John Wiley & Sons, Inc., 1967.
17. Bennich H, Ishizaka K, Johansson SGO, Rowe DS, Stanworth DR, Terry WD: Immunoglobulin E: A new class of human immunoglobulin. Bull WHO 38:151, 1968.
18. Bennich H, Johansson SGO: Structure and function of human immunoglobulin E. In Dixon FJ, Kunkel HG (eds): "Advances in Immunology." Vol. 13, New York: Academic Press, 1971.
19. Bennich H, Dorrington K: Structure and confirmation of immunoglobulin E. In Ishizaka K, Dayton DH (eds): "Proceedings of a Conference on the Biological Role of the Immunoglobulin E System." Bethesda: US Department of Health, Education, and Welfare, Public Health Service, NIH, 1972.
20. Bennich H, von Bahr-Lindström H: Structure of immunoglobulin E. In Brent L, Holborow J (eds): "Progress in Immunology II." Vol. 1, Amsterdam: North-Holland Publishing Co., 1974.
21. Berg T, Johansson SGO: IgE concentrations in children with atopic diseases. A clinical study. Int Arch Allergy Appl Immunol 36:219, 1969.
22. Berg T, Johansson SGO: Allergy diagnosis with the radioallergosorbent test: A comparison with the results of skin and provocation test in an unselected group of children with asthma and hay fever. J Allergy Clin Immunol 54:209, 1974.
23. Berglund G, Finnström O, Johansson SGO, Möller KL: Wiskott-Aldrich syndrome. Acta Paediatr Scand 57:89, 1968.
24. Bos JD, Hamerlinck F, Cormane RH: Antitreponemal IgE in early syphilis. Br J Vener Dis 56:20, 1980.
25. Brehm G: Verhalten von Immunoglobulin E bei ausgewählten Dermatosen. Arch Dermatol Forsch 248:329, 1974.
26. Brocklehurst WE: Slow reacting substance and related compounds. In Waksman BH, Kallós P (eds): "Progress in Allergy." Vol. 6, Basel: S. Karger AG, 1962.
27. Brown WR, Lee EH: Studies on IgE in human intestinal fluids. Int Archs Allergy Appl Immunol 50:87, 1976.
28. Brown GL, Corby DG, Lima JE, DiBella NJ, Nelson JK, Gray MR: IgE-IgM kappa gammapathy associated with lymphocytic lymphoma: Immunological evaluation. Milit Med 142:921, 1977.
29. Buckley RH, Wray BB, Belmaker EZ: Extreme hyperimmunoglobulinemia E and undue susceptibility to infection. Pediatrics 49:59, 1972.
30. Buckley RH, Fiscus SA: Serum IgD and IgE concentrations in immunodeficiency diseases. J Clin Invest 55:157, 1975.
31. Buckley RH, Becker WG: Abnormalities in the regulation of human IgE synthesis. In Möller G (ed): "Immunological Reviews." Vol. 41, Copenhagen: Munksgaard, 1978.
32. Cass RM, Anderson RR: The disappearance rate of skin-sensitizing antibody. J Allergy 42:29, 1968.
33. Ceska M, Lundkvist U: A new and simple radioimmunoassay method for the determination of IgE. Immunochemistry. 9:1021, 1972.
34. Chai H, Farr RJ, Froehlich LA, Mathison DA, McLean JA, Rosenthal RR, Scheffer AL, Spector SL, Townley RG: Standardization of bronchial challenge procedures. J Allergy Clin Immunol 56:323, 1975.
35. Conrad DH, Bazin H, Sehon AH, Froese A: Binding parameters of the interaction between rat IgE and rat mast cell receptors. J Immunol 114:1688, 1975.
36. Conrad DH, Froese A: Characterization of the target cell receptor for IgE. II. Poly-

acrylamide gel analysis of the surface IgE receptor from normal rat mast cells and from rat basophilic leukemia cells. J Immunol 116:319, 1976.

37. Coombs RRA, Gell PGH: Classification of allergic reactions responsible for clinical hypersensitivity and disease. In Gell PGH, Coombs RRA (eds): "Clinical Aspects of Immunology," 2nd ed. Chapter 20, Philadelphia: F. H. Davis Company, 1968.

38. Creyssel R, Bouvier M, Daumont A: Myélome IgE. Un nouveau cas. Nouv Presse Med 6:962, 1977.

39. Dammacco F, Miglietta A, Tribalto M, Mandelli F, Bonomo L: The expending spectrum of clinical and laboratory features of IgE myeloma. La Ricerca Clin Lab 10:583, 1980.

40. Dolovich J, Hargreave FE, Chalmers R, Shier KJ, Gauldie J, Bienenstock J: Late cutaneous allergic responses in isolated IgE-dependent reactions. J Allergy Clin Immunol 52:38, 1973.

41. Dorrington KJ, Bennich H: Structure-function relationships in human immunoglobulin E. In Möller G (ed): "Immunological Reviews." Vol. 41, Copenhagen: Munksgaard, 1978.

42. Eidinger D, Wilkinson R, Rose B: A study of cellular responses in immune reactions utilizing the skin window technique. I. Immediate hypersensitivity reactions. J Allergy 35:77, 1964.

42a. Endo T, Okumura H, Kikuchi K, Munakata J, Otake M, Nomura T, Asakawa H: Immunoglobulin E (IgE) Multiple Myeloma. Am J Med 70:1127, 1981.

43. Fishkin BG, Orloff N, Scaduto LE, Borucki DT, Spiegelberg HL: IgE multiple myeloma: A report of the third case. Blood 39:361, 1972.

44. Foucard T: A follow-up study of children with asthmatoid bronchitis. I. Skin test reactions and IgE antibodies to common allergens. Acta Paediatr Scand 62:633, 1973.

45. Fujita Y, Wicher K, Wypych JI, Reisman RE, Arbesman CE: *In vitro* reaction of antibodies to ragweed. II. Quantitative determination of non-IgE antibodies interfering in a radioallergosorbent test. Int Arch Allergy Appl Immunol 49:636, 1975.

46. Geha RS, Rappaport JM, Twarog FJ, Parkman R, Rosen FS: Increased serum immunoglobulin E levels following allogeneic bone marrow transplantation. J Allergy Clin Immunol 66:78, 1980.

47. Gerrard JW, Horne S, Vickers P, MacKenzie JWA, Goluboff N, Garson JZ, Maningas CS: Serum IgE levels in parents and children. J Pediatrics 85:660, 1974.

48. Gerrard JW, Geddes CA, Reggin PL, Gerrard CD, Horne S: Serum IgE levels in white and Metis communities in Saskatchewan. Ann Allergy 37:91, 1976.

49. Gleich GJ, Averbeck AK, Swedlund HA: Measurement of IgE in normal and allergic serum by radioimmunoassay. J Lab Clin Med 77:690, 1971.

50. Gleich GJ, Yuninger JW, Stobo JD: Laboratory methods for studies of allergy. In Middleton E Jr, Reed CE, Ellis EF (eds): "Allergy Principles and Practice." St. Louis: C. V. Mosby Co., 1978.

51. Gleich GJ, Adolphson CR, Yuninger JW: The mini-RAST: Comparison with other varieties of the radioallergosorbent test for the measurement of immunoglobulin E antibodies. J Allergy Clin Immunol 65:20, 1980.

52. Green RL, Scales RW, Kraus SJ: Increased serum immunoglobulin E concentrations in venereal diseases. Br J Vener Dis 52:257, 1976.

53. Grundbacher FJ: Causes of variation in serum IgE levels in normal population. J Allergy Clin Immunol 56:104, 1975.

54. Hoffman DR: Estimation of serum IgE by an enzyme-linked immunosorbent assay (ELISA). J Allergy Clin Immunol 51:303, 1973.

55. Hogarth-Scott RS, Johansson SGO, Bennich H: Antibodies to Toxocara in the sera of visceral larva migrants patients: The significance of raised levels of IgE. Clin Exp Immunol 5:617, 1969.

56. Ishizaka K: Cellular events in the IgE antibody response. In Dixon FJ, Kunkel HG (eds): "Advances in Immunology." Vol. 23, New York: Academic Press, 1976.
57. Ishizaka K, Ishizaka T: Human reaginic antibodies and immunoglobulin E. J Allergy 42:330, 1968.
58. Ishizaka T, Ishizaka K, Conrad DH, Froese A: A new concept of triggering mechanisms of IgE-mediated histamine release. J Allergy Clin Immunol 61:320, 1978.
59. Ishizaka T, Ishizaka K: Biologic function of immunoglobulin E. In Ishizaka K, Dayton DH Jr (eds): "Proceedings of a Conference on the Biological Role of the Immunoglobulin E System." Bethesda: US Department of Health, Education, and Welfare, Public Health Service, NIH, 1972.
60. Ishizaka T, Ishizaka K: Biology of immunoglobulin E. Molecular basis of reaginic hypersensitivity. In Kallos P, Waksman BH (eds): "Progress in Allergy." Vol. 19, Basel: S. Karger, 1975.
61. Ishizaka K, Ishizaka T: Immunology of IgE-mediated hypersensitivity. In Middleton E Jr, Reed CE, Ellis EF (eds): "Allergy Principles and Practice." St. Louis: C. V. Mosby Co., 1978.
62. Ishizaka K, Newcomb RW: Presence of γE in nasal washings and sputum from asthamatic patients. J Allergy Clin Immunol 46:197, 1970.
63. Ishizaka K, Ishizaka T, Hornbrook MM: Physicochemical properties of reaginic antibody. IV. Presence of a unique immunoglobulin as a carrier of reaginic activity. J Immunol 97:75: 1966.
64. Ishizaka K, Ishizaka T, Hornbrook MM: Allergen-binding activity of γE, γG, and γA antibodies in sera from atopic patients: *In vitro* measurements of reaginic antibody. J Immunol 98:490, 1967.
65. Ishizaka T, Soto CS, Ishizaka K: Mechanisms of passive sensitization. III. Number of IgE molecules and its receptor sites on human basophil granulocytes. J Immunol 111:500, 1973.
66. Ito K, Wicher K, Arbesman CE: Comparison of two myeloma IgE by monkey antiserum to human IgE. Int Arch Allergy Appl Immunol 39:178, 1970.
67. Johansson SGO: Raised levels of a new immunoglobulin class (IgND) in asthma. Lancet ii:951, 1967.
67a. Johansson SGO: Serum IgND levels in healthy children and adults. Int Arch Allergy Appl Immunol 34:1, 1968.
68. Johansson SGO, Bennich H: Immunological studies of an atypical (myeloma) immunoglobulin. Immunology 13:381, 1967.
69. Johansson SGO, Foucard T: IgE in immunity and diseases. In Middleton E Jr, Reed CE, Ellis EF (eds): "Allergy Principles and Practice." St. Louis: C. V. Mosby Co., 1978.
70. Johansson SGO, Bennich H, Wide L: A new class of immunoglobulin in human serum. Immunology 14:265, 1968.
71. Johansson SGO, Mellbin T, Vahlquist B: Immunoglobulin levels in Ethiopian preschool children with special reference to high concentrations of immunoglobulin E (IgEND). Lancet i:1118, 1968.
72. Johansson SGO, Bennich H, Berg T: The clinical significance of IgE. In Schwartz RS (ed): "Progress in Clinical Immunology." Vol. 1, New York: Grune and Straton, Inc., 1972.
73. Jones VE, Edwards AJ, Ogilvie BM: The circulating immunoglobulins involved in protective immunity to the intestinal stage of *Nippostrongylus brasiliensis* in the rat. Immunology 18:621, 1970.
74. Jones HE, Reinhardt JH, Rinaldi MG: Immunologic susceptibility to chronic dermatophytosis. Arch Dermatol 110:213, 1974.

75. Juhlin L, Johansson SGO, Bennich H, Högman C, Thyresson N: Immunoglobulin E in dermatoses. Arch Dermatol 100:12, 1969.
76. Kay AB, Stechschulte DJ, Austen KF: An eosinophil leukocyte chemotactic factor of anaphylaxis. J Exp Med 133:602, 1971.
77. Kazimierczak W, Diamant B: Mechanisms of histamine release in anaphylactic and anaphylactoid reactions. In Kallos P, Waksman BH (eds): "Progress in Allergy." Vol. 24, Basel: S. Karger, 1978.
78. Kikkawa Y, Kamimura K, Hamajima T, Sekiguichi T, Kawai T, Takenaka M, Tada T: Thymic alymphoplasia with hyper-IgE-globulinemia. Pediatrics 51:690, 1973.
79. Kjellman N-IM: Predictive value of high IgE levels in children. Acta Paediatr Scand 65:1, 1976.
80. Kjellman N-IM, Johansson SGO, Roth A: Serum IgE levels in healthy children quantified by a sandwich technique (PRIST). Clin Allergy 6:51, 1976.
81. Knedel M, Fateh-Moghadam A, Edel H, Bartl R, Neumeier D: Multiples Myelom mit monoklonaler IgE-Gammopathie. Dtsch Med Wochenschr 101:496, 1976.
82. Kraft D, Roth A, Mischer P, Pichler H, Ebner H: Specific and total serum IgE measurements in the diagnosis of penicillin allergy. A long-term follow-up study. Clin Allergy 7:21, 1977.
83. Kulczycki A Jr, Metzger H: The interaction of IgE with rat basophilic leukemia cells. II. Quantitative aspects of the binding reaction. J Exp Med 140:1676, 1974.
84. Landaas TØ, Grimmer Ø, Heier HE, Godal T: Increased serum IgE in Hodgkin's disease is of polyclonal origin. Acta Pathol Microbiol Scand [C] 87:377, 1979.
85. Levine BB: Genetic factors in reagin production in mice. In Austen KF, Becker EL (eds): "Biochemistry of the Acute Allergic Reactions." Oxford: Blackwell Scientific Publications, 1971.
86. Levine BB, Vaz NM: Effect of combinations of inbred strain, antigen, and antigen dose on immune responsiveness and reagin production in the mouse: A potential mouse model for immune aspects of human atopic allergy. Int Arch Allergy Appl Immunol 39:156, 1970.
87. Levy DA: Histamine and serotonin. In Weissmann G (ed): "Mediators of Inflammation." New York: Plenum Publishing Corp., 1974.
88. Levy DA, Widra M: A microassay for studying allergic histamine release from human leukocytes using an enzymic-isotopic assay for histamine. J Lab Clin Med 81:29, 1973.
88a. Lewis RA, Austen KF, Drazen JM, Clark DA, Marfat A, Corey EJ: Slow reacting substances of anaphylaxis: Identification of leukotrienes C-1 and D from human and rat sources. Proc Natl Acad Sci USA 77:3710, 1980.
89. Lichtenstein LM: Allergy. In Bach FH, Good RA (eds): "Clinical Immunobiology." Vol. I, New York: Academic Press, 1972.
90. Lichtenstein LM, Osler AG: Studies on the mechanisms of hypersensitivity phenomena. IX. Histamine release from human leukocytes by ragweed pollen antigen. J Exp Med 120:507, 1964.
91. Ludwig H, Vormittag N: "Benign" monoclonal IgE gammopathy. Br Med J 281:539, 1980.
92. Maia LCS, Vaz NM, Vaz EM: Effect of soluble antigen on IgE responses in the mouse. Int Arch Allergy Appl Immunol 46:339, 1974.
93. Marsh DG, Bias WB, Ishizaka K: Genetic control of basal serum immunoglobulin E level and its effect on specific reaginic sensitivity. Proc Natl Acad Sci USA 71:3588, 1974.
94. Marsh DG, Hsu SH, Hussain R, Meyers DA, Freidhoff LR, Bias WB: Genetics of human immune response to allergens. J Allergy Clin Immunol 65:322, 1980.

95. Mathur S, Goust J-M, Horger III EO, Fudenberg HH: Immunoglobulin E anti-Candida antibodies and Candidiasis. Infect Immun 18:257, 1977.
96. Metzger H: Effect of antigen binding on the properties of antibody. In Dixon FJ, Kunkel HG (eds): "Advances in Immunology." Vol. 18, New York: Academic Press, 1974.
97. Michel FB, Bousquet J, Greillier P, Robinet-Levy M, Coulomb Y: Comparison of cord blood immunoglobulin E concentrations and maternal allergy for the prediction of atopic diseases in infancy. J Allergy Clin Immunol 65:422, 1980.
98. Middleton E Jr, Reed CE, Elliot EF (eds): "Allergy Principles and Practice." Section C/Pharmacology, Chapters 23–30 (multiple authors), St. Louis: C. V. Mosby Co., 1978.
99. Miller DL, Hirvonen T, Gitlin D: Synthesis of IgE by the human conceptus. J Allergy Clin Immunol 52:182, 1973.
100. Mills RJ, Fahie-Wilson MN, Carter PM, Hobbs JR: IgE myelomatosis. Clin Exp Immunol 23:228, 1976.
101. Morgan CR, Lazarow A: Immunoassay of insulin: Two-antibody system. Plasma insulin levels of normal subdiabetic and diabetic rats. Diabetes 12:15, 1963.
101a. Murphy RC, Hammarström S, Samuelsson B: Leukotriene C: A slow-reacting substance from murine mastocytoma cells. Proc Natl Acad Sci USA 76:4275, 1979.
102. Newcomb RW, Ishizaka K: Physicochemical and antigenic studies of human IgE in respiratory fluid. J Immunol 105:85, 1970.
103. Newman SA, Rossi G, Metzger H: Molecular weight and valence of the cell surface receptor for immunoglobulin E. Proc Natl Acad Sci USA 74:869, 1977.
104. Nordbring F, Johansson SGO, Espmark A: Raised serum levels of IgE in infectious mononucleosis. Scand J Infect Dis 4:119, 1972.
105. Norman PS: In Vivo methods of study of allergy. In Middleton E Jr, Reed CE, Ellis EF (eds): "Allergy Principles and Practice." St. Louis: C. V. Mosby Co., 1978.
106. Ogawa M, Kochwa S, Smith C, Ishizaka K, McIntyre OR: Clinical aspects of IgE myeloma. N Engl J Med 281:1217, 1969.
107. Ogawa M, Berger PA, McIntyre OR, Clendenning WE, Ishizaka K: IgE in atopic dermatitis. Arch Dermatol 103:575, 1971.
108. Okumura K, Tada T: Regulation of homocytotropic antibody formation in the rat. VI. Inhibitory effect of thymocytes on the homocytotropic antibody response. J Immunol 107:1682, 1971.
109. Ooi BS, Pesce AJ, First MR, Pollack VE, Bernstein IL, Wellington J: IgE levels in interstitial nephritis. Lancet i:1254, 1974.
110. Orange RP, Austen KF: The immunological release of chemical mediators of immediate type hypersensitivity from human lung. In Amos B (ed): "Progress in Immunology I." New York: Academic Press, 1971.
110a. Örning L, Hammarström S, Samuelsson B: Leukotriene D: A slow reacting substance from rat basophilic leukemia cells. Proc Natl Acad Sci USA 77:2014, 1980.
110b. Orr TSC: In Daems WTh, Quanjer PhH, Reerink-Brongers EE (eds): "The Mast Cell in Relation to Allergic Mechanisms." Leusden: Netherlands Asthma Foundation, 1977.
110c. Parwaresch MR: "The Human Blood Basophil." New York: Springer-Verlag, 1976.
111. Patterson R, Fink JN, Pruzansky JJ, Reed C, Roberts M, Slavin R, Zeiss CR: Serum immunoglobulin levels in pulmonary allergic aspergillosis and certain other lung diseases, with special reference to immunoglobulin E. Am J Med 54:16, 1973.
112. Patterson R, Lieberman P, Irons JS, Pruzanski J, Melam HL, Metzger WJ, Zeiss CR: Immunotherapy. In Middleton E, Reed CE, Ellis EF (eds): "Allergy Principles and Practice." Vol. II, St. Louis: C. V. Mosby Co., 1978.
113. Penn GM, Sanders WH, Ryan T: IgD and IgE: The untypable M proteins. Am J Clin

Pathol 58:93, 1972.

114. Perelmutter L, Phipps P, Potvin L: Viral infections and IgE levels. Ann Allergy 41:158, 1978.

115. Plaut M, Lichtenstein LM: Cellular and chemical basis of the allergic inflammatory response. In Middleton E Jr, Reed CE, Ellis EF (eds): "Allergy Principles and Practice." St. Louis: C. V. Mosby Co., 1978.

116. Polmar SH, Waldmann TA, Terry WD: IgE in immunodeficiency. Am J Pathol 69:499, 1972.

117. Polmar SH, Waldmann TA, Balestra ST, Jost MC, Terry WD: Immunoglobulin E in immunologic deficiency diseases. J Clin Invest 51:326, 1972.

118. Prausnitz C, Küstner H: Studien uber die Überempfindlichkeit. Zentralbl. F. Bacteriologie, Parasitenkunde, Infectionskrankheiten und Hygiene. 86(1):160, 1921. Translated from German by Carl Prausnitz, In Gell GH, Coombs RRA (eds): "Clinical Aspects of Immunology." Oxford: Blackwell Scientific Publ., 1962, pp 808–816.

119. Rogers JS, Spahr J, Judge DM, Varano LA, Eyster ME: IgE myeloma with osteoblastic lesions. Blood 49:295, 1977.

120. Rosenberg RB, Whalen GE, Bennich H, Johansson SGO: Increased circulating IgE in a new parasitic disease—human intestinal capillaries. N Engl J Med 238:1148, 1970.

121. Rowe DS: Radioactive single radial diffusion: A method for increasing the sensitivity of immunochemical quantitation of proteins in agar gel. Bull WHO 40:613, 1969.

122. Rowe DS, Tackett L, Bennich H, Ishizaka K, Johansson SGO, Anderson SG: A research standard for human serum immunoglobulin E. Bull WHO 43:609, 1970.

123. Rubinstein E, Sokal JE, Reisman RE, Arbesman CE: Relationship of serum total IgE and cell-mediated immunity in patients with Hodgkin's disease. Int Arch Allergy Appl Immunol 55:439, 1977.

124. Salmon SE, Mackey G, Fudenberg HH: "Sandwich" solid phase radioimmunoassay for the quantitative determination of human immunoglobulins. J Immunol 103:129, 1969.

125. Scherr MS, Grater WC, Baer H, Berman BA, Center G, Hale R: Report of the committee on standardization. I. Method of evaluating skin test response. Ann Allergy 29:30, 1971.

126. Schild HO, Hawkins DF, Mongar JL, Herxheimer H: Reactions of isolated human asthmatic lung and bronchial tissue to a specific antigen: Histamine release and muscular contraction. Lancet ii:376, 1951.

127. Schopfer K, Baerlocher K, Price P, Krech U, Quie PG, Douglas SD: Staphylococcal IgE antibodies, hyperimmunoglobulinemia E and *Staphylococcus aureus* infections. N Engl J Med 300:835, 1979.

128. Shirakura T, Takekoshi K, Umi M, Kanazawa K, Okabe H, Inoue T, Imamura Y: Waldenström's macroglobulinemia with IgE M-component. Scand J Haematol 21:292, 1978.

129. Solley GO, Gleich GJ, Jordon RE, Schroeter AL: The late phase of the immediate wheal and flare skin reaction. J Clin Invest 58:408, 1976.

130. Stechschulte DJ: Slow-reacting substances. In Weissmann G (ed): "Mediator of Inflammation." New York: Plenum Publishing Corp., 1974.

131. Stefani DV, Mokeeva RA: Two occurrences of the rare forms of myeloma illness (D and E) (in Russian). Probl Haematol USSR 17:44, 1972.

132. Stokes CR, Hosking CS, Turner MW, Johansson SGO: Urinary IgE: A reappraisal. Eur J Immunol 3:241, 1973.

133. Tada T, Ishizaka K: Distribution of IgE forming cells in lymphoid tissues of the human and monkey. J Immunol 104:337, 1970.

134. Tada T, Okumura K: The role of antigen-specific T-cell factors in the immune response. In Dixon FJ, Kunkel HG (eds): "Advances in Immunology." Vol. 28, New York:

Academic Press, 1979.

135. Takatsu K, Ishizaka K: Reaginic antibody formation of the mouse. VII. Induction of suppressor T cells for IgE and IgG antibody responses. J Immunol 116:1257, 1976.

136. Thomas MR, Steinberg P, Votaw ML, Bayne NK: IgE levels in Hodgkin's disease. Ann Allergy 37:416, 1976.

137. Tse KS, Wicher K, Arbesman CE: Effect of immunotherapy on appearance of antibodies to ragweed in external secretions. J Allergy Clin Immunol 51:208, 1973.

138. Vaerman JP: A new case of IgE myeloma (Des) ending with renal failure. J Clin Lab Immunol 2:343, 1979.

139. Vervloet D, Fujita Y, Wypych JI, Reisman RE, Arbesman CE: The inhibitory effect of serum factors on measurement of the IgE Aspergillus antibody by RAST. Clin Allergy 4:359, 1974.

140. Vladutiu AO, Kohli RK, Prezyna AP: Monoclonal IgE with renal failure. Am J Med 61:957, 1976.

141. Waldmann TA, Bull JM, Bruce RM, Broder S, Jost MC, Balestra ST, Sver ME: Serum immunoglobulin E levels in patients with neoplastic disease. J Immunol 133:379, 1974.

142. Waldmann TA, Iio A, Ogawa M, McIntyre OR, Strober W: The metabolism of IgE. Studies in normal individuals and in a patient with IgE myeloma. J Immunol 117:1139, 1976.

143. Weltman JK, Frackelton AR, Szaro RP, Rothman MB: A galactosidase immunosorbent test (GIST) for total and ragweed specific IgE antibodies. J Allergy Clin Immunol 58:426, 1976.

144. Weiner E, DiCamelli R, Showel J, Osmand AP, Sassetti RJ, Gewurz H: IgE myeloma presenting with classical myeloma features. J Allergy Clin Immunol 58:373, 1976.

145. Wicher K, Ishikawa T, Arbesman CE: Direct immunofluorescent staining of IgE containing cells in tissues of human and monkey. Proceedings of VII International Congress of Allergology, Florence, Italy, 1970. Excerpta Medica International Congress series no. 211, p 17.

146. Wide L, Porath J: Radioimmunoassay of proteins with the use of Sephadex coupled antibodies. Biochim Biophys Acta 130:257, 1966.

147. Wide L, Bennich H, Johansson SGO: Diagnosis of allergy by an in vitro test for allergen antibodies. Lancet ii:1105, 1967.

148. Winkelmann RK, Gleich GJ: Chronic acral dermatitis. JAMA 225:378, 1973.

149. Wittig HJ, Belloit J, DeFillippi I, Royal G: Age-related serum immunoglobulin E levels in healthy subjects and in patients with allergic disease. J Allergy Clin Immunol 66:305, 1980.

150. Wütrich B, Kopper E: Ergebnisse der IgE Serumspiegel-Bestimmung und ihre klinische Bedeutung. Schweiz Med Wochenschr 104:1437, 1974.

151. Yoshitake J, Hiramatsu S, Komatsubara Y, Matsubara R, Fujita T, Akutagawa H, Mori Y, Kondo K, Inai S, Senda N: A case of IgE myeloma. Acta Haematol Jap 39:862, 1976.

152. Yunginger JW, Gleich GJ: Seasonal changes in serum and nasal IgE concentrations. J Allergy Clin Immunol 51:174, 1973.

153. Zavazal V, Sach J, Rozprimova L, Brumelova V: An unusual case of IgE myeloma. Allergol Immunopathol (Madr) VI:423, 1978.

154. Buckley RH, Sampson HA: The Hyperimmunoglobulinemia E syndrome. In Franklin EC (ed): "Clinical Immunology Update—Review for Physicians." New York: Elsevier Publ., 1981, pp 147–167.

155. Johansson SGO: The Clinical significance of IgE. In Franklin EC (ed): "Clinical Immunology Update—Review for Physicians." New York: Elsevier Publ., 1981, pp 123–145.

Index

A. *lumbricoides,* 318
AMP, cyclic (cAMP), 334–335
Abortion, septic, 173
α-Acid glycoprotein, 36, 53, 57
Active site
   antibody, 193
   constant domain, 275–282
   localization
      IgA activities, 256–258
      with IgG, 235–242
      IgD activities, 266–267
      IgE activities, 270–272
      IgM activities, 262
      therapeutic implications, 282
Adenocarcinoma, 70
Agarose slides, 100, 102
Albumin, 35, 44, 59, 69, 77
   bovine serum, as internal standard,
      93–94
   fetal, 73
   two-dimensional patterns, 72–73,
      81–85
Allergic disease, 194, 258, 270
   therapy, 337–342
Amaloidosis, 201
Amniocentesis, 81
Amniotic fluid, 104
   electrophoresis of, 66, 69, 81–82
Anaphylaxis reaction, 324, 330–337
Anemia, 39, 282
Ankylosing spondylitis, 201
Antibody(ies)
   active site, 193
   IgE serum, 319–320, 320–326
   circulating, 322–326
   diversity, 212, 214–216
   monoclonal, 86
   vs. prostatic fluid, 77

therapeutic, 282
Antibody-dependent cell-mediated
   cytotoxicity, 240–242, 252, 258,
   263, 273, 282
Antichymotrypsin, 44, 60, 72–73, 77
Antigen(s)
   Australia, 23
   characterization with CFA, 121
   excess, 103, 136
   hepatitis-associated, 108
   HLA, 269–275, 311
   thymus-dependent, 266–267
Antiserum
   monospecific, 93
   monovalent, 100–101, 110
   polyvalent, 97–100
α₁-Antitrypsin, 103
   comparative data, 133–134
   genetic variants, 30
   in HRE, 44–46, 53, 59–61
   two-dimensional pattern, 72–73
Arthritis, rheumatoid, 77, 194, 201, 282
Asthma, 234, 317
Ataxia, marie-Sanger-Brown, 53, 103
Autoimmune hemolytic anemia, 39

B lymphocytes, 194, 210, 216, 266, 268,
   278
BASIC (computer language), 160–161
Bence Jones L chains (proteins), 20,
   105, 109–110, 197, 200–202
Binding regions, 281–282
Blotting, electrophoretic, 85–86
Bovine serum albumin as internal
   standard, 93–94

Cancer detection, 70
Candida albicans, 318